LASERS IN CARDIOVASCULAR DISEASE: CLINICAL APPLICATIONS, ALTERNATIVE ANGIOPLASTY DEVICES, AND GUIDANCE SYSTEMS

Second Edition

Lasers in Cardiovascular Disease:
Clinical Applications, Alternative Angioplasty Devices, and Guidance Systems

Second Edition

RODNEY A. WHITE, M.D.
Associate Professor of Surgery
UCLA School of Medicine
Los Angeles, California
Chief, Vascular Surgery
Harbor-UCLA Medical Center
Torrance, California

WARREN S. GRUNDFEST, M.D.
Assistant Clinical Professor of Surgery
UCLA School of Medicine
Assistant Director of Surgery
Cedars-Sinai Medical Center
Los Angeles, California

YEAR BOOK MEDICAL PUBLISHERS, INC.
Chicago • London • Boca Raton

1 2 3 4 5 6 7 8 9 0 PR 93 92 91 90 89

Library of Congress Cataloging-in-Publication Data

Lasers in cardiovascular diseases : lasers, alternative angioplasty
devices, and guidance systems / [edited by] Rodney A. White, Warren
S. Grundfest. — 2nd ed.
      p.   cm.
    Includes bibliographies and index.
    ISBN 0-8151-9259-2
    1. Cardiovascular system—Laser surgery. 2. Laser angioplasty.
3. Cardiovascular system—Laser surgery—Instruments. 4. Laser
angioplasty—Instruments. I. White, Rodney A. II. Grundfest,
Warren S.
    [DNLM: 1. Cardiovascular Diseases—therapy. 2. Lasers—
-therapeutic use.   WG 166 L343]
RD597.L37   1989
617.4'1059—dc20
DNLM/DLC
for Library of Congress   89-5721
                                                                        CIP

Sponsoring Editor: Nancy E. Chorpenning
Associate Managing Editor, Manuscript Services: Deborah Thorp
Production Project Coordinator: Carol Reynolds
Proofroom Supervisor: Barbara M. Kelly

This book is dedicated to the hope of improving the quality _____
of patient care through an interdisciplinary approach,
without doing any harm.

19 39 06 72

CONTRIBUTORS

GEORGE S. ABELA, M.D.
Associate Professor of Medicine
Division of Cardiology
University of Florida College of Medicine
Gainesville, Florida

LOUIS ADLER, M.D.
Director Vascular Radiology
Attending Radiologist
Cedars-Sinai Medical Center
Los Angeles, California

WILLIAM B. ANDERSON, B.S.
Physicist, Optics and Delivery Systems
Advanced Interventional Systems
Irvine, California

YVON BARIBEAU, M.D.
Research Fellow
Cardiovascular Laser Surgery
Beckman Laser Institute and Medical Clinic
University of California at Irvine
Irvine, California

MICHAEL W. BERNS, PH.D.
Professor of Surgery and Cell Biology
Beckman Laser Institute and Medical Clinic
University of California at Irvine
Irvine, California

ALBERT K. CHIN, M.S., M.D.
Cardiovascular Research Staff
Sequoia Hospital
Redwood City, California

PHILIP D. COLMAN, M.B., B.S.,
  F.R.A.C.S.
Fellow in Vascular Surgery
Harbor-UCLA Medical Center
Torrance, California

EDWARD B. DIETHRICH, M.D.
Medical Director
Arizona Heart Institute
Chief of Cardiovascular Surgery
Chairman, Department of Cardiovascular
  Services
Humana Hospital
Phoenix, Arizona

D. LYNN DOYLE, M.D., F.R.C.S. (C)
Clinical Assistant Professor
Department of Surgery
University of British Columbia
Health Sciences Center Hospital
Vancouver, British Columbia

JOHN EUGENE, M.D.
Assistant Professor of Surgery
Beckman Laser Institute and Medical Clinic
University of California at Irvine
Irvine, California

THOMAS J. FOGARTY, M.D.
Director of Cardiovascular Surgery
Sequoia Hospital
Redwood City, California

JAMES S. FORRESTER, M.D.
Professor of Medicine
UCLA School of Medicine
Director, Cardiovascular Research
Cedars-Sinai Medical Center
Los Angeles, California

ROY M. FUJITANI, M.D.
Research Associate
Senior Surgical Resident
Harbor-UCLA Medical Center
Torrance, California

TSVI GOLDENBERG, PH.D.
Vice President
Optics and Delivery Systems
Advanced Interventional Systems
Irvine, California

WARREN S. GRUNDFEST, M.D.
Assistant Clinical Professor of Surgery
UCLA School of Medicine
Assistant Director of Surgery
Cedars-Sinai Medical Center
Los Angeles, California

CAROL GUTHRIE, M.D.
Research Associate
Surgical Resident
Harbor-UCLA Medical Center
Torrance, California

LISA HESTRIN, M.P.H.
Patient Coordinator
Laser Angioplasty Program
Cedars-Sinai Medical Center
Los Angeles, California

ANN HICKEY, M.D.
Associate Cardiologist
Division of Cardiology
Cedars-Sinai Medical Center
Los Angeles, California

YORK N. HSIANG, M.B., CH.B.,
    M.HS., F.R.C.S.(C)
Clinical Instructor
Department of Surgery
Division of Vascular Surgery
Health Sciences Center Hospital
University of British Columbia
Vancouver, British Columbia

GEORGE E. KOPCHOK, B.S.
Biomedical Engineer
Director Experimental Laser Laboratory
Harbor-UCLA Medical Center
Torrance, California

SHARON KUPFER, B.S.
Optical Engineer
Optics and Delivery Systems
Advanced Interventional Systems
Irvine, California

JAMES B. LAUDENSLAGER, PH.D.
Vice President, Laser Development
Advanced Interventional Systems
Irvine, California

FRANK LITVACK, M.D.
Assistant Professor of Medicine
UCLA School of Medicine
Associate Director
Cardiac Catheterization Laboratory
Cedars-Sinai Medical Center
Los Angeles, California

LOUANN W. MURRAY, PH.D.
Adjunct Assistant Professor of Pediatrics
Department of Pediatrics
Harbor-UCLA Medical Center
Torrance, California

SHI-KAUNG PENG, M.D., PH.D.
Professor of Pathology
Department of Pathology
Harbor-UCLA Medical Center
Torrance, California

THOMAS L. ROBERTSON, M.D.
Chief, Cardiac Diseases Branch
Division of Heart and Vascular Diseases
National Heart, Lung, and Blood Institute
National Institutes of Health
Bethesda, Maryland

DAVID ROSENBAUM, M.D.
Research Associate
Harbor-UCLA Medical Center
Torrance, California

TIMOTHY A. SANBORN, M.D.
Associate Professor of Medicine
Director, Interventional Cardiology
Research and Laser Angioplasty Program
Department of Medicine
Division of Cardiology
Mount Sinai Medical Center
New York City, New York

MICHELE SARTORI, M.D.
Methodist Hospital Cardiology Section
Houston, Texas

JAMES M. SEEGER, M.D.
Associate Professor of Surgery
Department of Surgery
University of Florida College of Medicine
Chief, Vascular Surgery
Veteran's Medical Center
Gainesville, Florida

JACOB SEGALOWITZ, M.D.
Fellow, Department of Surgery
Cedars-Sinai Medical Center
Los Angeles, California

TAKANOBU TOMARU, M.D.
Research Fellow
Division of Cardiology
University of Florida College of Medicine
Gainesville, Florida

JERRY W. VLASAK, M.D.
Research Associate
Surgical Resident
Harbor-UCLA Medical Center
Torrance, California

GEOFFREY H. WHITE, M.D.
Assistant Professor of Surgery
UCLA School of Medicine
Los Angeles, California
Vascular Surgeon
Harbor-UCLA Medical Center
Torrance, California
Chief, Vascular Surgery
Veterans Administration
Wadsworth Medical Center
Los Angeles, California

RODNEY A. WHITE, M.D.
Associate Professor of Surgery
UCLA School of Medicine
Los Angeles, California
Chief, Vascular Surgery
Harbor-UCLA Medical Center
Torrance, California

PREFACE TO THE SECOND EDITION _____

The second edition of this book follows the first edition by 2 years. Half of the chapters are new and, all have been updated; only three remain without substantial revision or lengthy addition of new material. These changes reflect the rapid accumulation of clinical data and an attempt to define the role of lasers in cardiovascular diseases, as well as the development and use of ancillary devices.

At the time of the first edition, lasers were solely a research tool; their role in clinical vascular interventions was only speculative. Since then, there has been an explosion in the use of laser for angioplasty, with two manufacturers having FDA-approval for their devices, and approval rapidly approaching for many more manufacturer's devices. The number of cases has been estimated at nearly 20,000 in more than 600 centers that have devices. Although the technique remains experimental, evidence is accumulating that substantiates benefit from therapy in at least a segment of the patients, and if improvement in devices and guidance methods continues, the laser techniques may dramatically change the treatment of vascular disease in a significant segment of the population.

Accompanying these rapid developments is an unrealistic depiction, particularly in the media, of the new devices as panaceas for cure of hopeless cases. Consumer awareness, patient demand, and a mystical appeal of the laser methods have created substantial economic pressures for physicians to at least know the methods, and to have the technique available if patient volumes are to be maintained. Controversies regarding indications for use and involvement of surgeons, cardiologists, and radiologists in applying the technology have led to unfortuante in-fighting in institutions where collaboration is not initiated early. It is our strong conviction that collaborative efforts yield better patient care and case selection. For these devices, defining the indications for use requires careful follow-up evaluation of several hundred cases. The rush to prove that one device is better than another must give way to the understanding that time, experience, and knowledge regarding case selection are required to appropriately assess the role of each device.

This book addresses the state of the art in applications of lasers in cardiovascular disease by reviewing the current theory of laser-tissue interactions, providing a review of all available experimental and clinical data, and detailing the limitations and future research needs. Considering the interest and controversy surrounding this topic, we have attempted to provide a detailed review of all pertinent issues from several perspectives so that the readers can draw their own conclusions based on the spectrum of available information and opinions.

Rodney A. White, M.D.
Warren S. Grundfest, M.D.

PREFACE TO THE FIRST EDITION

The use of lasers in medicine and surgery has generated significant interest. The initial enthusiasm was based mainly on the fascination for a "star-wars" concept, which ascribes mystical powers to this unique form of energy. The idea that a laser can be used as a surgical instrument to cut tissue, destroy tumors, and open obliterated atherosclerotic arteries triggered a degree of speculation and enthusiasm that preceded the reality that scientists and physicians have been trying to determine. This effort has required the development of a unique collaboration among physicists, engineers, biologists, and clinicians. To the pleasant surprise of all, many of the speculations regarding the potential uses of lasers in medicine are rapidly developing into applications.

The adaptation of lasers as therapy for cardiovascular diseases is in its infancy, but the use of lasers to treat difficult clinical problems and improve overall care of patients is coming close to reality. The ability to selectively ablate abnormal tissues and atherosclerotic lesions and enhance the technical accuracy and healing of vascular repairs is now more than an appealing concept.

The objective of this book is to convey a basic understanding of laser physics, safety, and laser-tissue interactions, and to describe the current state-of-the-art and eminent developments to physicians, allied health professionals, and those interested in the frontiers of medicine. It will become evident that the current laser applications are not the cure-all that the extensive publicity may lead one to believe; in a curious way the field is developing in a manner that adds credence to some of the early speculations regarding the use of laser surgery.

Rodney A. White, M.D.
Warren S. Grundfest, M.D.

ACKNOWLEDGMENTS ⸺⸺⸺⸺⸺

We wish to thank the contributors for their timely assistance in the preparation of this book. Special thanks are given to Gloria Stevens who provided expert assistance in manuscript preparation and word processing. Special recognition is also given to our colleagues, research associates, and support personnel at Harbor-UCLA and Cedars-Sinai Medical Centers who consistently provided help and encouragement. We also thank Carol Reynolds, Deborah Thorp, Nancy Chorpenning, and Beth Caldwell of Year Book Medical Publishers for their help and support.

Rodney A. White, M.D.
Warren S. Grundfest, M.D.

CONTENTS _____

PART III   ANGIOPLASTY GUIDANCE SYSTEMS AND ANCILLARY DEVICES   181

Color Plates

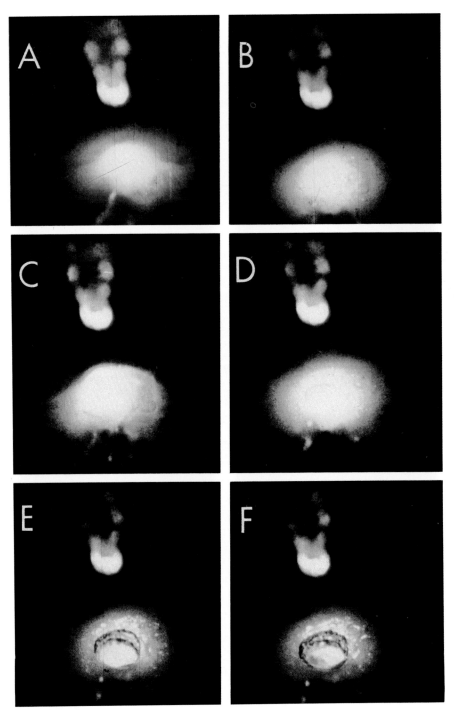

Plate 1.—See legend at top of facing page.

←

Plate 1.—A, this frame is obtained from the high-speed filming of Nd:YAG ablation of athero-sclerotic tissue at 30 W delivered via a 400-μm fiber. The white light is the aiming light of the laser. The laser irradiation begins, and approximately 0.25 seconds later the tissue begins to turn white. **B,** at 0.4 seconds a small crater begins to form. As the crater enlarges, one can see material melt and boil. **C,** boiling can sometimes occur explosively as deeper and deeper layers of tissue are heated. Note that laterally the tissue is thermally injured and it blanches and turns white. **D,** as all molten material evaporates, temperature rises and pyrolysis begins. The crater is easily visible, with sharply defined margins. However, denaturation of the protein laterally turns the tissue from pink to gray. **E,** as pyrolysis continues, carbonization begins and the crater walls turn black. **F,** as temperatures rise laterally, molten material pours back into the crater, now filling the base of it. As the crater cools, lateral thermal effects extend outward.

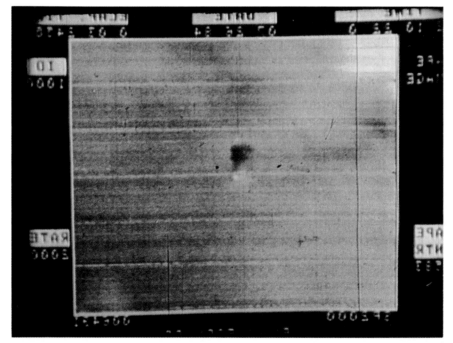

Plate 2.—This frame is taken from the high-speed filming of 308-nm excimer laser ablation of atherosclerotic tissue. The beam is directed from the laser output mirror and is 0.4 × 0.8 mm. Pulse duration is 80 nanoseconds. The area of tissue ablation is also 0.4 × 0.8 mm. The ambient light is coming in at a 45-degree angle. No debris is observed escaping from the crater, and the incision has extremely sharp, precisely cut edges. There are no surrounding tissue effects. The color or the texture of the tissue do not change.

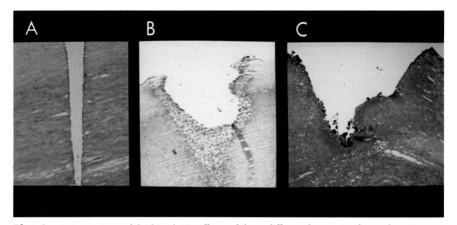

Plate 3.—A comparison of the histologic effects of three different lasers on atherosclerotic aorta. **A** shows a cut made with an excimer laser from a fiberoptic waveguide. This cut is in human atherosclerotic aorta. The thickness of the aorta here is approximately 2.2 mm. The width at the very top is 0.4 mm, and the average width is approximately 0.35 mm. The crater walls are sharp, without carbonization or blast damage. A 2-μm rim of eosinophilic tissue is present, but adjacent tissue is not affected. **B** shows the effects of an Nd:YAG laser, again ablating atherosclerotic tissue that is only minimally calcified. The fiberoptic waveguide is aimed perpendicular to the intimal aortic surface. Spot size was 0.9 mm in diameter. The crater is 2.1 mm in diameter by approximately 1.8 mm in depth; note the surrounding zone of vacuolized tissue, carbonized edges, and loss of tissue architecture. **C** shows a histologic section of human cadaver atherosclerotic aorta after irradiation with an argon laser using a 0.4-mm fiberoptic waveguide with the energy set at 8 W, spot size 0.5 mm. The crater created was 2.2 mm in diameter by approximately 1.6 mm in depth. Note the carbonization and lateral coagulation injury. (From Grundfest WS, Litvak F, Glick D, et al: Current status and future prospects for angioscopy and laser angioplasty. *J Vasc Surg* 1987; 5:667–672. Reproduced by permission.)

Plate 4.—This is a four-panel histologic comparison of the ablation effects at four wavelengths. **A** shows the effect of Nd:YAG ablation at 1,060 nm at 7 nanoseconds (nsec), 100 mJ/sq mm. There is significant charring and surrounding blast damage to the tissue. **B** shows the effect of 532 nm, or green light, similar to that from the argon laser, but pulsed at 7 nsec at 65 mJ/sq mm. This wavelength produced variable effects and significant blast damage and, in some cases, shredded the tissue. At higher energy densities both of these lasers were able to cut tissue. However, the energy was so high that it cut the quartz plates used to hold the tissue as well. **C** shows the effect of 353 nm at 7 nsec, 45 mJ/sq mm. Note that there are visible thermal effects at this wavelength. However, they are small compared with the continuous-wave lasers; the edges are not as smooth as those obtained in the shorter wavelength. **D,** in contrast, shows 266 nm at 7 nsec, 11 mJ/sq mm, which produced extremely precise edges with minimal thermal damage. The shorter the ultraviolet wavelength, the more precise the ablative process for this particular tissue. (From Grundfest WS, Litvak F, Goldenberg T, et al: Pulsed ultraviolet lasers and the potential for safe laser angioplasty. *Am J Surg* 1985; 150:220–226. Reproduced by permission.)

$\longrightarrow$

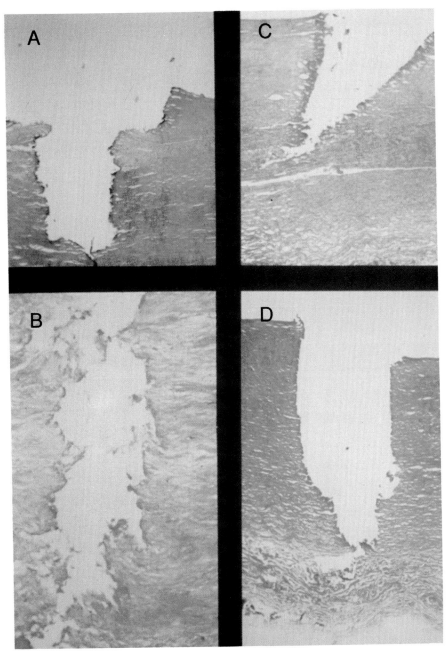

Plate 4.—See legend at foot of facing page.

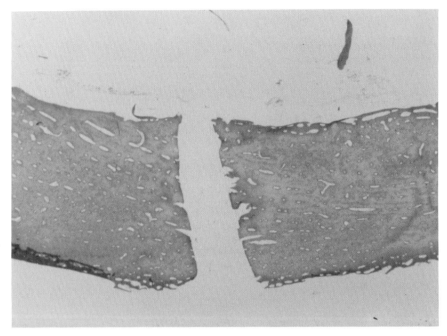

Plate 5.—This 4-mm-thick section of bovine femur was irradiated at 308 nm output from a 1.0-mm fiberoptic waveguide, carving a 1-mm channel. This channel was created in approximately 1 minute 45 seconds with a laser operating at 20 Hz. Fiberoptic output was 75 mJ/sq mm. (From Litvak F, Grundfest WS, Beeder C, et al: Laser angioplasty: Status and prospects. *Semin Intervent Radiol* 1986; 3:75–81. Reproduced by permission.)

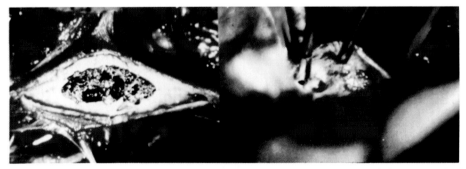

Plate 6.—Continuous-wave irradiated aorta demonstrating carbonization and thermal destruction of adjacent tissue *(left)*, while excimer-irradiated specimens show no gross evidence of thermal injury *(right)*.

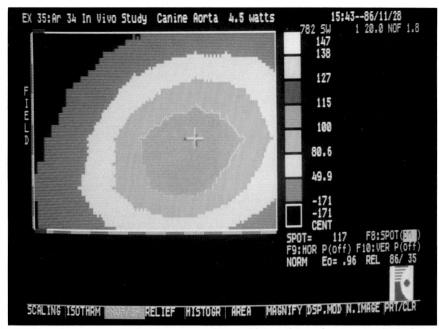

Plate 7.—Computer-generated color thermogram of argon ablation of normal canine aorta (intimal surface). The red area is the hottest, the blue, the coolest. The crosshairs in the frame denote the maximum temperature of 117°C.

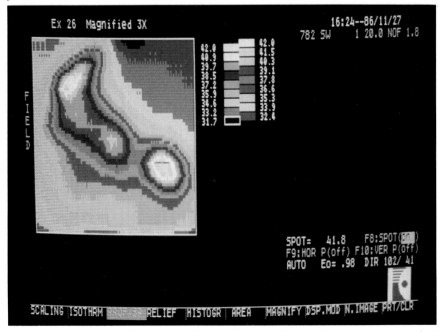

Plate 8.—Computer-generated thermogram shows excimer irradiation at 31.5 mJ/sq mm per pulse. The maximal temperature in this frame was 41.8°C; three consecutive pulses are visible, with the last pulse having the highest temperature.

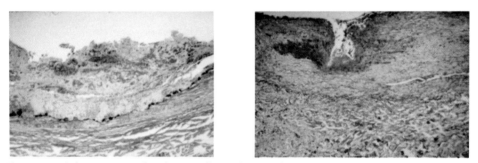

Plate 9.—At 3 days, argon-irradiated aortas all revealed mural thrombus with an inflammatory infiltrate visible on histologic examination *(left)*, while excimer-irradiated aortas showed minimal thrombus, no inflammatory response, and new islands of endothelial cells (hematoxylin-eosin, ×40).

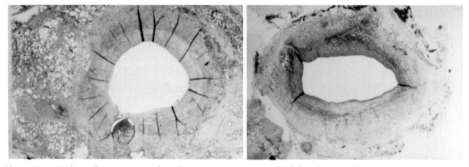

Plate 10.—At 4 weeks, argon-irradiated aortas were surrounded by dense inflammatory response and showed evidence of minimal hyperplasia, with disorganization of endothelial components *(left)*. Excimer-irradiated aortas were grossly similar to controls, with a normally reconstituted endothelium and an intact elastic lamina (hematoxylin-eosin, ×4).

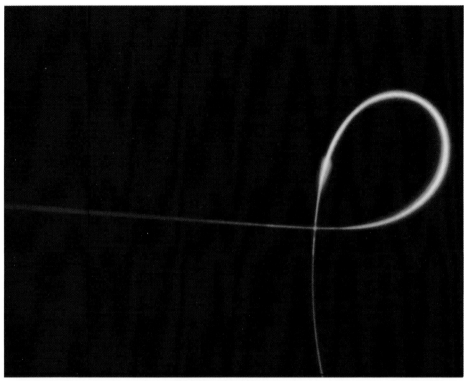

Plate 11.—Energy loss in a 400-μm fiber due to bending.

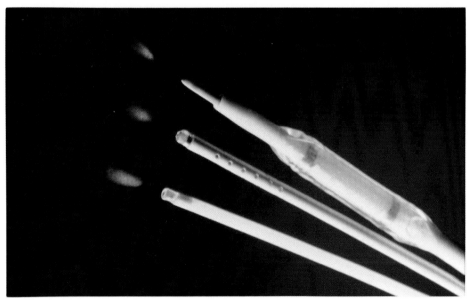

Plate 12.—A variety of new excimer laser systems are under development. The *top* system shows a specially designed, large lumen 7 F balloon angioplasty catheter. A central lumen accommodates a laser fiber. The *middle* catheter consists of 7 ×300 μm fibers arranged circumferentially around a 0.018-in. guidewire. This system permits distal dye injection and ablates a 2.2-mm channel. The *bottom* system is a highly flexible 12-fiber design for coronary applications.

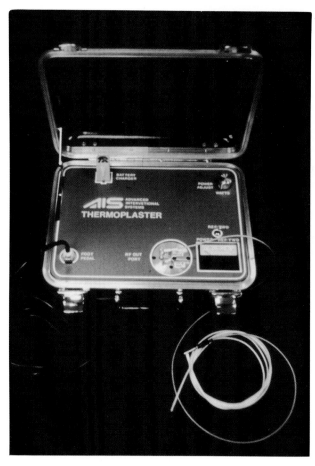

Plate 13.—Portable battery-powered radiofrequency hot-tip unit.

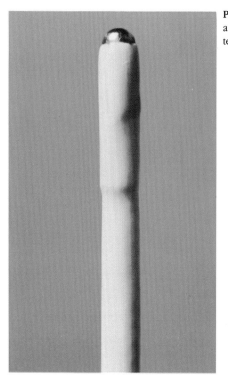

Plate 14.—Gold-tipped radiofrequency hot-tip catheter with a high temperature plastic insulation that limits the shaft temperature to 90°C.

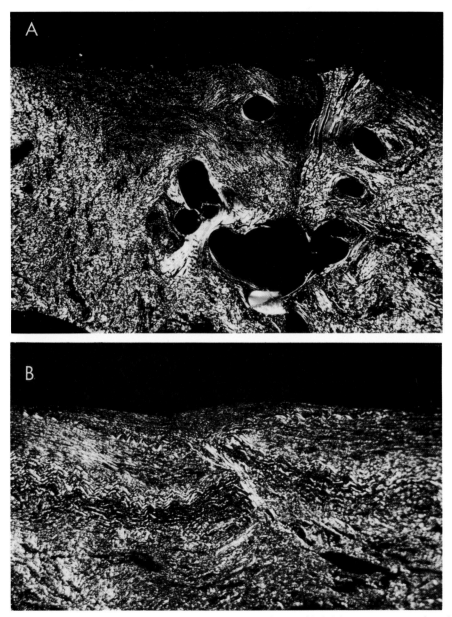

Plate 15.—Histologic appearance of sutured (**A**) and argon laser-welded (**B**) arteriotomies at 4 weeks. The disorientation of the collagen, elastin, and cellular matrix in the sutured repair in contrast to the near-normal restoration of the arterial wall architecture in the laser-welded specimen is highlighted by a Sirius red stain viewed under polarized light (× 40). (Histologic sections and photographs compliments of James Anderson, M.D., Ph.D., Case Western Reserve University, Cleveland.)

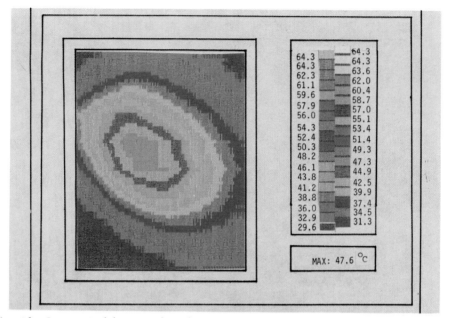

Plate 16.—Computerized thermographs at the anastomotic line during laser welding at 0.50 W, demonstrating the effect of saline irrigation. In this instance, the tissue heated to 47.6°C with application of laser light.

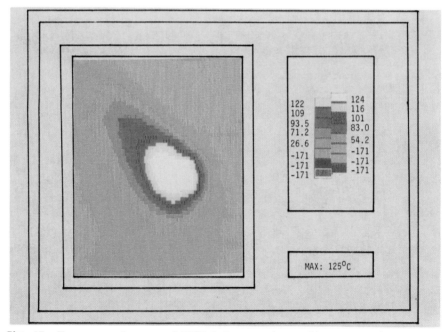

Plate 17.—Temperatures in excess of 125°C during argon laser welding without saline irrigation at 0.50 W power.

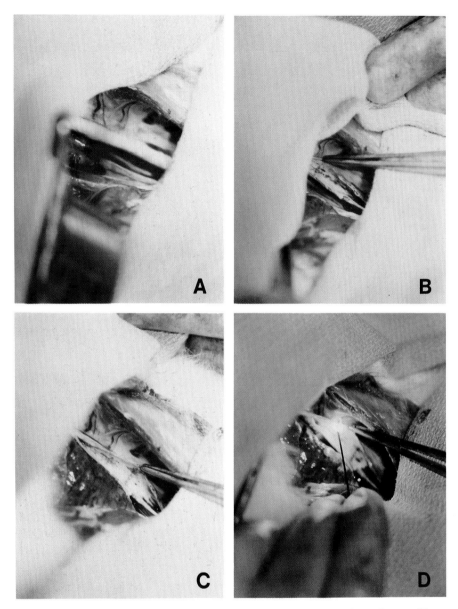

Plate 18.—Argon ion laser endarterectomy in an atherosclerotic rabbit. **A,** an atherosclerotic rabbit aorta. The aorta is markedly thickened and discolored chalk white. **B,** a longitudinal arteriotomy is made to expose an atheroma. **C,** lines of laser craters have been created at one end of the atheroma. **D,** individual argon ion laser exposures are being used to create lines of laser craters at the other end of the atheroma. (From Eugene J, McColgan SJ, Hammer-Wilson M, et al: Laser endarterectomy. *Lasers Surg Med* 1985; 5:265–274. Reproduced by permission.)

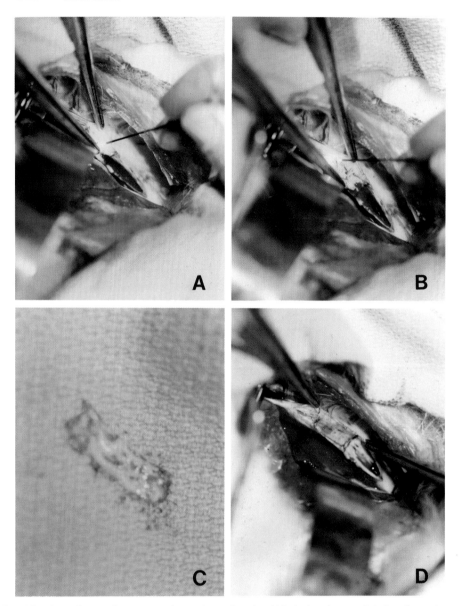

Plate 19.—Argon laser endarterectomy in an atherosclerotic rabbit. **A,** the atheroma is being elevated away from the aorta by continuous argon ion laser radiation. **B,** the cleavage plane is being developed within the media by continuous argon ion laser radiation. **C,** the atheroma has been removed from the artery. **D,** the completed endarterectomy has a smooth, glistening surface with proximal and distal end points welded in place. (From Eugene J, McColgan SJ, Hammer-Wilson M, et al: Laser endarterectomy. *Lasers Surg Med* 1985; 5:265–274. Reproduced by permission.)

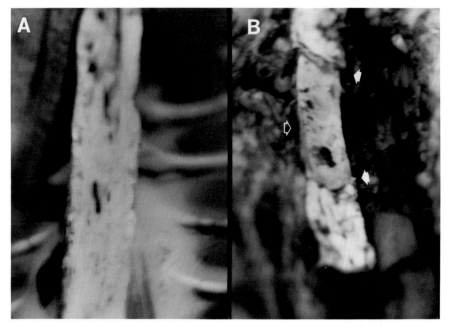

Plate 20.—The luminal surface of an atherosclerotic aorta 48 hours after injection of Photofrin II, 5 mg/ kg. **A,** the porphyrin-laden atherosclerotic plaque fluoresces salmon-pink when photographed under ultraviolet light. **B,** following open laser endarterectomy with an argon ion laser, the endarterectomy surface *(open arrow)* lacks gross fluorescence, whereas the residual plaque beyond the end points *(closed arrow)* retains fluorescence.

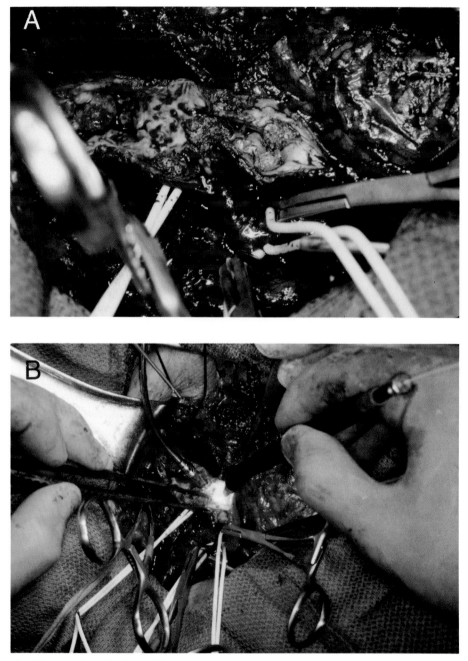

Plate 21.—See legend at foot of facing page.

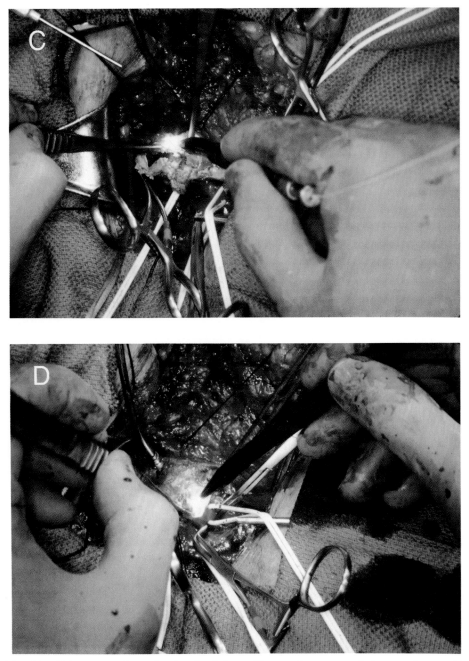

Plate 21.—Right common femoral and profunda femoral laser endarterectomy. **A,** the artery is opened to expose the arteriosclerotic plaque. **B,** argon ion laser radiation is delivered to separate the plaque from the media. **C,** argon ion laser radiation is delivered to dissect the plaque out of the artery. **D,** argon ion laser radiation is directed at the profunda to weld the distal end point in place.

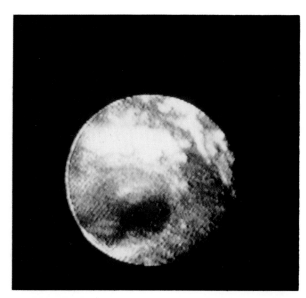

Plate 22.—Angioscopic visualization of a thermal laser probe recanalization of an occlusion in the superficial femoral artery.

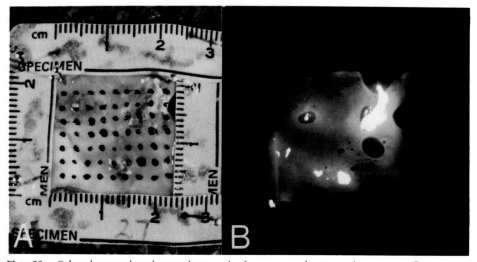

Plate 23.—Color photograph and x-ray photograph of a segment of aorta used to generate fluorescence maps. **A**, the aortic segment has been open flat on a corkboard. The black spots at 2.5-mm intervals are india ink marks corresponding to the fluorescence collection sites and are identified in the x,y axis by the paper rulers glued to the arterial margins. Lipid-rich areas of the intimal surface appear with more intense pink colors because the photograph has been taken after staining the artery with Sudan IV. **B**, soft x-ray photograph at the same magnification as **A**. Areas of calcification appear as bone dense structures. (From Sartori M, Weilbaecher D, Henry P: Laser induced autofluorescence of human arteries, *Circ Res*, 1988; 63:1053–1059. Used by permission.)

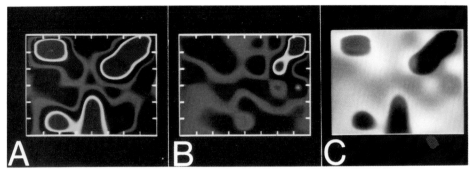

Plate 24.—Autofluorescence maps of the human aorta described in Figure 5. **A,** map obtained by digitizing the ratio of the peak at 550 to 520 nm. All the areas of atherosclerotic tissue (lipid and calcified) appear as yellow and red color. Normal regions are blue. **B,** map derived by digitizing the intensity of the peak at 520 nm. Only the calcified plaque at the right top corner is visualized. **C,** map obtained by overlapping **A** and **B**. The result is a three color map in which the normal tissue appears in purple, the lipid-rich regions in blue and the calcified region in black. (From Sartori M, Weilbaecher D, Henry P: Laser induced autofluorescence of human arteries, *Circ Res,* 1988; 63:1053–1059. Used by permission.)

Introduction

Overview of Administrative and Safety Considerations

George Kopchok, B.S.

Rodney A. White, M.D.

The recent development of lasers for use in medicine and surgery has created a new frontier with numerous potential cardiovascular applications. Among the questions to consider while exploring this new technology are (1) Why use lasers to treat cardiovascular disease? and (2) What are the special considerations required for choosing appropriate instrumentation, assuring facility safety, and conducting personnel training?

Lasers are expensive equipment that have unique space and facility requirements. Unless they fulfill a need in our armamentarium that is not available by current, less expensive technologies, the use of lasers in cardiovascular medicine is not appropriate. As outlined in the remainder of this text, there are several advantages that lasers offer to the cardiovascular surgeon, cardiologist, and radiologist. Specific ablation of intracardiac and intravascular lesions, disobliteration of totally occluded small internal diameter arteries, augmentation of current clinical techniques such as percutaneous balloon dilatation, and laser welding of vascular tissue are current applications that may soon find significant clinical utility. The initial studies using percutaneous transluminal balloon angioplasty were performed less than a decade ago, but this technique is now used widely for rapidly expanding indications. Laser vascular surgery appears to have the same potential for broad applicability and development.

CHOICE OF MEDICAL LASER SYSTEMS

In most cases the lasers that are currently available in hospitals are improperly designed or have inadequate power ranges to make them easily adaptable to cardiovascular applications. Because of the expense of purchase, installation and maintenance of lasers, hospitals are obviously concerned with maximizing the use and cost-effectiveness. A new laser system that is to be used primarily for cardiovascular applications should, if possible, have the broadest applicability to multiple specialties. The desirability of any particular instrument directly increases with its versatility.

Conceptually, the ideal laser should be an instrument that can be dialed over a wide power range (watts), is tunable over the entire spectrum of wavelengths, permits fiberoptic transmission and is designed to accommodate any future demands that would be placed on the instrument. Unfortunately, at the present state of technology, lasers that meet these specifications are not available. Dye lasers use various organic dyes as lasing media to produce a tunable characteristic over the range of approximately 300 to 1,000 nm, although they are currently far from ideal. Each dye provides wavelengths over a narrow range. The dyes are cumbersome to use, and some dyes are unstable. The free electron laser is a theoretical solution to this problem as it may be tunable over all wavelengths and produce a wide range of power, but it requires a very large and expensive particle separator for operation.[1] Currently, carbon dioxide (CO_2) (10,600 nm), neodymium:yttrium-aluminum-garnet (Nd:YAG) (1,060 nm), and argon (488 to 515 nm) are the clinical lasers available at most hospitals. The CO_2 lasers have power outputs of a few hundred milliwatts to 100 W and are used for cutting or ablation of soft tissue. The Nd:YAG lasers are most reliable between 1 and 60 W and are used by general surgeons and gastroenterologists for tissue coagulation. Argon lasers provide a steady output from the milliwatt to 15-W level and are used primarily in ophthalmology and dermatology to coagulate pigmented lesions. The argon and Nd:YAG lasers are transmitted through flexible quartz optic fibers, while CO_2 can only be transmitted via mirrors and articulating arms or potentially by a hollow tubular waveguide. Although other promising laser prototypes are at various stages of experimental development, none of them at present are commercially available for cardiovascular applications. Throughout this interval of rapid development, one must keep in mind the current availability of lasers and separate that from what may be state-of-the-art in the future.

ORGANIZATION/PERSONNEL

In order to make rational decisions regarding lasers, establishment of laser safety protocols and laser acquisition should be scrutinized and controlled by a hospital laser technology committee. Key individuals who should be involved in the laser committee activities are administrative personnel, the hospital safety officer, a representative from the hospital mechanical services and nursing, and a representative from each of the medical and surgical subspecialties that have interest in laser applications. Frequent meetings of this group are necessary to assess the current state of laser applications within the hospital, to evaluate the priorities in laser program development, and to assess the utility and cost-effectiveness of proposed new purchases.

An administrative representative to the laser committee is obviously essential to evaluate the cost-effective use of instrumentation and to represent the fiscal responsibilities and priorities in hospital program development. It is also administrative responsibility to address billing for laser procedures. Most of the cardiovascular laser applications are still considered experimental, and third-party payers may decline payment on this basis. Some of these procedures are done as adjuncts to other standard procedures, such as laser-assisted balloon angioplasty. The technology is also being used in combination with, or as a substitute for, standard procedures in the operating room. In this instance, the laser procedures may significantly reduce the cost of therapies that currently pay a substantial diagnosis-related group (DRG) fee.

At present, several billing mechanisms exist, primarily because the methods of reimbursement vary among states. A few institutions that do large volumes of cardiovascular

TABLE 1–1.
Credentialing Standards

A. Laser safety standards and practices should be developed by a hospital laser technology committee. The primary responsibility for laser safety should be organized by an individual designated by the institution and approved by the committee as the laser safety officer.
B. Department chairmen or their selected representative within the department or divisions hold the basic responsibility to ensure that the use of lasers on their service is performed by competent personnel. Staff members shall petition for permission to use laser through their department chairman or department/divisional representative.
C. Staff members desiring to utilize the laser must be trained in the use, care, and physics of the laser and have fulfilled the following criteria:
    1. The candidate has demonstrated proficiency, knowledge, and safety in the use of lasers through previous use, which is common knowledge of the department chairmen or his representative and the laser safety committee.
    2. The candidate may present certification of approved training sessions indicating that the staff member has completed a laser course of at least 4 hrs of didactic and 2 hrs of "hands-on" experience. The applicant should also demonstrate proficiency specific to that physician's specialty by observation of a departmental preceptor for two or more procedures, if necessary, based on the preceptor's decision. Documentation of the preceptor's approval should be kept on file.
D. The department chairman will forward all approved laser use requests to the chairman of the laser technology committee for proficiency verification and activation to user status.
E. "Active laser use status" staff members will receive a copy of the laser safety guidelines and will acknowledge their reading and understanding of these guidelines by signing a copy that will be kept on file in the office of the department chairman and/or the laser technology committee chairman, and in the facility where the laser is being used (i.e., operating room, etc.).
F. Each department chairman by generating a list of laser treatments within his specialty, will document which procedures the petitioning physician will have permission to perform. When appropriate, privileges that are limited to the use of particular type(s) of laser(s) should be noted. The laser technology committee has the final responsibility for ensuring appropriate and safe use of laser devices.

laser procedures have negotiated payment schedules from appropriate carriers but, in general, a uniform payment schedule has not been developed. It is likely that codes will be assigned by the insurance industry in the near future.

The laser safety officer or his designee fulfills an important role on the laser committee by establishing laser safety protocols for the institution and by ensuring that instrumentation, new programs, and new facilities fulfill these requirements and are accompanied by the necessary approvals.[2–5] A representative from mechanical services is needed to evaluate the power and plumbing requirements for new instrumentation and to expedite facility construction. Nursing plays a key role in space planning, training programs, equipment maintenance, and oversight of the safe use of the lasers.

CREDENTIALING

The final responsibility for laser safety and for determining appropriate requirements for credentials to use the lasers rests with the institutional laser technology committee. Physicians can demonstrate proficiency by either previous experience or by certification by an approved training program. Each department chairman should generate a list of approved laser treatments and decide in conjunction with the laser technology committee which procedures a particular physician can perform. Table 1–1 displays a sample format for credentialing standards.

Considerable concern exists regarding credentialing criteria for cardiovascular applications of lasers, in particular, laser angioplasty. The appropriate use and monitoring of these new, rapidly developing devices and techniques generate interest in most institutions because many of the new cardiovascular laser procedures are being used by multiple subspecialties, i.e., surgeons, radiologists, and cardiologists. For this reason, the primary factor in establishing appropriate guidelines in any institution is a cooperative effort among the interested specialties to deal with all appropriate concerns and to prevent "in-fighting" over the technology. We encourage collaboration and find that each group learns from the expertise of the other, i.e., surgeons benefit from the percutaneous and catheter techniques of the radiologists and cardiologists, and the success of the radiologists and cardiologists is enhanced by the vascular surgeons' understanding of arterial pathology derived from direct observation and intraoperative skills.

For individuals applying for privileges on the basis of a course certificate, the course should consist of 4 to 6 hours of lecture that outlines all pertinent safety information, clinical data, etc. and also includes 2 to 4 hours of hands-on experience. The didactic material is quite well standardized. Controversy exists regarding what constitutes adequate hands-on training. In most instances, hands-on training is limited to use of the instruments in animal models on an in vitro and occasionally in vivo basis. Animal models of arterial diseases have limited availability and are not useful except for preliminary training. For this reason, the best approach is to combine the course requirement with a specified number of proctored minimal-risk cases.

It is likely that most specialties will develop their own guidelines for laser use. When this document exists, it should be used for the specialty that develops the document but not be used to exclude other subspecialties requesting similar privileges. Ultimately, we must rely on the Board of each specialty and the training programs to provide trainees with knowledge of the new procedures so that credentialing can be based on the Board Certificate. As an example, 90% of the vascular surgery training programs now include balloon angioplasty experience, and the majority are adding laser angioplasty and angioscopy. In general, we recommend that patients undergoing percutaneous procedures should be evaluated before the procedure by a physician with "bed privileges" so that hospitalization and care for complications can be accomplished readily.

In most cases, laser surgery, including laser angioplasty, is credentialed by an institutional committee primarily because it is a major safety issue not only for patients, but also for hospital personnel. Aside from requirements for course training and proctoring, the new technologies can be introduced into clinical practice with minimal risk.

LASER SAFETY

Establishment of a laser safety protocol, facility specifications, approvals, in-service training, and continuing education for personnel are essential to maintain a safe environment. Personnel training regarding operating procedures and precautions to prevent personal injury and property damage must be given to all laser users. Only certified personnel should be permitted to set up, use, and discontinue use of laser equipment. Although laser radiation can cause eye damage, skin burns, and combustion of flammable materials, these hazards can easily be averted by a carefully planned program.

The physician and all key operating room personnel should be fully versed with an understanding of laser physics, appropriate nomenclature regarding laser energy, and laser tissue interactions.[2, 6] The physician user is ultimately responsible for selecting the wattage and appropriate lens or fiber for each procedure. However, a laser safety officer or his designee should be present at all cases (American National Standard for the Safe Use of Lasers in Health Care Facilities, ANSI Z136.3, 1988).

Laser procedure and operating rooms must have all windows covered with nontransparent barriers to prevent inadvertent passage of laser light (Fig 1-1). All doors must be

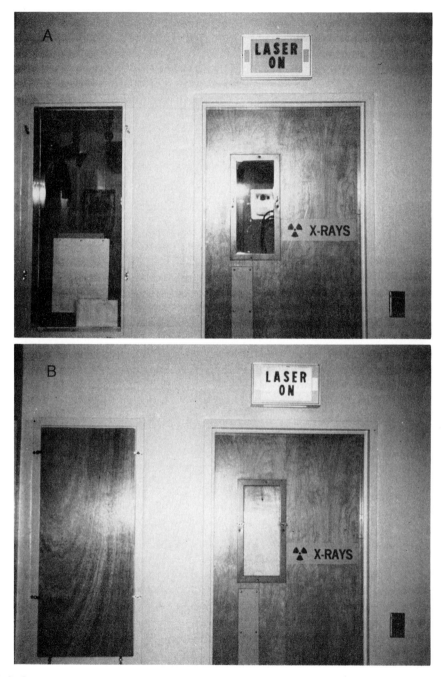

FIG 1–1.
Windows of the operating rooms **(A)** are covered by nontransparent barriers to prevent passage of laser light **(B)**. Clearly visible flashing lights are also activated during procedures to help control access to the room.

closed and access to the room should be restricted while the laser is activated. Clearly visible warning signs with flashing lights to signify that the system is activated are mandatory. The laser should remain in the off position or with the safety shutter closed until ready for use. Control of laser emission by a foot pedal and direction of the beam by hand control greatly enhance the safety. Laser energy should be directed and activated only when it is aimed at a specific target. Control of fiberoptic laser delivery is similar to the use of electrocautery in that the system is activated only when it is in contact with the tissue being treated. Reflective surgical instruments should be avoided and reflective surfaces in the laser procedure room minimized. Moist sponges in the operating field can prevent combustion of dry or paper material.

Laser energy can affect different parts of the eye depending upon which structure absorbs that particular wavelength. The three areas of most concern are cornea, lens, and retina. Laser energy outside the visible range (<350 nm and >1,400 nm) is absorbed by the cornea and lens. Exposure to this energy can produce cataracts and corneal scarring. Laser energy in the visible wavelength is focused by the cornea and lens onto the retina, leading up to 100,000 times amplification of radiant exposure.[3] Careless misdirection of the laser light even at low powers can result in instantaneous burning of the retina and consequent blindness in the visual field corresponding to the burn spot. Everyone in the operating room, including the patient, must have appropriate eyewear during the procedures (Fig 1–2). For the CO_2 laser, clear plastic or glass lenses are adequate, and wet gauze can be used to protect the patients' eyes. Green lenses (nontransparent to 1,060 nm) are recommended for the Nd:YAG laser, and amber lenses (nontransparent to 488 to 515 nm) are necessary to absorb the green or blue light of the argon laser. Other lasers

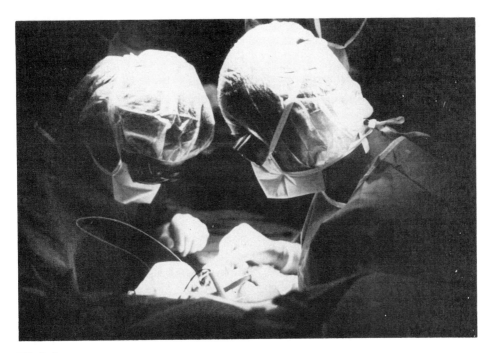

FIG 1–2.
Appropriate eyewear, which is non-transparent to the particular wavelength laser energy being used, is required for everyone in the room where the procedure is being performed to prevent eye injury.

TABLE 1–2.

Laser Standards of Practice

THIS FORM IS USED TO PROVIDE WRITTEN VERIFICATION THAT THE USER HAS BEEN ADVISED OF ALL SAFETY PRECAUTIONS AND OPERATIONAL HAZARDS. LASER OPERATORS ARE RESPONSIBLE FOR ASSURING THAT THE OPERATIONAL REQUIREMENTS DESCRIBED IN THIS DOCUMENT ARE FOLLOWED DURING PROCEDURES.

I. Operational guidelines
   A. Prior to beginning any laser procedure, the laser safety officer and the user must be sure that:
      1. There are no flammable chemicals in the room.
      2. Opaque barriers are intact to prevent propagation outside the controlled access area.
      3. There is adequate ventilation to eliminate laser plume and hazardous concentration of by-products if plastics or combustibles are used in the procedure.
      4. Warning signs on the entrance door and laser, and English labels on laser controls, are intact.
      5. The entrance door to the controlled area is secured.
   B. During procedures
      1. Appropriate protective eyewear must be worn by all personnel and by the patient.
      2. User must be sure that laser beam path is free of specularly reflective surfaces and combustible materials and that the beam is terminated in a noncombustible, nonreflective barrier.
      3. Lasers are to be activated, when possible, by foot-pedal control and directed to the operative site by handpieces to maximize accuracy and safety.
   C. Following laser operative procedures
      1. Laser is to be turned off before controlled access entrance is opened.
      2. Key to the laser control is to be removed when the laser is not in use to prevent unauthorized operation.
      3. Laser operating entrance is to be locked at all times when the facility is not in use, or the instrumentation must be secured in some way to prevent unauthorized use.

User Signature

---

with different wavelengths require specific lenses for eye protection as recommended by the manufacturer of the instrumentation.

Lasers are classified according to their potential to cause biologic injury. The parameters used for laser classification are laser power, wavelength, exposure duration, and beam spot size at the area of interest. Lasers are stratified into four classes. Class I, or exempt lasers, produce no hazard under normal operating conditions. The total amount of energy produced is less than the maximum permissible exposure level established by ANSI, and therefore no special facility or safety precautions are needed. Class II lasers are low power lasers that do not present a visual hazard due to normal aversion response. The eye normally closes in approximately 0.25 second when exposed to a noxious stimulus. This response avoids eye damage from a Class II laser. Class IIIa lasers operate with maximum power output ≤5 mW and power density ≤2.5 mW/cm. These lasers present a hazard if viewed through any collecting optics, but present no hazard if viewed momentarily with the unaided eye. Class IIIb lasers can damage the eyes if viewed directly but present no hazard to the skin. Class IV denotes high power laser systems that are hazardous to the eyes, skin, and flammable material from a direct and/or diffusely reflected beam. Facility requirements vary with the class of laser being used. Generally Class IV lasers are used in cardiovascular surgical applications and therefore operating facilities must be set up in accordance with requirements for this classification.[2, 4]

The most frequent cause of laser injury in industrial environments is accidents involving electricity. Activation of the laser systems frequently requires high current; thus the electric outlets should be carefully positioned when the room is designed. Adequate warning signs and in-service training are essential to prevent inadvertent accidents. Maintenance is to be performed by trained technicians only. Laser use and maintenance records must be kept from the date of installation. The laser system should be stored so that components and ignition key are secured when the laser is not being used. Table 1–2 summarizes the pertinent guidelines and procedures that should be included in a standard of practice for lasers.

Although the risk of airborne contaminants with cardiovascular laser applications is minimal, users should be aware that precautions must be implemented to prevent exposure and inhalation of laser plume. There is still a controversy whether laser plume contains viable cancer and/or mutagenic cells or whether laser exposure destroys these organisms. A closed system smoke evacuator should be used if exposure to laser plume is likely to occur. Dangerous by-products may be released from many inorganic materials also. Plastic bottles, drapes, instruments, and tubing may emit poisonous gases if exposed to laser energy or ignited. Polytetrafluoroethylene (PTFE) vascular grafting material emits hydrogen fluoride and perfluorocarbon olefins at temperatures above 350°C.[7, 8]

REFERENCES

1. Robinson AL: Free electron laser success explained. *Science* 1987; 235:27–29.
2. *American National Standard for the Safe Use of Lasers.* New York, American National Standards Institute, 1980, ANSI #Z-136.1.
3. *Laser Safety Guide.* Toledo, Ohio, Laser Institute of America, 1986.
4. *A Guide for the Control of Laser Hazards.* Cincinnati, American Conference of Governmental Industrial Hygienists, 1981.
5. *Occupational Health and Environmental Controls: Nonionizing Radiation,* title 29, chapter 17, part 1926 54. Washington, DC, Occupational Safety and Health Administration (OSHA).
6. Arndt KA, Noe JM, Northam BC, et al: Laser therapy: Basic concepts and nomenclature. *J Am Acad Dermatol* 1981; 5:649–654.
7. McCluren ME, McHaney JM, Colone WM: *Physical Properties and Test Methods for Expanded Polytetrafluoroethylene (PTFE) Grafts,* special technical publication 898. American Society for Testing and Materials, Philadelphia, 1987.
8. *Health and Safety Aspects of "Fluon" Polytetrafluoroethylene,* technical services note F10, ed 2. Imperial Clinical Industries Ltd, 1978.

Chapter 2

Laser Fundamentals

James B. Laudenslager, Ph.D.

The word *laser* is an acronym for *l*ight *a*mplification by *s*timulated *e*mission of *r*adiation. To most people a laser is a device that generates a highly directional beam of monochromatic light (i.e., a single color), and this beam of laser light can produce intense power densities on a target at considerable distances from the laser source. These characteristics of a laser beam are quite different from those of light generated from conventional sources, such as incandescent lights, fluorescent lights, or the light produced by chemical combustion reactions in a candle flame or an oil lamp. Conventional light sources, although ideal for illumination, produce light with a wide distribution of frequencies or colors, and the light scatters in all directions; consequently, the light energy reaching a target at a distance drops off inversely as the square of the distance between the target and the light source.

Lasers currently used in medical applications cover wavelength regions in the ultraviolet, visible, and infrared portions of the electromagnetic spectrum (Fig 2–1), which are nonionizing to tissue. The history of laser devices is recent, although the fundamental principles of lasers are based on the development of quantum theory in the early 1900s. The first laser demonstrated was the visible ruby laser by Maiman in 1959,[1] followed by the helium-neon (He-Ne) laser by Javan et al. in 1961,[2] the visible argon ion laser,[3] metal ion laser,[4] and infrared carbon dioxide (CO_2) laser in 1964,[5] and the ultraviolet discharge excimer (meaning excited dimer) laser in 1975,[6–8] to list only a few. Historically, a laser device has had a 9- to 10-year development period from the time it is first demonstrated until the time it is adequately engineered and packaged into a reliable system for various applications. This long gestation period is one reason for the recent increased utilization of lasers in medical applications, particularly for argon ion, neodymium:yttrium-aluminum-garnet (Nd:YAG) and CO_2 lasers, which have had the most extensive engineering period.

Common features of lasers currently used by medical practitioners[9] are (1) they are expensive; (2) the devices are complex and require specialized maintenance; (3) the laser technology is in a constant state of evolution and improvement; and (4) medical lasers (>1 W) require specialized power outlets and water cooling, consume an appreciable amount of valuable operating room space for all the associated equipment, and require protective eye measures to shield personnel from the laser radiation. Despite these factors, the use of controlled laser light has found important applications in many disciplines of

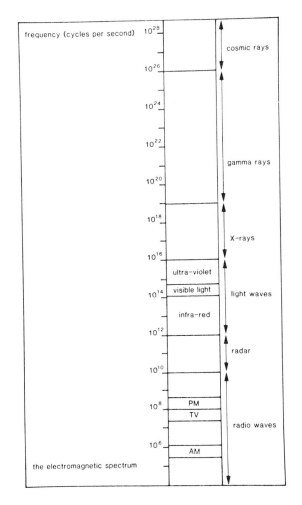

FIG 2–1.
The electromagnetic spectrum. The frequency region for laser radiation is from 10^{12} to 10^{16} cps.

medical treatment. The following chapters will present several emerging applications for laser treatment of cardiovascular disease.

Often, a physician will ask why scientists and engineers cannot eliminate these negatives from laser devices, particularly the high costs. Why is a laser that is powerful enough to cut through bone not reduced to the size of a wristwatch or hand calculator, as is often depicted in movies? The technical reasons for the size and for the requirements of water cooling and specialized power will be better understood once the principles of the laser device are explained. The high cost of medical lasers is due in part to the relatively short time span the laser has been available for use in medical treatment coupled with the lengthy period required for engineering these devices for reliable usage. Also, the lack of understanding of the interaction of laser radiation with tissue has led to improper choice of laser parameters for a variety of medical applications. Because of these factors, there is not yet a large demand for lasers; hence, they are manufactured in limited numbers, a major hindrance to lower prices.

One barrier to the wider use of lasers in medicine, as well as other areas of laser application, is the tendency to associate the laser device with the application in a generic manner without understanding the nature of the laser energy interaction on the material or tissue being irradiated. Even researchers who deal with laser development often use the term *laser* generically instead of identifying the parameters of the beam of light used for the particular application in terms of (1) power density, (2) wavelength, (3) spatial and temporal properties, and (4) total accumulated energy dosage.

To illustrate, precise ablation of atherosclerotic plaque has been demonstrated using an ultraviolet xenon chloride (XeCl) excimer laser with fiber delivery without thermal damage to surrounding tissue.[10] The common assumption is that the use of an XeCl excimer laser with fiberoptic delivery is the key to achieving the desired clinical result. However, this is not the case! The key factors in achieving precise cutting without thermal damage are the application of pulsed ultraviolet laser with optimal parameters. Careful studies in our laboratory have shown that this can be achieved with pulsed ultraviolet lasers delivered through a fiberoptic with (1) a pulse duration on the order of 200 nanoseconds (a nanosecond [nsec] is one billionth of a second) but less than 1 μsec; (2) an energy density or fluence at the distal end of the fiber of greater than 35 mJ/sq mm per pulse but less than 100 mJ/sq mm; (3) a wavelength near 300 nm; and (4) a pulse repetition frequency of 20 pulses per second (pps). If the same XeCl excimer laser were used under different operating conditions with a pulse energy of less than 5 mJ/sq mm of energy exiting from the distal end of the fiber, the tissue would show signs of thermal damage with irregular rather than precisely cut edges, even though it was the same laser at the same wavelength. Additionally, if the pulse energy from the XeCl laser were the same as in the favorable case but the pulse width were only 10 nsec, the fiberoptic would be easily damaged, even though the same energy density was used. If a continuous wave (CW) laser operating in this ultraviolet wavelength region were used at a power level that would cut the tissue and would be transmitted through the fiber, one would produce severe thermal damage to the tissue even though the wavelength was still in the ultraviolet. If a high pulse repetition rate of 500 pps or very high focused energy density of 1 J/sq mm were used to irradiate the tissue, it would produce severe blast damage. For each laser procedure and tissue, an optimal set of parameters must be defined!

For these reasons there is no universal laser device or set of laser light parameters for effective treatment of all medical diseases, just as there is no universal drug for all human disorders.

Therefore, greater acceptance of lasers for medical treatment will come with better understanding of the proper choice of laser light energy values needed to perform a specific treatment. When this knowledge is identified from careful scientific studies in the research laboratory, a safely packaged laser device and delivery system operated within the appropriate range of conditions will greatly increase the acceptance of lasers for clinical applications.

LASER FUNDAMENTALS

A laser device inefficiently converts electrical energy into light energy. Energy in the form of a laser beam of light energy has certain special characteristics compared with other forms of energy. Before understanding the laser device, one requires an understanding of some properties and characteristics of light. Light is electromagnetic radiation that has a frequency, phase, and amplitude. Light also has particle characteristics, and a beam of light consists of discrete packets of energy called photons. To understand medical laser applications it is important to understand that light is a form of radiant energy that is convertible into other forms of energy, such as electrical, heat, chemical, and kinetic energy. From quantum theory, the energy of a photon of light is related to its frequency of oscillation in the electromagnetic spectrum, which is in the range of 10^{12} to 10^{16} cps. These frequencies are so high that they are extremely difficult to measure experimentally, and therefore another wave property, the wavelength, or the distance between wave crests of the wave, is measured, as depicted in Figure 2–2. The wavelength is related to the speed of light *(c)* and the frequency of the electromagnetic radiation by the relationship $\lambda = c/v$, where λ is the wavelength expressed in units of length, typically angstroms (10^{-8} cm), nanometers (10^{-9} m), or microns (10^{-6} m). The energy carried by a photon of light is given by the relationship $E = hv$ or $E = hc/\lambda$, where E is a unit of energy, typically in joules, and h (Planck's constant) is 6.6×10^{-34} joule-seconds. To achieve a better understanding of the relationship between laser wavelength, energy of a photon, frequency, and the form of energy emanating from lasers used in medical research, Table 2–1 lists several commonly used lasers with these relationships. From the relationships in this table one can see that when the frequency of light increases, the energy per photon increases and the wavelength decreases.

Interaction of Laser Radiation With Matter

Light interacts with matter by the processes of absorption, transmission, reflection, refraction, diffraction, and several types of scattering. From common experience, we visualize objects that do not emit light of their own but reflect light from some other source of illumination, such as the sun or a lamp. Visible light covers the wavelength region from 400 to 700 nm, and white light is made up of a distribution of wavelengths in this range. When an object appears colored under illumination by white light, it is due to selective absorption of light of the colors other than that observed. The absorption of light of the other frequencies is most often converted into heat in the absorbing material.

Atoms and molecules are the chemical building blocks of matter and can exist in many different energy states. An atom has translational energy or energy of motion that

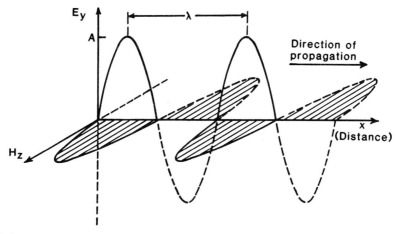

FIG 2–2.
The instantaneous electric (E_y) and magnetic (H_z) field strength vectors of a light wave with wavelength (λ) as a function of position along the axis of propagation (x). A is the amplitude of the electric field.

TABLE 2–1.
Various Medical Lasers and Their Properties

Laser	Wavelength, μm	Frequency, cps	Energy/Photon		Photons/W (J/sec)
			J	eV	
CO_2	10.6	2.8×10^{13}	1.9×10^{-20}	0.12	3.7×10^{19}
Nd:YAG	1.06	2.8×10^{14}	1.9×10^{-19}	1.2	5.3×10^{18}
Second harmonic	0.532	5.6×10^{14}	3.6×10^{-19}	2.3	2.7×10^{18}
Third harmonic	0.353	8.4×10^{14}	5.6×10^{-19}	3.5	1.8×10^{18}
Fourth harmonic	0.266	1.1×10^{15}	7.5×20^{-19}	4.7	1.3×10^{18}
Argon ion	0.514	1.1×10^{14}	3.8×10^{-19}	2.4	2.6×10^{18}
Excimer					
XeCl	0.308	9.7×10^{14}	6.5×10^{-19}	4.0	1.6×10^{18}
XeF	0.351	8.6×10^{14}	5.6×10^{-19}	3.5	1.8×10^{18}
KrF	0.248	1.2×10^{15}	8×10^{-19}	5.0	1.3×10^{18}
ArF	0.193	1.6×10^{15}	1.0×10^{-18}	6.4	9.7×10^{17}

is characteristic of the temperature of the environment wherein the atom is located. Atoms also have various electronic energy states in which they can exist where the electrons orbiting around the positive nucleus can be excited to higher energy orbits by absorption of a photon of radiation or by collision with a fast-moving particle such as an electron. Molecules have similar energy states of translational motion as well as numerous electronic energy states but they also absorb energy into rotational and vibrational motion, as depicted in Figure 2–3. From quantum theory, the energy levels of rotation and vibration of molecules and the electronic energy levels of atoms and molecules can have only certain discrete energy values, whereas translational motion energy can have a continuum of values. Each discrete energy level is unique to the particular atom or molecule and is the basis of the characteristic chemical properties of atoms and molecules. For an atom or molecule to absorb a photon of light to transfer it from one optically allowed energy level to another, excited energy level, the frequency of the photon must be in resonance or correspond to the exact energy difference between two energy levels in the molecular or atomic species. The majority of atoms and molecules have optical energy resonances only in the infrared and ultraviolet region of the electromagnetic spectrum. Resonances in the visible region lie between 1.5 and 3 eV, which is too high an energy for molecular rotation and vibration and too low an energy for most electronic excitation. However, there are certain complicated organic and inorganic molecules that do have visible resonances, and these compounds are usually designated dye molecules or pigments. Table 2–2 lists various energy transitions of atomic and molecular species with the typical magnitude of the difference between two types of energy levels and their corresponding energy spectral resonances.

Therefore, absorption of light by an irradiated material results directly in increasing the energy content of the material. This increased energy can be eliminated by reradiation of the absorbed photon; if the photon emitted has the same energy as the photon absorbed, there is no net increase in the energy of the material. If the absorbed photon is not reemitted or a photon with less energy than that absorbed is reemitted, as is usually the case, some energy remains, which is usually converted into thermal motion or heat in the absorber. For most surgical applications of laser light, the absorption process is most critical to the desired treatment.

Refraction and Reflection of Light

If a beam of light is not absorbed in a material or reflected from its surface, it is transmitted through the medium, but its path may be deviated and dispersed. When light encounters an interface between two transparent media in which the velocity is different

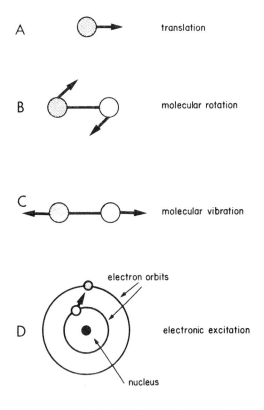

FIG 2–3.
Pictorial view of the types of energy on atomic and molecular levels. **A** through **C** are examples of thermal motion of the molecule. **D** shows how electronic excitation can, in a molecular system, lead to direct fragmentation of chemical bonds.

(i.e., materials having different values of the index of refraction, such as an air-glass interface), a portion of the beam of light is reflected, and that portion that is transmitted can undergo a change in direction or is said to be refracted. We make use of this property when we focus a laser beam by means of a lens or when we disperse wavelengths using a prism. The amount of light reflected vs. transmitted is wavelength dependent and is also dependent on the angle of incidence to the medium. For example, a beam of visible light impinging perpendicular to a glass window will have a 4% reflection loss at each air-glass interface or suffer an 8% loss of beam intensity on passing through a transparent window or lens. If the same beam of light is incident at a glancing angle, the reflection loss may be less than 4% per surface, with the minimum reflection loss being defined as Brewster's angle, which is about 54 degrees for visible wavelengths incident on an air-glass interface.

TABLE 2–2.
Characteristics of Molecules at Different Energy Levels

Energy Transition	Typical Energy Separation, eV	Spectral Region	
		μm	Frequency Range
Electronic	≥2.5	≤0.496	Visible → ultraviolet
Vibrational	0.12	10.3	Infrared
Rotational	1.2×10^{-3}	1,033	Radar
Translational (1 kT at 300°K)	2.6×10^{-2}	47.7	Infrared

Light incident on a surface can also be reflected. When the reflected portion is a substantial portion of the incident light, the surface is called a mirror. Specular reflection occurs at a smooth surface, and the reflected light returns at an angle equal to the angle of incidence of the light beam on the mirror surface. Diffuse reflection occurs at irregular surfaces, and the reflected light is dispersed in an angular distribution proportional to the cosine of the angle of incidence. This type of scattering is called lambertian scattering, after Lambert's cosine law.

Absorption and Scattering of Light

When light is absorbed, the absorbing medium is increased in energy content by the energy contained by the total number of photons that were absorbed. This usually results in raising the temperature of the absorbing medium. The relationship between the absorption and transmission of monochromatic light by any homogeneous, isotroptic medium obeys the Beer-Lambert formula: $I = I_0 \exp(-\mu x)$, where I is the intensity of light transmitted through a dilute homogeneous medium of length x, with an attenuation coefficient of μ, and I_0 is the incident intensity of the light beam. The ratio of I/I_0 is the transmittance through a medium; a ratio of 1 would indicate a totally transparent medium with no absorption (this neglects reflection losses at the container surface). The formula states that for the conditions specified above for an absorbing medium, the attenuation of light is exponential, with the proportion of light absorbed per unit of length being constant.

Scattering of a beam of light by a medium does not always result in increasing the energy content of the medium and raising its temperature. Scattering of light by particles smaller than the wavelength of the light beam is called Rayleigh scattering, and its effect on a parallel beam of light is to disperse a portion of the beam in other directions. This type of scattering is strongest for shorter wavelengths, such as the ultraviolet. This scattering is symmetric in both forward and backward directions to the line of propagation of the light beam. If the scattering particles are larger in size than the characteristic of the wavelength of light (e.g., for green light, 0.4-μm diameter), the scattering is called Mie scattering and depends on the size and the shape of the particles as well as the wavelength of light. Forward scattering predominates for Mie scattering. For a laser beam propagating across a room, Rayleigh scattering is produced by the molecules of air, whereas Mie scattering results from dust or particulates in the room. When the particles are much larger than the wavelength of light, Mie scattering and diffraction dominate over Rayleigh scattering. For this reason, when smoke is placed in a laser beam path, it allows the observer to photograph its propagation across a room.

Since a laser produces energy in the form of a beam of light, the propagation of this form of energy through various media is very important in determining the effect of the light energy when it is finally incident on a tissue surface. To get a beam of light from a laser to the tissue site for a medical procedure, the process of reflection is used to steer the beam from the source to the target. Refraction or reflection from a curved surface is used to focus or defocus the spot size of the laser beam to either increase or decrease the energy and power density on the target. Fiberoptic transmission is another form of light beam propagation through an optical fiber guide by means of total internal reflection. Once the beam is delivered and shaped by the various optical elements, the processes of absorption and scattering in the target and any fluid media surrounding the target are of utmost importance in understanding the therapeutic effect of light energy.

In actuality, the simple formulas of Beer's law and Mie and Rayleigh scattering do not hold rigorously for high-energy light densities as are often used in laser procedures on tissue. First, tissue is heterogeneous, and scattering phenomena can be multiple rather

LIGHT ABSORPTION AND STIMULATED EMISSION

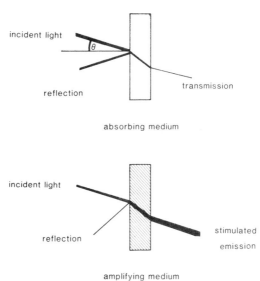

FIG 2–4.
The upper figure displays the typical effects of a beam of light incident on an absorbing medium. The lower figure shows the process when the medium is activated to produce stimulated emission.

than single, as occurs for low-density absorbing and scattering medium. Additionally, the high peak power generated by pulsed laser radiation often produces nonlinear absorption processes that do not occur when low-power light sources are used. For cardiovascular applications inside a blood vessel, not only may a beam of laser light be very strongly absorbed by blood itself, but the red blood cells will scatter the light or tend to defocus it by Mie scattering and diffraction. On the other hand, infrared laser beams will be strongly attenuated by water absorption and will not propagate through any aqueous media.

Stimulated Emission

Figure 2–4 shows the typical processes of light reflection, absorption, and transmission through a medium. Stimulated emission, the basis for laser action, is a special case where incident light on a specially prepared active medium results in an amplified or more intense beam of collimated light as it propagates through this amplifying medium. What Figure 2–4 does not show is the other energy source that must be used to take a normal transmitting or absorbing medium into an amplifying state. The deposition of raw electrical energy into a medium to produce an optical amplifier is the basis for a laser generator.

To illustrate the physics underlying a laser gain medium, we will consider a gaseous laser medium, although liquid, solid, and plasma media are also suitable for laser action. The various energy values pertinent to a gaseous molecule have been listed previously (see Table 2–2). When a gaseous system is contained at a particular temperature and does not have any input from any other energy source, the molecules will reside in the lowest energy levels consistent with the temperature of the gas. At this equilibrium

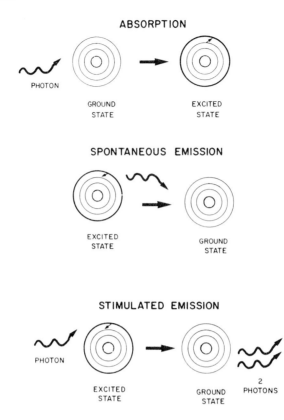

FIG 2–5.
The upper figure shows a typical atomic absorption process for a photon resulting in excitation of an electron to a higher energy level. The atom will lose the energy in collision with another species, increasing the thermal energy, or reemit the energy by spontaneous emission. Stimulated emission occurs when a photon encounters an excited state and induces the excited level to a lower level, with the emission of a photon with the same energy, phase, and direction as the incident photon.

temperature, the ratio of the number of molecules in an excited state 1 to that in a lower energy state 0, with an energy difference between the two states of ΔE $(E_1 - E_0)$, is given by the formula

$$n_1/n_0 = g_1/g_0 \exp - (\Delta E/KT)$$

where g_1 and g_0 are the degeneracies of each energy state. Considering the energy levels in Table 2–2, at room temperature, the fraction of molecules existing in an excited electronic energy level is 10^{-41}, for vibrational energy the ratio is 10^{-2}, and for rotational it is 0.95. At room temperature, the probability of finding any molecules in an excited electronic state are extremely small; about 1% of the molecules reside in the first excited vibrational state, and there is almost an equal population between the lowest and next higher rotational energy states.

Possible interactions of a photon with an atom or molecule are depicted in Figure 2–5. When a photon whose energy is in resonance between two energy levels of molecular species passes through the gas, it will most probably be absorbed, since at equilibrium almost all the molecules are in the lower energy state. Therefore, the interaction of the photon with molecules in the lower energy state is to excite molecules in this lower energy state to the higher state. This process results in energy deposition into the gas. This excited species can lose this absorbed energy by reemitting a photon in a random direction. This process is called spontaneous emission. However, if by some means one can excite the gas so that there is a greater population in the excited energy level than in the lower energy level, then when the photon passes through this excited gas medium it will stimulate the emission of a photon in phase and in the same direction as the incident photon to cause the excited molecule to return to the lower energy level. This process, stimulated emission, will continue as long as a critical population difference remains between the number of molecules in the excited state and the number in the lower state. However, as stimulated emission or laser action begins, it removes molecules from the upper level and increases the population of the lower level. At some point the population difference between the two levels will decrease and the probability of a photon being absorbed will increase and cease laser action. To prevent the laser action of the gain medium from being terminated, either some means must be found to pump the lower level to the upper level at a rate faster than the depopulation by stimulated emission to the lower level, or some means is needed to depopulate the lower level at a rate faster than it is being produced by the lasing action.

Thus, the process of producing laser action is to excite a gain medium to produce either a continuous population inversion between an excited energy level and a lower energy state or a temporary inversion between two levels for pulsed operation. As shown in Figure 2–6 for a three- and four-level pumping scheme, it is much easier to produce and maintain a population inversion in a multilevel system than in a two-level system, with the lower level being the ground level because the ground level is highly populated.

Figure 2–7 illustrates the processes occurring in a laser when this population inversion is produced. A gain medium is terminated with a totally reflective mirror and a partially reflective mirror. Next, energy is deposited into the gain medium to produce a high population of energetically excited species. The excited species try to lose this extra energy either by degradation of the absorbed energy into thermal motion or heat or by reradiation of the excess energy from the excited state to the lower state by spontaneous emission, which occurs with a random phase and in a random direction. Some of this spontaneously emitted light will propagate in line with the optical cavity axis and be returned through the gain medium. If the photons emitted are incident on a gas molecule in the lower energy level, they will be absorbed and more excited molecules will be

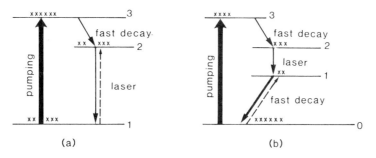

(a)   (b)

FIG 2–6.

A, schematic diagram of a three-energy-level laser pumping scheme, where a population inversion between levels 2 and 1 is required for lasing; if the pumping rate from 1 to 3 is not greater than the deactivation rate of 2 to 1, absorption as depicted in the dashed line will terminate the laser action. B, a four-energy-level pumping scheme, where a population inversion between levels 2 and 1 must be maintained.

EVENTS IN A LASER RESONATOR

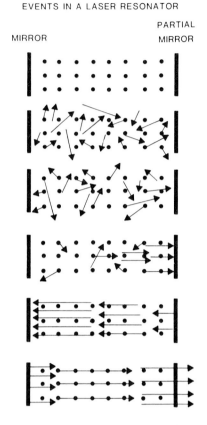

FIG 2–7.
Events in a laser resonator consist of excitation of an active medium. The randomly generated spontaneously emitted photons are fed back through the gain medium in an optical cavity with a partially transmitting mirror output to produce a directional laser beam.

produced. However, if they encounter molecules in the excited state, they will stimulate them to emit photons in the same direction, with the same energy and the same phase as the incident photons. If the pumping means maintains this excited condition, the stimulated emission process will build an intense beam of collimated light that will compete with the spontaneous emission process and the thermal degradation mechanism for deexcitation of the excited state. Essentially, the laser action is initiated from the spontaneous emission process and, rapidly using optical feedback, builds to be the dominant process for removal of excited species from the gain medium. To produce infrared laser action, a population inversion must be established between two vibrational-rotational levels, whereas to produce a visible or ultraviolet laser action, a population inversion must be produced between two electronic energy levels.

LASER DEVICES

Argon Ion Lasers

The argon laser has been used extensively for medical procedures and is a well-developed laser system. It operates on a CW basis and is capable of average powers up to approximately 20 W. The laser emits radiation at a variety of wavelengths, but the wavelengths most commonly selected for medical use are in the blue-green spectral region at 488 to 514 nm. The population inversion in argon gas is produced by passing a very high electric discharge current through the gas. Figure 2–8 shows the energy level diagram for producing a population inversion in electronic states of argon ion. In this case, the discharge in the argon gas produces high-energy electrons that collide with argon atoms to excite and ionize the atom. Note that the upper laser level requires 35 eV of energy to produce the upper laser level in the singly charged argon ion. This upper level radiates to a lower energy level of argon ion with the emission of a photon at 514 nm, which has an energy of only 2.5 eV. Therefore, the ultimate theoretical efficiency of this laser device is 2.5/35 × 100%, or 7%, but in reality the overall efficiency is much less than this because of the low probability of electron impact producing the upper state and because of low optical extraction efficiency. In practice, the overall efficiency of an argon ion laser is only about 0.1%, which means that the power supply has to produce 20 kW of power to generate 20 W of green laser light.

The lower laser level in the argon ion transition radiates spontaneously away in the vacuum ultraviolet wavelength region. This is typical of multilevel visible and ultraviolet laser transitions. To create a population inversion between electronic energy levels, the laser transition must be of lower energy than the transition from the lower level to its next lower energy state. This condition requires that the rate of energy loss by collision or radiation be proportional to the magnitude of energy transition difference between the two levels. Therefore, visible and ultraviolet lasers are inherently much more inefficient converters of electrical to light energy, since they operate on a multiple-level transition scheme. Since 99.9% of the 20 kW of electrical power ends up as heat in the laser gain medium, this thermal energy must be removed or the high temperatures will rapidly destroy the laser tube. The need to remove large quantities of heat adds significant cooling requirements, which further complicate laser design.

The blue-green light of the argon ion laser is primarily absorbed by chromogens and hemoglobin and it penetrates tissue to a greater extent than ultraviolet and far-infrared light. The absorption of focused high-power argon radiation leads to heating of the

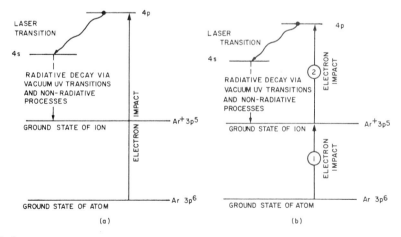

FIG 2–8.
Energy level diagram for a singly ionized argon *(Ar)* laser. There are two electron excitation mechanisms: **A**, a single excitation from the ground level of Ar to the upper level of Ar⁺; and **B**, a two-step electron excitation process. *UV* indicates ultraviolet; *s* and *p* are spectroscopic designators for orbits of the excited electrons.

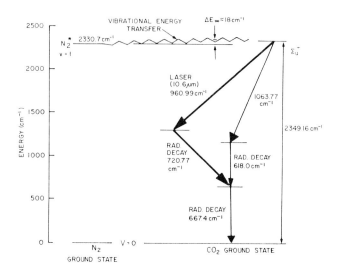

FIG 2-9.
Energy level diagram showing the transfer of energy from vibrationally excited metastable nitrogen (N_2^*) to the upper level of vibronically excited carbon dioxide (CO_2), which produces lasing at 10.6 μm. v indicates vibrational quantum number; RAD, radiative; $\Delta E\infty$, energy separation between metastable N_2^* and the upper laser level state of CO_2; Σ_u^+ spectroscopic symbol for energy level of CO_2.

irradiated area. If chromophores are present, argon laser energy is useful for applications that require selective localized heating of tissue. However, the excessive penetration into most tissue with the concomitant lateral scattering and large heat-affected zone preclude CW irradiation using this wavelength for controlled applications. In fact, the use of CW argon laser for angioplasty has been hindered by the lack of control of ablation and by deep heating of the vessel wall.[11] Considerable improvement in the use of this laser for angioplasty has been achieved by converting the laser energy into heat at a metal cap and using the laser in essence as an electrocautery device to minimize the depth of heat penetration into the blood vessel wall.[12] Since the visible wavelength is readily transmitted by glass optical fibers, this laser energy can easily be delivered in medical procedures.

The CO_2 Laser

The CO_2 is an infrared laser operating on a molecular vibrational energy transition and lases at 10.6 μm. The laser can be operated at high power levels on a CW basis, on a radio frequency (RF) excited basis, and as a high peak power pulsed transversely excited (TEA) laser. Although each type of operation mentioned still produces a laser beam at 10.6 μm, the nature of the laser device is different, and the beam of 10.6-μm radiation from each type of CO_2 laser device can produce substantially different effects on tissue, although they all go by the name CO_2 laser.

The active medium in the CO_2 laser is CO_2, but additions of nitrogen (N_2) and He are important for its operation. Figure 2-9 shows the energy diagram for the laser transition. Note that for an infrared laser it is easier to operate at energy levels close to the ground level, providing for a more favorable efficiency. In this laser, an electric discharge is established in the gas mixture and the N_2 is raised to an excited vibrational level by collisions with electrons in the discharge. Because the N_2 molecule is symmetric and has no permanent dipole, it does not lose the excited vibrational energy by radiation;

in effect it is trapped in a metastable state and transfers its excess energy in a collision with a CO_2 ground-state molecule, which rises to an excited vibrational level of CO_2 in close energy resonance with the excited N_2 molecule. The CO_2 molecule, however, does have a dipole-allowed radiation transition at 10.6 μm; therefore, once the energy deposited in N_2 from the electric discharge is transferred from excited N_2 to CO_2, laser action can occur and the intermediate CO_2 energy levels are rapidly depopulated by radiation and collisions with He. The He gas also rapidly removes heat from the system so that the lower levels in the CO_2 transition do not become heavily populated. The CO_2 laser can be very efficient, on the order of 10%.

It is much easier to produce a population inversion between vibrational-rotational levels than electronic levels. However, the limitation of this argument is that the pump source, which in this case is an electrical discharge, tends to decompose molecular species, which limits the utility of the laser gain medium unless the gas mixture is continually replaced. For the CO_2 laser, the discharge dissociates the CO_2 molecule, producing CO and O_2, which are detrimental to laser action. It is the inability of the gain medium to regenerate itself that limits the types of practical laser devices that have been demonstrated for molecular infrared lasers.

The CO_2 laser wavelength is strongly absorbed by water vapor, and since most tissue has a large water content, the penetration depth of this wavelength is small, and only local superficial heating is produced, in contrast to the visible and near-infrared wavelengths. This wavelength is good for local heating, microsurgery, and surface coagulation. However, the particular procedures for this laser wavelength should be carefully evaluated for the choice of laser beam delivery (i.e., pulsed vs. CW) and the peak power of the pulsed laser application. Although the CO_2 laser has found a wide acceptance for use in medical procedures, its utility is limited by the lack of availability of suitable flexible fiberoptic delivery; it is usually delivered by means of awkward, flexible, articulated arms or short, hollow waveguide tubes. The CO_2 has been used for intraoperative coronary laser angioplasty, but the laser energy has had to be delivered through a short, hollow, metal waveguide.[13] The CW or RF excited CO_2 lasers, which are compact, simple devices, may not be as appropriate for cardiovascular surgery as use of a higher-powered pulsed TEA CO_2 laser, especially if calcified material needs to be removed without extensive heat deposition into surrounding tissue.

Solid-State Lasers: the Nd:YAG

This laser is an example of a solid-state laser gain medium instead of the gaseous lasers discussed before. Solid-state lasers are optically pumped either by incoherent broad spectral radiation produced by a flashlamp or by another laser. Figure 2–10 shows the method of optical pumping. Electrical energy is passed through a gas discharge flashlamp, producing excited species that radiate the excited energy by spontaneous emission. A solid laser rod intercepts some of the randomly emitted flashlamp radiation, and a portion of the broad spectral output is absorbed into an excited energy state. Figure 2–11 shows the energy level diagram for the Nd:YAG laser. Excited levels of Nd are produced when radiation in only the 0.73- and 0.8-μm wavelength regions is absorbed from the flashlamp. Since only a portion of the laser rod is pumped by the flashlamp and only a fraction of the output of the flashlamp is emitted in the appropriate wavelength regions, the efficiency of the laser is only about 1% overall. The Nd:YAG laser is a four-level laser transition, which facilitates maintaining a population inversion. This laser can be run either CW or pulsed. One advantage of a solid-state laser gain medium is that more active species for

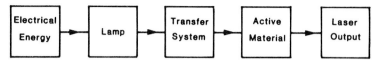

FIG 2–10.
General scheme of an optically pumped laser system. Each box is coupled with a certain energy transfer efficiency. The total laser efficiency is the product of the individual efficiencies.

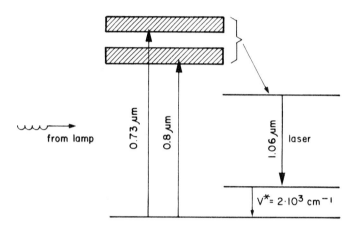

FIG 2–11.
Simplified level schematic for neodymium:YAG laser transition. Note the upper starting laser levels are produced by absorption of narrow bands in the 0.7- to 0.8-µm region from the broad spectral output of the flashlamp.

the upper laser population can be produced than in a gas or liquid per unit volume of the gain region, owing to the increased density in a solid matrix. Additionally, the upper excited laser state can be stored before the stimulated emission process is initiated, and the energy can be released as short intense optical pulses by an optical feedback mechanism. This technique, called "Q-switching" the laser, produces high-peak-power pulses in the range of 10 nsec and less from a pulsed Nd:YAG laser. These high-power Q-switched pulses can be used for nonlinear second harmonic generation in a suitable crystal host to convert substantial fractions (40% to 50%) of the 1.06-µm radiation into the green at 0.532 µm. Additional frequency conversion to produce 0.352 and 0.266 µm can be done but with decreasing efficiency. The efficient generation of the various harmonics of the Nd:YAG laser is peak-power dependent; therefore, the harmonics are best produced with short pulses at high peak power produced by a Q-switched laser.

The disadvantage of solid-state lasers, as in most lasers, is still the low laser efficiency, about 1%; the rest of the pump energy is rapidly degraded into heat in the solid host. Heat can damage the expensive laser rod and also cause the laser beam to be distorted in passage through the laser gain medium if a temperature gradient exists. Other types of optically pumped solid-state lasers are the alexandrite laser, which lases at 0.760 µm, the ruby laser at 0.68 µm, and the erbium (Er):YAG and Er:YLF lasers, which radiate near 3.0 µm.

The 1.06-µm radiation of the Nd:YAG laser is readily transmitted through silica fiberoptics. This laser can operate at high average powers CW and high peak powers for pulsed applications, and its output can be converted to shorter wavelengths. This makes this laser a very versatile tool. The 1.06-μm radiation has deep penetration into tissue, causing heat generation beyond the surface of irradiation, and is used for coagulation and tumor necrosis. To localize the heating produced by CW laser irradiation at 1.06 μm, sapphire tips have been used. As with the argon laser probe with a metal cap at the end of the fiberoptic, this turns the laser into a heating probe similar to an electrocautery device. Microablation using the shorter-wavelength harmonics of Nd:YAG is possible but suffers from the decreased laser efficiency when the frequency is changed and from difficulty in transmitting high-peak-power pulses through fiberoptics even though the fibers are transparent to these wavelength. Since high-peak-power pulses are necessary to produce the other wavelengths, this may present a problem for efficient fiber delivery.

The Er:YAG laser is of considerable interest for microsurgical applications because the strong water absorption at 3.0 μm makes this laser similar to the CO_2 laser for small penetration into tissue. Although this laser is not as well developed or as versatile as the CO_2 laser, it does have efficient fiberoptic transmission, which the CO_2 laser lacks. However, other aspects of fluoride infrared fibers, such as low flexibility, brittleness, and poor strength, make them less applicable than plastic or silica fibers. For many medical procedures, if one cannot get the laser radiation conveniently to the target, in most cases by fiberoptics, then the laser will have limited use.

Dye Lasers

Dye lasers are another example of an optically pumped laser system. Either a flash-lamp or another laser is used to pump the liquid dye solution. Depending on the dye chosen, laser emission can be obtained in a particular portion of the wavelength spectrum from the near ultraviolet through the near infrared. These lasers can be operated in either a CW or a pulsed mode. The dye laser is very useful as a general-purpose laser to determine the optimum wavelength for a medical procedure. However, these laser systems are complicated since the dye must be circulated through a chamber, since dye lifetime is rather short, and since the dye solution must be replaced regularly. As discussed previously, except for pigments that selectively absorb visible light, strong absorption by tissue occurs in either the infrared or the ultraviolet, where dye lasers do not operate efficiently.

Excimer Lasers

The excimer gas laser is one of the few lasers that operate directly in the ultraviolet spectral region, and it only operates in a pulsed mode of operation (i.e., it does not operate CW). The word *excimer* stands for excited dimer, and there are a variety of excimer lasers that operate in regions of the ultraviolet from 0.193 to 0.351 μm. The laser is produced by chemical reaction induced by generating a high-voltage, transverse-pulsed electric discharge on a high-pressure gas mixture containing several atmospheres of an inert gas, such as He, Ne, or argon, and several percent of another inert gas, such as Xe or krypton (Kr), and a much smaller percentage, around 0.1%, of a halogen compound such as hydrogen chloride or fluorine (F_2). The excimers, or rare-gas halide lasers, are unusual lasers as they are a two-level energy system and the gas is very good at regenerating itself between pulses to the original starting species, allowing for long sealed operation, in particular for the Cl lasers. The electric discharge ionizes and causes electronic excitation of the minor inert gas species, such as Xe, in the discharge. At the same time, the electrons in the discharge produce negative halogen ions, such as Cl^-.

The Xe$^+$ ion is strongly attracted to the negative halogen ion to produce an ionically bound molecule in an excited state (i.e., XeCl), which is similar in electronic structure to salts such as sodium chloride. When this excimer molecule radiates, it goes to the lower ground level of XeCl, which is covalently bonded very weakly, as the Xe atom has returned to its inert gas electronic configuration. This lower energy state of the XeCl molecule rapidly separates to the individual atoms. Therefore, the lower laser molecular level is lost as soon as it is formed, and there is very little population in this level to stop laser action.

Excimer lasing actions from ArF at 0.193 μm, KrCl at 0.222 μm, XeCl at 0.308 μm, and XeF at 0.351 μm are examples of a class of intense pulsed laser sources of ultraviolet radiation. Since these lasers are relatively new devices, their use in the medical field is rather recent. The output pulse width obtainable from these devices ranges from under 10 nsec to several hundred. Descriptions of the excimer laser kinetics and laser design are found in the literature.[14, 15]

The advantage of the excimer laser for medical applications is the strong absorption by tissue in the ultraviolet range, which minimizes penetration heating and provides for microsurgical procedures. The ArF laser, at 0.193 μm, has the strongest absorption but has been used mostly for corneal applications, since this wavelength is difficult to transmit through present fiberoptics. The XeCl laser and the XeF laser are readily transmitted through high-purity silica-based fiberoptics, provided the pulse width of the laser is long enough to keep the power density on the fiber below its destruction level. Precise ablation of calcified and fatty plaque using long-pulse 0.308-μm radiation through a fiberoptic has been demonstrated.[10] At present, the XeCl laser is the most appropriate laser source for pulsed ultraviolet angioplasty since it is (1) a very efficient laser device (1% to 4%), (2) has the most benign long-lived gas mixture of all the excimer lasers, and (3) is readily transmitted through fiberoptics when operated at pulse widths greater than 100 nsec.

For microsurgical applications there is a requirement for strong absorption by the laser wavelength to limit the ablation area and volume per pulse. Either infrared or ultraviolet wavelengths are needed for tissues that do not possess a strong visible chromophore or pigment. In the infrared, the CO$_2$ laser is hampered by the lack of an adequate fiberoptic delivery system, and the newer Er:YAG and Er:YLF lasers need more development for both the laser and the fiberoptic delivery system, but there is promise that these engineering issues may be solved. The excimer lasers have not been as extensively refined for use in the medical environment, but there is no major engineering problem to prevent achievement of a proper medical design. Fiberoptic delivery is possible for long-pulse-width XeCl and XeF laser radiation at 0.308 and 0.351 μm. Besides proper system engineering, questions regarding possible mutagenic effects of the ultraviolet wavelength have to be addressed. Adequate fiberoptic delivery at the shorter ultraviolet wavelengths, such as 0.193 and 0.248 μm, has yet to be demonstrated satisfactorily. The main promise for the use of ultraviolet wavelengths is the high efficiency for ablation of most materials owing to the direct photochemical molecular dissociation mechanism[16] vs. rapid heating, as is the mechanism for infrared ablation. In addition, the ultraviolet does not require a water absorption mechanism to transfer the light energy to the tissue; therefore, it is possible to pass some ultraviolet wavelengths through fluid media, such as saline solutio.ı, with limited attenuation. Obviously, further work is necessary to study the differences between ablation from the two wavelength regions in the ultraviolet and infrared.

LASER-TISSUE INTERACTION

The fundamentals of how laser light is produced by the laser device have been presented, but the physician is dealing with the effects of that laser radiation on tissue. To understand tissue response to laser light radiation, several optical variables must be specified. These are the irradiance level, the energy fluence, and the exposure time, which provide the total light energy dosage. Therefore, these variables of laser light must always be specified: (1) the energy delivered per unit of time at the target, (2) the spot size of the target area irradiated, and (3) the time of irradiation and, if pulsed laser is used, the duration of the laser pulse. There are two types of laser light power designations, average power and peak power, when a pulsed laser is used. Average power is the energy delivered per unit of time, whereas peak power is the energy contained in a single laser pulse divided by its pulse width. The pulse width is typically measured using a fast photodetection-oscilloscope combination, and for a symmetric pulse shape the width is defined as the width at half the maximum of the peak of the pulse. The average power delivered by a pulsed laser is the total energy delivered per unit of time, which equals the number of pulses per second from the laser times the individual pulse energy. These two forms of average power level, one for a pulsed laser and the other for a CW laser, usually produce distinctly different effects on tissue even when the total energy dosage is the same and the wavelength is the same. Designating average power without knowing the other characteristics of the laser, especially if used in a pulsed manner, is insufficient for understanding the procedure. In all cases, the irradiance or power per unit area is the important characteristic for understanding a laser procedure. For example, if a pulsed laser produces pulses with energy of 100 mJ at 100 pulses per second with a 10-nsec pulse duration in a 1-sq cm spot size, its average power density is 100 mJ times 100 pulses per second per square centimeter or 10 W/sq cm average power, but the peak power is 100 mJ $\div$ 10 $\times$ 10^{-9} sec/sq cm, or 10 megawatts (MW)/sq cm. For pulsed lasers, both the average as well as peak power density or irradiance values are important. For CW lasers, the irradiance is equal to the laser power output from the laser divided by the laser beam cross section at the tissue site, and its unit is watts per square centimeter.

The primary uniqueness of energy in the form of laser light is the ability to concentrate the light energy both spatially as well as temporally to cause very high levels of local energy deposition, which cannot be easily achieved using other sources or forms of energy. The energy fluence is the energy per pulse divided by the beam spot area and is expressed in joules per square centimeter. For a CW laser the energy fluence is given by the laser output power in watts times the exposure time in seconds divided by the area irradiated.

Once these parameters of the laser light are measured, the next important effect is absorption and scattering of the light energy by the tissue, which is typically wavelength dependent. The three basic mechanisms of absorption of laser light are shown in Figure 2–12. The most common for CW lasers or pulsed lasers in the visible and infrared is the conversion of the absorbed photons into heat or thermal motion of the molecules that compose tissue. As heat is deposited into an irradiated area, there is thermal conduction by the tissue to its surrounding area. To minimize the lateral spread of this heat conduction, either a pulsed laser with a pulse duration shorter than the characteristic thermal conduction time of the tissue is used or a very small area is irradiated. As the absorbed laser energy is converted into heat, the temperature of the tissue rises, causing cell necrosis. The temperature of the tissue continues to rise until it reaches the level where water vaporization occurs, and then the temperature rises until tissue vaporization occurs. This thermal absorption process occurs with both CW and pulsed laser sources when the pulse duration is greater than the thermal diffusion time for the tissue or the energy per pulse is below ablation threshold.

The other two absorption mechanisms in medical applications are predominantly produced by high-peak-power pulsed laser sources. The photoplasma mechanism is somewhat independent of laser wavelength and can occur in materials normally transparent to the laser wavelength at low power levels. Very high-peak-power laser radiation produces a very intense local electric field, causing dielectric breakdown of material and heating of liberated electrons, which avalanche to produce a local plasma. The sudden expansion of vaporized material produces a shock wave, causing localized rupture of the tissue. This process is used in ophthalmology where the laser beam can be focused into the eye. At the focal spot, the power density is high enough to produce tissue ablation by means of dielectric breakdown. This mechanism works on materials that are normally transparent to the laser wavelength at low intensity; this mechanism can also destroy optics and solid laser rods if any high laser power densities are incident on the optical elements. The third mechanism only pertains to short-pulse ultraviolet wavelengths and is called photochemical ablation. The energy of an ultraviolet photon if absorbed by a molecule can rupture the molecular bonds directly, causing a change of a large molecule to smaller fragment molecules, which then leave the substrate in a rapid expansion. This is a very efficient tissue ablation mechanism and produces clean incisions with minimal thermal heat retention in the nonirradiated tissue when short-pulsed ultraviolet laser sources are used (10 nsec to 1 μsec). This process requires a strong absorption of the laser wavelength by the tissue in the ultraviolet, and for pulsed ultraviolet sources, multiphoton processes may occur as well as single photon absorption for the photochemical bond-breaking mechanism.

Figure 2–13 is a general material processing graph[17] for pulsed lasers. The effects of laser light at a given wavelength can produce different effects depending on the power density and pulse duration used. The aspect of absorption depth is not contained in this graph. Note that if a pulse of laser energy is applied over a long time, then that laser

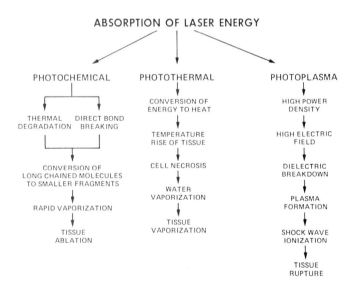

FIG 2–12.
Schematic of three types of energy deposition mechanisms in tissue following absorption of laser energy.

PULSED LASER MATERIAL PROCESSING

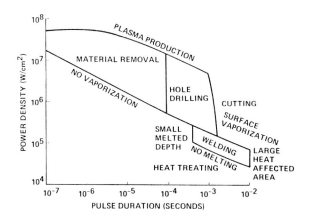

FIG 2–13.
Generalized schematic of laser power density and pulse duration suitable for material processing applications. This schematic will vary with target material and laser wavelength. (From Ready JF: *Industrial Application of Lasers.* New York, Academic Press, 1978. Used by permission.)

pulse will have a lower power density then the same energy delivered in a shorter pulse duration to the same spot size. To melt a material for welding, one needs to heat the material to a certain depth and not have it cool too rapidly or have the material rapidly vaporize. One can see that this process requires the energy to be delivered over a longer period or at lower power densities than for vaporization. If the power density level is low, heating without vaporization occurs because the absorbed heat is conducted away too rapidly to allow the material temperature to reach its vaporization level. Therefore, for efficient welding of tissue, the appropriate wavelength for the desired penetration depth is used, and the power density must be in a narrow region to prevent excess vaporization. If vaporization for material removal is required, the laser energy must be delivered at a higher power density. If the power density exceeds dielectric breakdown level, plasma production occurs. The control of the value of power density is achieved by varying the pulse duration of a non-CW laser and/or the energy by changing the area of the spot size, as shown in Figure 2–14. The smaller the spot size, the higher the power density and energy density. Note that the control of spot size using a focusing lens strongly depends on the focal length of the lens and position of the lens from the tissue surface.

The high power densities produced by laser radiation on small areas provide very localized photobiologic effects on tissue, and there is a specific minimum energy dosage required to effect tissue change on a given volume of tissue. If the laser radiation is just converted into thermal energy and subsequent heating of the tissue, the biologic effects of heat are nonspecific to the laser wavelength. The choice of laser wavelength just determines the depth of penetration of the energy deposition and extent of scattering into the tissue. The use of short pulses temporarily to concentrate the laser power density further can yield substantially different biologic effects on tissue. The wavelength in the case of the photoablation mechanism needs to be in the ultraviolet.

In conclusion, when performing a laser procedure it is best to think of the laser device as only an optical power generator and carefully consider the combination of laser wavelength, irradiance, and energy fluence used. The same type of laser, if operated in a different output mode, can cause considerably different tissue effects even though the

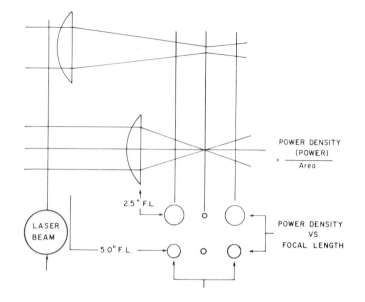

FIG 2–14.
Power density vs. focal length (F.L.) for a focused laser beam showing the relationship between laser spot size and power density with distance from the lens.

wavelength is the same. It is important to understand the nature of the interaction of the light energy with the tissue for each procedure. The necessity for the large size of the laser device with its associated heat exchangers and power supplies is due to the inefficiency of converting electric energy into the precise controlled energy in the form of a collimated, coherent laser beam. For certain medical procedures the therapeutic effect of this form of energy more than compensates for the cost and complexity of medical laser devices.

REFERENCES

1. Maiman TH: Stimulated optical radiation in ruby. *Nature* 1960; 187:493–494.
2. Javan A, Bennett WR Jr, Herroit DQ: Population inversion and continuous optical laser oscillation in a gaseous discharge containing a He-Ne mixture. *Phys Rev Lett* 1961; 6:106–110.
3. Bridges WB: Laser oscillation in singly ionized argon in the visible spectrum. *Appl Phys Lett* 1964; 4:128–130.
4. Bell WE: Visible laser transitions in Hg^+. *Appl Phys Lett* 1964; 4:34–35.
5. Patel CKN: Continuous wave laser action on vibrational-rotational transitions of CO_2. *Phys Rev* 1964; 136:A1187–A1193.
6. Burham R, Harris NW, Djeu N: Xenon fluoride laser excitation by transverse electric discharge. *Appl Phys Lett* 1976; 28:86–87.
7. Wang CP, Mirels H, Sutton DG, et al: Fast-discharge-initiated XeF laser. *Appl Phys Lett* 1976; 28:236–238.
8. Laudenslager JB, Pacala TJ, Wittig C: Electric discharge pumped nitrogen ion laser. *Appl Phys Lett* 1976; 29:580–582.
9. Fuller TA: Fundamentals of lasers in surgery and medicine, in Dixon JA (ed): *Surgical Applications of Lasers.* Chicago, Year Book Medical Publishers, 1983, pp 11–28.

10. Forrester JS, Litvack F, Grundfest WS: Laser angioplasty and cardiovascular disease. *Am J Cardiol* 1986; 57:990–992.

11. Ginsburg R, Wexler L, Mitchell RS, et al: Percutaneous transluminal laser angioplasty for treatment of peripheral vascular disease: Clinical experience with 16 patients. *Radiology* 1985; 156:619–624.

12. Sanborn TA, Faxon DP, Haudenschild CC, et al: Experimental angioplasty: Circumferential distribution of laser thermal energy with a laser probe. *J Am Coll Cardiol* 1985; 5:934–938.

13. Livesay JJ, Leachman DR, Hogan PJ, et al: Preliminary report on laser coronary endarterectomy in patients, abstracted. *Circulation* 1985; 72(suppl 3):III–302.

14. Brau CA: Rare gas halogen excimers, in Rhodes CK (ed): *Excimer Lasers.* New York, Springer-Verlag New York, 1979.

15. Laudenslager JB: Ion-molecule processes in lasers, in Ausloos P (ed): *Kinetics of Ion-Molecule Reactions.* New York, Plenum Publishing Corp, 1978.

16. Grundfest WS, Litvack F, Doyle L, et al: Comparison of in vitro and in vivo thermal effects of argon and excimer lasers for laser angioplasty, abstracted. *Circulation* 1986; 74(suppl 2):204.

17. Litvack F, Doyle L, Grundfest W, et al: In vivo excimer laser ablation: Acute and chronic effects on canine aorta, abstracted. *Circulation* 1986; 74(suppl 2):360.

Chapter 3

Laser-Tissue Interactions: Considerations for Cardiovascular Applications*

Warren S. Grundfest, M.D.

Frank I. Litvack, M.D.

D. Lynn Doyle, M.D., F.R.C.S.(C.)

James S. Forrester, M.D.

The objectives of this chapter are to review laser-tissue interactions as functions of type of laser, components of tissue, and mode of energy delivery. Though there are many types of lasers, the one common denominator is their ability to deliver intense, monochromatic radiation to a small area of tissue. The incident laser energy may be reflected with minimal effect on the tissue. The energy may be absorbed, and, depending on the wavelength, the depth of penetration, and the absorption characteristics of the tissue, the incident energy may be converted to heat, may be emitted as fluorescence, or may directly photoactivate chemical bonds. At very high intensities (>1 megawatt), the laser energy forms an expanding ''plasma'' in the tissue and generates an explosive shock wave. This ''explosion'' may lead to tissue removal. Each of these processes leads to fundamentally different outcomes.

The choice of laser depends on the application. Results of the laser-tissue interaction can be predicted if the following information is known:

1. The wavelength of the laser energy.

*This experimental work is supported in part by the Imperial Grand Sweepstakes, the Grand Sweepstakes, and the Medallion Funds of Cedars-Sinai Medical Center. This work is also supported in part by Specialized Centers of Research in Ischemic Heart Disease of the National Heart, Lung, and Blood Institute grant #HL-17651. Doctors Grundfest and Litvack are recipients of NHLBI clinical awards #HL-01522 and #HL-01381 respectively.

2. The time span and intensity of the delivered light.
3. Absorption characteristics of the tissue. If the energy is reflected, there will be little effect; if the energy is absorbed at the tissue surface, only those cells irradiated may be affected. However, if the light scatters and penetrates deeply into the tissue, the effects of this energy may occur at some site distant from the point of irradiation.

Attempts to produce mathematical models of the laser-tissue interaction are complicated by the great heterogenicity of tissue and the changes that occur during irradiation. Any model must account for optical scattering, absorption, and reflection. These parameters change during the irradiation, making all but the simplest models very complex and difficult to use. When additional factors such as tissue heterogeneity, thickness, and boundary layers are considered, accurate modeling with differential equations becomes mathematically complex and difficult, if not impossible, to solve.

TYPES OF LASER-TISSUE INTERACTIONS

Physical Processes

The choice of laser radiation depends on the desired outcome of the absorption and transmission of the energy. Energy that is not absorbed at the surface of the tissue can be scattered and absorbed at areas remote from the site of irradiation. The effect of the scattered energy depends on the depth of penetration of energy and the presence of absorbing molecules (chromophores). If the energy is delivered in short, intense pulses, or if boiling and ejection of material occur, acoustic transients can be set up within tissue, causing cavitation. Cavitation can lead to loss of tissue architecture. A "photoplasma" explosion can vaporize tissue and cause disruption in the surrounding zone adjacent to the explosion.

Thermal Process

When the absorbed energy is dissipated primarily as heat, tissue changes occur along a predictable continuum as the heat increases. Tissue welding by lasers occurs at relatively low temperatures. Heating of the tissue from 43 to 50°C may allow for the uncoiling and annealing of collagen helices so that apposed tissue edges may be fused by reforming covalent bonds. As the tissue temperature increases, between 50 and 60°C, irreversible protein denaturation and subsequent cell death occur.[1] Beyond 60°C, cell death is inevitable. As temperatures reach 90 to 100°C, the underlying collagen and elastin structures begin to degrade. At temperatures greater than 100°C, melting, boiling, ablation, and pyrolysis occur, resulting in tissue ablation. Ablation temperatures for calcified tissues may exceed 500°C.

When laser energy is converted to heat in the tissues, thermal diffusion begins. Diffusion of heat through the tissue depends on the thermal properties of the irradiated material. Vascular tissue tends to have thermal diffusion constants in a range of 1 to 10 μm/sec.[2] Pulses longer than several microseconds will allow thermal energy to diffuse over 10 to 100 μm in a few milliseconds. Pulses in the millisecond range are sufficiently long to allow for heat generated to diffuse between 100 and 1,000 μm away from the zone of irradiation. The thermal relaxation (cooling) phenomenon is influenced by (1) the thermal coefficient of the tissue, (2) the properties of the surrounding tissue or fluids, and (3) the temperature differential between the irradiated and nonirradiated tissue.[3]

Photochemical Processes

Photochemical change can occur as a result of direct excitation of electronic bonds by the laser energy and is one of the proposed mechanisms of action of pulsed, ultraviolet lasers. Electronic excitation by laser is not 100% efficient; therefore, heat is also generated during this process. The physical chemistry of pulsed tissue ablation is as yet not well defined. Two potential mechanisms appear to operate.[4] At shorter wavelengths, tissue components, proteins, and lipids absorb photons and become electronically excited. This "photoexcitation" leads to rupture of molecular bonds and formation of molecular fragments. These molecular fragments then undergo a process known as photochemical desorption and are ejected from the irradiated surface in less than 1 μ/sec. The ejected fragments carry with them much of the energy that was initially deposited within the tissue to generate the fragments. This electronic excitation occurs before conversion to heat or thermal diffusion occurs. A second possible mechanism to explain this phenomenon is very high-speed, localized absorption, which leads to formation of a very small area of vaporized photoproducts. These products expand rapidly away from the tissue surface, again carrying away the incident energy. The result of optimal pulsed ultraviolet ablation is tissue removal with minimal thermal damage to adjacent structures.

Fluorescent Phenomena

Fluorescence occurs when photons of light are absorbed by tissue and reemitted at a longer wavelength. This rapidly occurring process (nanoseconds or less) is strongly affected by the electronic bond structure and the chemical composition of the irradiated matter. Fluorescence can be used to detect and monitor specific compounds that occur naturally or that have been added to the system. A particular wavelength fluorescence must be distinguished from the baseline autofluorescence that occurs in tissue. This can be done using various filters after identifying the specific wavelengths of the emitted (fluorescent) light. To date this work has primarily focused on photodetection of hematoporphyrin derivatives,[5, 6] tetracycline,[7] and carotenoids.[8]

Laser-induced fluorescence results when a portion of the laser light is absorbed and reradiated. Given the high intensity and monochromaticity of the laser beam, the reradiated light can be of sufficient intensity to permit detection and analysis. The returning fluorescent light pattern can act as a fingerprint for identification of certain compounds. Analysis of the fluorescent pattern is now under study as a means of differentiating normal from atherosclerotic tissue.[9, 10] This would permit target-specific laser angioplasty. Preliminary results are encouraging; however, the laser-induced fluorescence is so sensitive to chemical changes that irradiated or ablated tissue may give different signals than normal or atherosclerotic tissue.

QUANTITATION OF THE LASER-TISSUE INTERACTION

Our group uses high-speed filming, quantitative ocular micrometry, and tissue thermal analysis to characterize and quantitate the changes that occur during laser-tissue interactions. High-speed filming allows us to slow down events that happen too rapidly to be seen with the naked eye. Figure 3–1 displays a schematic of the high-speed filming apparatus. This arrangement permits the study of laser energy delivered either through a fiberoptic waveguide or directly from the output mirror to a tissue specimen mounted on a platform or immersed in fluid, usually saline solution. Quantitative ocular micrometry

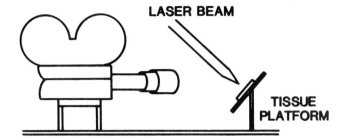

FIG 3–1.

Schematic diagram of the experimental apparatus for high-speed film analysis. The laser beam is carried either by a fiberoptic waveguide or directly from the output mirror and is aimed at the tissue platform containing atherosclerotic human aorta. The film or video moves at 500 to 6,000 frames per second, giving an expansion of time from 20:1 to 500:1.

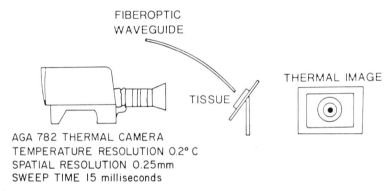

FIG 3–2.

To achieve a thermal map or picture of the heat generated, we use a thermal digital camera (AGA 782). This has a temperature resolution of 0.2°C, a spatial resolution of 0.2 mm, and a sweep time of 15 msec. The thermal camera is aimed at the target tissue, in vitro or in vivo, and real-time images are displayed on a monitor and stored on videotape. Selected frames are then transferred to a computer, where detailed analysis of the thermal image at any given time can be performed.

of histologic sections of irradiated tissue permits quantitation of the depth and width of the lesions created by the laser-tissue interaction. Temporal and spatial analysis of the thermal gradients generated at the tissue interface defines the role of tissue heating in the ablative process. These observations are made using an infrared thermal camera (AGA 782) (Fig 3–2). This camera allows for continuous high-resolution recordings of the heat generated at the tissue surface during the laser-tissue interaction. With the use of appropriate filters and standards, very accurate temperature measurements can be made. In addition, zones of temperature changes can be recorded and followed.

Using this methodology, we have observed that tissue responds to heating with a slight volume expansion. As heating proceeds above 50°C, protein denaturation occurs. Time exposure is critical since exposures of less than a microsecond may not result in cell death, whereas exposures of greater than a millisecond usually produce irreversible protein denaturation. As temperatures rise above 60°C, extracellular proteins and collagen fibers begin to denature. Such loss of structure is seen histologically as coagulation injury or hypereosinophilia of the tissue. As heating proceeds beyond 100°C, water begins to boil, leaving behind vacuoles within the remaining proteinaceous structure of the coagulated tissue. Vacuoles are telltale signs of temperatures in excess of 100°C. As temperatures rise above 125°C, complete oxidation of the protein and lipids occurs, leaving behind carbon particles. This carbonization or charring of the tissue surface indicates relatively high temperature processes. Explosive vaporization of water or transmission of shock waves induced by pulsed lasers is evidenced by development of vacuoles and loss of tissue architecture. Shock wave injury can be quite prominent and independent of thermal injury.

Continuous-Wave Laser-Tissue Interactions

We have performed a series of high-speed camera observations using continuous-wave neodymium:yttrium-aluminum-garnet (Nd:YAG), continuous-wave argon ion, and continuous-wave ultraviolet laser sources. High-speed filming of these processes is most informative (Plate 1). The first observation is that the tissue blanches as the chromophores are bleached. Second, the tissue begins to melt, and a molten pool of material appears immediately under the area of irradiation. Surrounding this molten pool, a small, raised crater rim develops and boiling begins. As heating continues, steam can be seen rising from the tissue surface. This is sometimes accompanied by ejection of relatively large particles. As the temperature deep to the tissue surface rises, explosive ejection of tissue fragments promptly follows. As all of the molten material evaporates, pyrolysis of the tissue occurs. Concentric zones of thermal injury develop and continue to expand as the ablative process continues. Deep to the crater surface, boiling continues. During this phase of ablation, material deep to the crater flows into the area being directly ablated. This material undergoes intense laser irradiation and is usually carbonized rapidly. The zone of thermal injury expands radially outward and beneath the tissue surface, and molten material from lateral heating continues to flow into the crater. In summary, continuous-wave lasers ablate tissue by a series of overlapping phases. Tissue first blanches due to protein denaturation and loss of hydration, then melts. As heating continues, boiling ensues, followed by pyrolysis and carbonization of the tissue concomitant with lateral thermal injury.

Pulsed Ultraviolet Laser-Tissue Interactions

Pulsed ultraviolet lasers, in particular those operating at wavelengths less than 337 nm, produce tissue ablation through a different process. High-speed film observations made during irradiation of atherosclerotic aortic tissue with a 308-nm excimer laser or with a pulsed frequency-tripled Nd:YAG laser at 266 nm have shown that the ablative process occurs with each pulse. These laser pulses range from 7 to 200 nanoseconds (nsec). Such intense pulses of energy have profoundly different effects on the tissue compared with those seen with the continuous-wave irradiation. The first three to four pulses appear to have little impact on the tissue, then ablation begins with each pulse. No lateral thermal effects are seen if the area is irradiated at or above ablation threshold limits. As irradiation proceeds, the ablated area corresponds precisely to the area irradiated at or above threshold limits (Plate 2).

Thermal injury can occur with pulsed lasers either at high repetition rates, in which there is insufficient time to allow for thermal relaxation of the tissue, or by irradiation at subthreshold levels. High repetition rates also tend to produce significant zones of blast injury. Quantitative ocular micrometry can quantify the extent of histologically observable laser-induced damage. This technique can also be used to compare and contrast the effects of different lasers on vascular tissue. As demonstrated in Plate 3, attempts to produce a 2-mm-deep zone of ablation can have widely variable results depending on the choice of laser. Predictable ablation is a critical factor in developing a safe laser angioplasty system. As seen in Figure 3–3, pulsed lasers appear to have an inherent advantage over continuous-wave lasers, since the ablation by pulsed lasers removes a defined depth of tissue.[11]

Ablation by 7-nsec pulsed irradiation at 532 nm (the second harmonic of YAG laser) tends to produce variable results in atherosclerotic tissue. We observed many different outcomes of pulsed 532-nm irradiation. Some tissues, particularly soft atheroma, appeared to undergo explosive ablation, as large particles were ejected from the tissue surface. Calcified tissue was relatively unaffected, and in some tissue specimens molten or liquid material filled the newly created hole, almost erasing all traces of irradiation. High-speed filming revealed tremendous scatter of the 532-nm radiation through the tissue. Similar processes were also observed at 1,040-nm irradiation. It should be pointed out that energies necessary to ablate calcified tissue at 532-nm energy pulses also destroy quartz plates. Therefore, it is indeed possible to ablate atheromatous tissue at 532 nm, but this is not a feasible solution for laser angioplasty since the energy density is in the gigawatt per square millimeter range and destroys all known fiberoptic schemes. In addition, such intense energies tend to produce severe blast injury within the tissues, causing complete loss of local tissue architecture (Plate 4). At shorter wavelengths, thresholds are lower and thermal and blast injury are minimized.

High-speed thermal analysis of the laser-tissue interaction has identified the temperatures at which tissue destruction occurs. Such thermal analysis is a relative measurement since it is not conducted under the conditions that occur in vivo. It does, however, allow us to predict the maximum temperatures that might occur in vivo. With this method of analysis, the thermal gradient and temperatures produced during the interaction of light with tissue can be studied and correlated with observed histologic findings. We see that irreversible protein denaturation (coagulation injury) occurs at temperatures in excess of

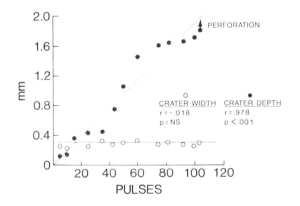

FIG 3–3.
Using ocular micrometry, a graph of the incision dimensions vs. the number of excimer pulses can be obtained. On the *y* axis is the depth or width in millimeters, and on the *x* axis is the number of pulses. This was done for 308-nm pulses at 30 mJ per pulse. There is a relatively linear relationship between depth and number of pulses. However, the width remains relatively constant. Precise control of depth without any change in width of a crater is possible and easily obtained, in contrast to the continuous-wave lasers, in which depth and width are only loosely correlated. (From Grundfest WS, Litvack F, Forrester JS, et al: Laser ablation of human atherosclerotic plaque without adjacent tissue injury. *J Am Coll Cardiol* 1985; 5:929–933. Used by permission.)

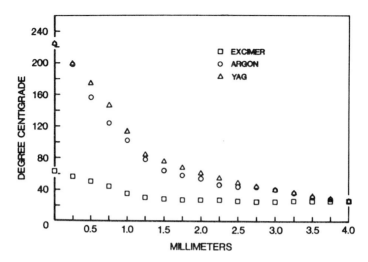

FIG 3–4.
Collating data, a graph of temperature vs. distance at 2 seconds for a given depth of ablation can be derived. On the x axis is distance from the crater center. The tissue has been set on the x and z axes extending into and out of the plane on the paper, and the laser is aimed on the y axis perpendicular to it. A crater 1 mm in diameter would have its edge at the 0.5 mm mark on this graph. For the neodymium (Nd):YAG and the argon lasers, at the tissue edge the temperature is in excess of 100°C, and even at 1.5 mm the temperature is above 60°C. In contrast to the excimer laser, the temperature at 0.5 mm is less than 50°C, and within 1 mm the tissue temperature drops below 40°C. It is important to note that the tissue temperature barely exceeds 60°C, even in the center of the ablative excimer beam. This is important since 60°C is a temperature at which irreversible protein denaturation occurs. Thus, the excimer laser ablates tissue at temperatures much lower than those of the Nd:YAG or argon lasers.

50 to 60°C. Above 100°C, blast injury becomes prominent. Above 125°C formation of carbon particles is seen. These processes, common to all continuous-wave lasers, are not seen when pulsed lasers are employed at optimal operating parameters.

During the analysis of pulsed 308-nm light with calcified atherosclerotic tissue, we observed a maximal temperature rise in vitro of 63.5°C. This was the maximum observed temperature in 395 specimens of excimer irradiated human cadaveric atherosclerotic aorta. In contrast, temperatures produced by argon, Nd:YAG, or continuous-wave ultraviolet sources exceeded 100°C in all cases (Fig 3–4). Figure 3–4 is a graph of the temperatures that occurred at 2 seconds during laser irradiation sufficient to produce a crater 1 mm deep. For continuous-wave Nd:YAG, argon, and ultraviolet lasers, temperatures always exceeded 125°C during the ablative process. In contrast, excimer ablation temperatures rarely exceeded 60°C. Laterally, only a small volume of tissue was heated above 50°C during excimer ablation. In contrast, a zone of tissue 1.5 to 2 mm in diameter was heated above 60°C during ablation with any of the continuous-wave sources.

Such widespread thermal heating accounts for the inability to control and precisely predict the events during direct continuous-wave radiation. Several schemes have been proposed to limit and confine thermal damage from continuous-wave sources. The most successful to date has been the use of the ''hot-tip,'' which radially distributes the thermal energy over the vessel surface. Other devices are under investigation, including optical shields, sapphire tips, and defined ablation areas with multiple fibers, with the primary goal of preventing perforation due to uncontrolled thermal injury. To achieve meaningful experimental results, any analysis must be repeated, with the diversity of tissue samples ranging from smooth, mildly atherosclerotic atheroma to heavily calcified irregular disease. Failure to carry out analysis over a broad spectrum of biologic specimens will lead to a series of inappropriate conclusions.

As detailed by our angioscopic observations in coronary arteries, there is enormous variability even within a few centimeters of the arterial tree.[12] One section of the atheroma can be smooth and white and in the next centimeter the atheroma can be hard and calcified, followed by ulcerated, pigmented atheroma. Such heterogeneity makes it difficult to choose lasers based on a particular tissue characteristic. Attempts to achieve ablation through chromophore enhancement are limited by the tissue's variability or lack of chromophore uptake within many segments. Fifty percent to 60% of all coronary and 60% to 70% of all peripheral atheromas contain calcium. Very hard calcified lesions are not uncommon in either peripheral or coronary circulation. Thus, when choosing the appropriate laser for ablative processes, we must consider the tissue heterogeneity. None of the continuous-wave lasers, including carbon dioxide, Nd:YAG, argon ion, and continuous-wave ultraviolet, was effective in ablating calcified material. In contrast, the 308-nm excimer laser and the Nd:YAG 266-nm harmonic were capable of effective ablation of calcified material. Though 353 nm can ablate calcified material, this is somewhat more difficult and is accompanied by thermal injury in the surrounding tissue. At 532 nm, ablation of calcified material was almost impossible except at energy densities that exceeded 2 gigawatts (GW)/sq mm. This level of energy is clearly not feasible for fiberoptic transmission and is therefore impractical. Plate 5 demonstrates excimer ablation of a bovine femur. This was done through a fiberoptic waveguide in a saline medium. Note the preservation of the local tissue architecture on the smooth, clean cut that was possible using excimer ablation. It should be noted that if the energy level is subthreshold, thermal injury will occur.

The three-phase analytical method outlined above has allowed us to define the optimal wavelength for laser angioplasty by direct ablation. The optimal parameters for direct ablation appear to be in the pulsed ultraviolet wavelength. We have not yet tested the pulse and wavelength characteristics of the 2.9-μm lasers. Given the extremely short depth of penetration, one would predict that, through multiphoton processes, a precise ablative mechanism might occur at selected infrared wavelengths. However, fiber, lasers, and delivery systems have yet to be optimized for this wavelength.

ANIMAL MODELS FOR LASER ANGIOPLASTY

The next step in optimizing the laser-tissue interaction in regard to laser angioplasty is to study the healing response to laser irradiation. This can be performed in a variety of ways. There is as yet no good model for atherosclerosis in animals that allows observation of the healing response. We have, however, carried out studies in normal canine arteries. In addition, several investigators, including Abela et al.[13] and Sanborn et al.,[14] have studied the effects of various continuous wavelengths on normal canine arteries as well as atherosclerotic arteries in rabbits. Each of these models has its advantages and disadvantages. The studies in normal arteries allow one to predict the human response for relatively normal human vasculature and look for thrombus formation and intimal proliferation resulting from endothelial cell injury. In addition, such normal models can be used to study the potential for aneurysm formation. However, these models are only relative predictors of the healing response that such lasers will have in man.

Experiments in atherosclerotic rabbits allow investigators to evaluate the ability of a particular laser to ablate soft, smooth, toothpastelike atheroma and to test for the potential of perforation, since rabbit arteries are very thin. However, rabbit atherosclerosis is a foam-cell disease. It is not directly comparable to the human atherosclerotic process. Several investigators have implanted excised human coronary arteries into dogs; however, the intense fibrotic reaction due to the foreign body makes study of healing responses difficult to interpret.[13] We have developed a different model that appears to simulate fibrotic human atherosclerosis.[15] This model permits one to assess the flexibility and ability of systems to recanalize vessels similar to coronary arteries. This model is too new, though, to permit the study of the laser-tissue interaction since it takes approximately 4 to 6 months for the atherosclerotic process to develop. Once the characteristics of this model have been quantified, it may allow for a better understanding of the healing processes that occur in the presence of smooth muscle cell proliferation.

COMPARISON OF IN VIVO THERMAL AND HISTOLOGIC EFFECTS OF ARGON AND EXCIMER

Previous research has demonstrated that 308-nm excimer laser light ablates vascular tissue with great precision and minimal thermal effect. However, lack of a fiberoptic delivery system has limited study of in vivo effect of excimer lasers.

To define acute and chronic histologic differences produced by excimer and argon ablation delivered by fiberoptics in living animals, and to correlate these histologic effects with thermal gradients produced by ablation in vascular tissue, we studied laser effects in vivo.[16, 17] In 25 anesthetized dogs, we employed a standardized method of aortic exposure through a midline incision. Through the midline incision, the abdominal aorta was controlled and the posterior intima exposed by a longitudinal aortotomy. Irradiation of a 125-sq mm area within a template was performed. Eight aortas were irradiated with argon laser and 13 aortas were irradiated with an excimer laser. In four control dogs the aorta was opened, exposed, and repaired but not irradiated. Aortic repair was performed with 6-0 polypropylene (Prolene) suture. A 308-nm excimer laser was delivered through a 600-μm core fiberoptic waveguide in contact with the tissue. Argon laser energy was transmitted by a 400-μm core fiber held 5 ± 2 mm from the intimal surface. Excimer spot size was 0.6 mm in diameter. Argon spot size was 0.6 to 0.7 mm in diameter. Energy density was 25 to 35 mJ/sq mm per pulse at 20 Hz for the excimer laser, or 0.5 to 0.7 J/sq mm/second. Argon energy was delivered at 5.1 to 15.5 J/sq mm/second. Irradiation was continued until the intimal surface in the template was ablated.

Three methods of analysis were used. First was immediate gross appearance as photographed, with the surface characterized as smooth, irregular, or carbonized. Second, during irradiation thermal gradients were recorded with a thermal camera (AGA 782). Third, serial histology was obtained from acute response to 4-week healing.

Acute continuous-wave irradiated aorta showed carbonization and thermal destruction of adjacent tissue. Excimer-irradiated specimens showed no gross evidence of thermal injury (Plate 6). Temperature measurement showed argon ablation occurring above 115°C (Plate 7). In contrast, excimer ablative temperatures did not exceed 48°C (Plate 8). At three days, argon-irradiated aortas all revealed mural thrombus with an inflammatory infiltrate visible on histologic examination (Plate 9). Excimer-irradiated aortas showed minimal thrombus, no inflammatory response, and new islands of endothelial cells.

The most striking difference occurred at 4 weeks (Plate 10). Argon-irradiated aortas were surrounded by dense inflammatory response and showed evidence of minimal hyperplasia, with disorganization of subendothelial components. Excimer-irradiated aortas were grossly similar to controls, with a normally reconstituted endothelium and an intact internal elastic lamina on histologic examination.

As the above study was performed in canine arteries, its relevance to atherosclerotic arteries is unclear. The available data suggest that the significant trauma to the vessel wall leads to platelet aggregation and a subsequent proliferative response. The magnitude of the "healing response" is in part due to the magnitude of injury. Thus, it seems likely that lasers that cut with minimal adjacent tissue damage will produce a surface less likely to cause restenosis and thrombosis. This remains to be tested in the clinical setting.

REFERENCES

1. Gorisch W, Boargen KP: Heat induced contraction of blood vessels. *Lasers Surg Med* 1982; 2:1–13.
2. Anderson RR, Parrish JA: Selective photothermolysis: Precise microsurgery by selective absorption of pulsed radiation. *Science* 1983; 220:524–527.
3. Hu C, Barnes FS: The thermal-chemical damage in biological material under laser irradiation. *IEEE Trans Biomed Eng* 1970; 17:220–231.
4. Srinivasan R: Ablation of polymers and biological tissues by ultraviolet lasers. *Science* 1986; 234:559–565.
5. Spears JR, Serur J, Shropstire D, et al: Fluorescence of experimental atheromatous plaques with hematoporphyrin derivative. *J Clin Invest* 1983; 71:395–399.
6. Litvack F, Grundfest WS, Forrester JS, et al: Effects of hematoporphyrin derivative and photodynamic therapy on arteriosclerotic rabbits. *Am J Cardiol* 1985; 56:667–671.
7. Abela GS, Barbieri E, Roxey T, et al: Laser enhanced plaque atherolysis with tetracycline, abstracted. *Circulation* 1986; 72(suppl 2):7.
8. Prince MR, Deutsch TF, Mathews-Roth MM, et al: Preferential light absorption in atheromas in vitro: Implications for laser angioplasty. *J Clin Invest* 1986; 78:295–302.
9. Cothren RM, Hayes GB, Cramer JR, et al: A multifiber catheter with an optical shield for laser angiosurgery. *Lasers Life Sci* 1987; 1:1–12.
10. Sartori MP, Bossaller C, Weilbacher D, et al: Detection of atherosclerotic plaques and characterization of arterial wall structure by laser induced fluorescence, abstracted. *Circulation* 1986; 74(suppl 2):7.
11. Grundfest WS, Litvack F, Forrester JS, et al: Laser ablation of human atherosclerotic plaque without adjacent tissue injury. *J Am Coll Cardiol* 1985; 5:929–933.
12. Forrester JS, Litvack F, Grundfest W, et al: A perspective of coronary disease seen through the arteries of living man. *Circulation* 1987; 75:505–513.
13. Abela GS, Normann SJ, Cohen DM, et al: Laser recanalization of occluded atherosclerotic arteries in vivo and in vitro. *Circulation* 1985; 71:403–411.
14. Sanborn TA, Faxon DP, Haudenschild C, et al: Experimental angioplasty–Circumferential distributions of laser thermal energy with a laser probe. *J Am Coll Cardiol* 1985; 5:934.
15. Doyle L, Litvack F, Grundfest W, et al: An in vivo model for testing laser angioplasty systems, abstracted. *Circulation* 1986; 74(suppl 2):361.
16. Grundfest WS, Litvack F, Doyle L, et al: Comparison of in vitro and in vivo thermal effects of argon and excimer lasers for laser angioplasty, abstracted. *Circulation* 1986; 74(suppl 2):204.
17. Litvack F, Doyle L, Grundfest W, et al: In vivo excimer laser ablation: Acute and chronic effects on canine aorta, abstracted. *Circulation* 1986; 74(suppl 2):360.

Chapter 4

Laser Delivery Systems

Tsvi Goldenberg, Ph.D.

William B. Anderson, B.S.

Sharon Kupfer, B.S.

Successful delivery of laser energy requires a carefully designed fiberoptic catheter. Size, flexibility, and steerability are important considerations for safe negotiation through coronary and peripheral arteries. Additionally, the laser angioplasty delivery catheter must safely direct the high-energy laser light and should create a clinically efficacious channel. This chapter explains the physics of light and energy transmission through optical fibers, addresses the problems encountered with designing a laser delivery system, and describes possible solutions for design of an optimal laser angioplasty catheter.

PHYSICS OF LIGHT TRANSMISSION IN OPTICAL FIBERS

An optical fiber consists of a transmissive core, a cladding, and an outer coating (Fig 4–1). The core and cladding serve to propagate light through the fiber. The outer coating is a protective jacket that maintains the natural strength of the two inner layers of the fiber to minimize breakage.

When light travels from one medium to another it bends, or refracts. This angle of refraction, θ_r, is governed by Snell's law:

$$n\sin\theta = n_1\sin\theta_r$$

The variable n, the index of refraction, is the ratio of the speed of light in a vacuum to the speed of light in a particular medium. For light entering a fiber, n equals the refractive index of the medium outside the fiber, n_1 equals the refractive index of the core of the fiber, θ equals the incident angle of the light and θ_r equals the refracted angle (Fig 4–2).

In order for light to propagate through the fiber, it must impinge on the fiber at an angle less than or equal to a maximum value of θ, θ_{max}. A light ray incident at θ_{max} will strike the interior wall of the fiber at the critical angle, θ_c. Entry at the critical angle

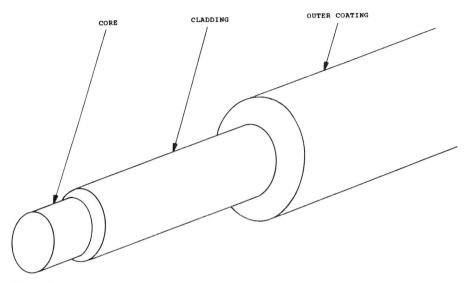

FIG 4–1.
Optical fiber construction.

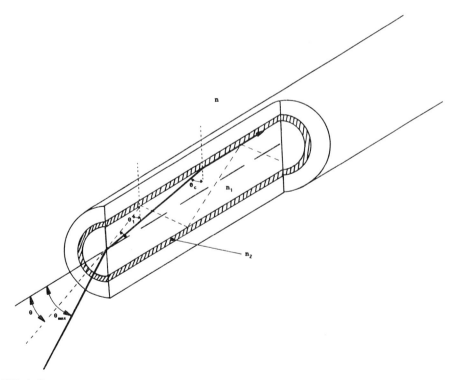

FIG 4–2.
Transverse cross section of an optical fiber.

results in a light ray that travels along the boundary of the core and the cladding, $\theta_2 = 90°$ (see Fig 4–2). Thus, for $\theta_2 = 90°$, $\sin\theta_2 = 1$, and Snell's law becomes

$$\theta_1 = \theta_c = \sin^{-1}\left(\frac{n_2}{n_1}\right)$$

where n_2 = refractive index of the cladding
$\quad\quad\ n_1$ = refractive index of the core, $n_1 > n_2$

Light entering the fiber at an angle *less than* θ_{max} results in a ray incident upon the core-cladding boundary at an angle that exceeds θ_c. For all refracted rays greater than the critical angle, light will undergo total internal reflection at the core-cladding interface, zig-zagging repeatedly through the optical fiber. Within the fiber, the incident and reflected angles are equal at each reflection, generally with a loss of less than 0.001% per reflection (see Fig 4–2). On the other hand, rays incident on the face of the fiber at an angle greater than θ_{max} strike the interior wall of the fiber at an angle less than θ_c and are only partially reflected at the core-cladding boundary. These rays will eventually leak out of the fiber and will not be effectively transmitted.

NUMERICAL APERTURE

The angle θ_{max} also determines the numerical aperture (NA) of an optical fiber. The numerical aperture defines the maximum divergence of the cone of light that enters and exits the fiber. Numerical aperture is defined as

$$NA = n\sin \theta_{max}$$

It is useful to rewrite the numerical aperture in terms of the refractive indices of the core and cladding. Making use of Snell's law and rearranging terms, the numerical aperture of an optical fiber can be expressed as:

$$n\sin\theta_{max} = NA = (n_1^2 - n_2^2)^{1/2}$$

Thus, the cone of light that an optical fiber can accept or emit is a function of the ratio of refractive indices of the core and the cladding of the fiber.

The numerical aperture of the fiber must be considered when designing an energy coupling device from the laser to the fiberoptic delivery catheter. The energy coupler focuses the laser beam so that it will be incident on the fiber within its accepting cone.

BENDING LOSSES

When a fiber bends, the angles of the light rays that internally reflect at the core-cladding interface change. If these rays are altered so that they strike the core-cladding boundary at an angle less than the critical angle, they leak out of the fiber (Fig 4–3). This phenomenon, bending loss, is of obvious concern in laser angioplasty because the fiberoptic delivery system must negotiate through tortuous bends. Plate 11 shows the energy losses of a 400-μm fiber due to bending.

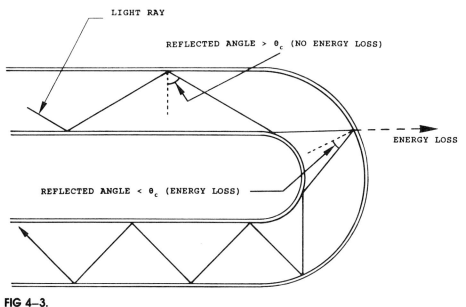

FIG 4–3.
Bending loss in an optical fiber.

It is difficult to determine how much loss will occur for a given set of bends with a given fiber. Therefore, it is not possible to predict how much energy is exiting a delivery system once it has been passed through a guide catheter and subsequent bends of the vasculature. Additionally, losses decrease the energy available for ablation and increase the chance of energy or power leakage into the surrounding environment. Thus, a fiber that minimizes bending losses is desired. A fiber with a high NA, and thus a large θ_{max}, will have a smaller critical angle than a fiber with a low NA. Hence, for a given energy input and bend radius, a fiber with a high NA yields lower losses than a fiber with a low NA.[1]

OUTER COATING

The outer coating of the fiber serves to protect the core-cladding from scratches and breakage and prevents laser energy leakage into the surrounding environment. In addition, the coating must be resistant to the high energy needed for plaque ablation. Coatings that have been investigated include silicone oils and rubbers, cellulosic lacquers, blocked urethanes, hot melt elastomers, polyimide, ultraviolet curable elastomers, and ultraviolet curable coatings.[2] Most of these materials are neither stable nor durable. Ultraviolet curable coatings and elastomers have successfully overcome these problems.[2–5] These coatings also have advantages when transmitting high-energy pulsed ultraviolet laser light in that the coating absorbs losses due to bending. Hence, the amount of energy that may potentially leak into the surrounding environment is minimized.

FIBER CHOICE

The ideal optical fiber is durable, minimizes energy loss during transmission, and has a large core to cladding ratio so as to reduce unused surface area. Highly pure silica

TABLE 4–1.
Laser Comparisons

Laser Medium	Type	λ(nm)	Fiber	Ablates Calcified Plaque	Causes Thermal Damage
KrF	Pulsed	248	Silica	Yes	No
XeCl	Pulsed	303	Silica	Yes	No
XeF	Pulsed	351	Silica	Yes	No
Argon ion	CW \} Pulsed \}	448,514.5	Silica Silica	No	Yes
Dye	Pulsed \} CW \}	300—1,000	Silica Silica	No No	Yes Yes
Nd:YAG	Pulsed \} CW \}	1,064	Silica Silica	No No	? Yes
Ho:YLF	Pulsed	2,060	Silica	?	?
Er:YAG	Pulsed	2,940	ZrF$_4$	Yes	No
CO$_2$	Pulsed \} CW \}	10,600	Halide Halide	Yes No	No Yes

core fibers have been found to be the most successful for most laser angioplasty applications.[6–8] Plastic-clad silica (trade name: PCS), Hard-clad silica (trade name: HCS), and core-clad silica fibers are among the fibers manufactured with a highly pure silica core and a large core-to-cladding ratio.[9–11] Studies have shown that both PCS and HCS fibers degrade with time when transmitting high energy ultraviolet light.[8] Core-clad silica fibers have been shown not to degrade at 100,000 pulses of a XeCl excimer laser.[12] Unfortunately, the fiber that provides the best transmission for most laser angioplasty applications, core-clad silica, has a relatively low NA (0.2). In contrast, PCS and HCS fibers have an NA of 0.37 to 0.47.[9, 10]

LASER-FIBEROPTIC INTERACTION

The lasers used for angioplasty are categorized as either pulsed or continuous wave (CW). It is generally easier to transmit ablative levels of continuous power from CW lasers than from pulsed lasers through optical fibers. However, the CW laser energy causes adjacent thermal tissue damage as well as vessel spasm.[13–16] Thermal damage occurs because the rate of energy delivery to tissue exceeds the rate of energy dissipation.

Pulsed lasers deliver an intense, short burst of energy. During the relaxation interval, the tissue dissipates excess laser energy.[17–21] The high peak power can also cause nonlinear absorption effects that can cause tissue ablation by nonthermal rupture of molecular bonds.[18] These nonlinear absorption effects also enable some pulsed laser energy to ablate hard calcified plaque that other systems cannot ablate. For example, the XeCl excimer laser ablates hard calcified plaque,[20] whereas the CW argon laser heats the same hard plaque without any significant material removal.[18–22] Table 4–1 compares characteristics of the various lasers used to remove atherosclerotic disease.[13, 16–28]

ENERGY LOSSES IN FIBEROPTICS

Losses in an optical fiber *L*(total), can be summarized by the following equation:

$$L(\text{total}) = L(s) + L(b) + L(c)$$

L(s) represents a 4% reflective loss in energy that occurs at both the input and output surface of any fiber. If the delivery system is subjected to bends of small radii, such as those found in coronary arteries, significant bending losses, *L(b)*, may occur. Bending loss can be minimized by choosing a fiber with a high numerical aperture. Absorption losses that occur due to the core of the optical fiber are represented by *L(c)*. The core of the fiber is comprised of a solid material, such as silica, that absorbs laser energy. Absorption can be high or negligible depending on the type of silica used and the wavelength[1] and energy density[24] of the transmitted light. It happens that the energy of laser systems that have the best tissue ablation characteristics also tend to be the most difficult to transmit through optical fibers.

An absorption loss that occurs in all fiber delivery systems, Rayleigh scattering, is due to small defects in the structure of the fiber core. The attenuation coefficient for this effect is inversely proportional to the fourth power of the energy wavelength. Thus, shorter wavelengths are more severely attenuated.[1] Absorption losses are more complicated in pulsed systems than CW systems due to nonlinear optical effects. Effects such as stimulated Brillioun scattering and Raman scattering occur at the high peak powers present in pulsed systems.[1, 29, 30] A detailed explanation of these effects is beyond the scope of this work; however, a good simplification is that the laser light energy is converted into thermal and acoustic energy within the fiber. The best means of minimizing absorption within an all-silica fiber is to select a substantially pure silica for the core with minimal defects.[31, 32] Stretching the pulse width of a pulsed laser system reduces the level of peak power per pulse. Reduction of peak power reduces nonlinear effects and subsequently raises the damage threshold of the fiber.[24]

INPUT SURFACE DAMAGE

To overcome losses that occur throughout an optical fiber, the input surface of a pulsed laser delivery system is subjected to high-energy density. As a result, it is usually the first part of the delivery system to fail due to laser damage.[7, 24, 31, 33, 34] In addition to high-energy exposure, the fiber input surface represents a discontinuity in a medium that has been mechanically prepared by polishing or cleaving. There is inevitably contamination embedded in the polished surface that can create an absorption center and invite laser or laser-induced thermal damage.[31] Additionally, a cleaved fiber may have a small chip or burr that will be vulnerable to laser damage. Thus, a means of producing an extremely clean and smooth surface at the input of the optical fibers must be achieved.[29, 31] Figure 4–4 illustrates input surface damage of an optical fiber.

LASER ENERGY COUPLING

All angioplasty systems require that the large-aperture, low-energy density beam that exits the laser be concentrated and funneled into the fiberoptic delivery system in order to achieve the high-energy densities necessary for plaque removal. The density of energy delivered to the optical fiber input surface should be adjustable so that the proper energy fluence can be delivered from the distal tip of the system. Energy coupling is generally accomplished by either a convex-lens–based apparatus or a tapered fiber that converges the laser beam to a sharp focal point. Additionally, the energy coupler serves to position

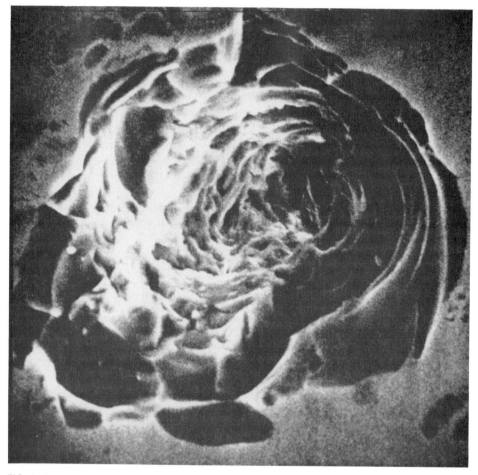

FIG 4–4.
Input surface damage of an optical fiber.

the optical fiber input surface precisely. Precise positioning of the input surface ensures that the delivered energy density does not change with time and that modularity is maintained. Modularity of an energy coupler maintains consistent output fluence while interchanging delivery systems. Figure 4–5 illustrates an energy coupler with these features.[35, 36]

The beam exits the laser and is focused by the lens. The fiber input surface can then be moved precisely into and away from the focal spot of the beam in order to adjust the energy density delivered to the input surface of the fiber. Exotic variations of this general theme such as a liquid energy coupler have been designed. This type of coupler keeps the input surface of the fiber submersed in an index of matching fluid in order to reduce damage to the input surface.[35]

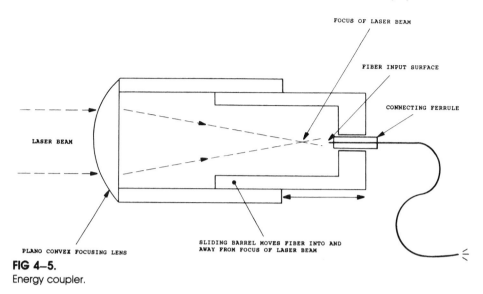

FOCUS OF LASER BEAM

FIBER INPUT SURFACE

CONNECTING FERRULE

LASER BEAM

PLANO CONVEX FOCUSING LENS

SLIDING BARREL MOVES FIBER INTO AND
AWAY FROM FOCUS OF LASER BEAM

FIG 4–5.
Energy coupler.

SURFACE DAMAGE OF FIBER OUTPUT

In CW systems, the intense heat that develops at the distal end of the delivery system tends to damage the optical fiber output surfaces.[37] Output surface damage has been reduced in the CW systems by attaching specialized tips, such as metal and sapphire, to the fiberoptic in order to protect it.[37, 38]

At the output surface of fibers in pulsed systems, reflection and other surface effects cause enhancement of the intense electric fields present.[31] If the electric fields become strong enough, the molecules of the silica fiber may be torn apart. The best way to eliminate output surface damage in pulsed systems is to reduce the energy density exiting the delivery system. For example, the XeCl excimer laser with pulse width of approximately 200 nanoseconds ablates calcified plaque at 50 mJ/sq mm.[17] Gross output surface damage does not occur until the output energy density approaches 100 mJ/sq mm.[29]

BULK FIBER DAMAGE

Bulk damage occurs when a fiber shatters in the core of the fiber. One cause of bulk damage is contamination or voids in the core, which occur when the quality of the fiber is not carefully controlled during manufacture. If the void or the contaminant is large enough, it will absorb enough laser energy to initiate a thermal stress crack.[31] Once this crack is exposed to the high-density laser energy, it will spread and destroy the fiber at this point. Raman and Brillioun scattering, involving the transformation of energy into heat and sound waves, can also lead to bulk damage if the energy densities are high enough.[30]

An interesting effect that can raise energy densities above the damage threshold of the fiber is called self-focusing or self-trapping.[30, 39] When strong electric fields induced by the electromagnetic laser radiation are present in a dielectric, its index of refraction can be altered. The altered index of refraction acts as a focusing lens inside the core of the fiber. The laser beam traveling through the fiber gets continually focused until the energy density exceeds damage threshold. An indication of this type of damage is linear destruction along the axis of the fiber.[29, 30]

MULTIPLE-FIBER TRANSMISSION AND FLEXIBILITY

Mechanical perforation of blood vessels is a serious problem when a single bare fiber of 300-μm core diameter or greater is used.[25, 38, 40] Multiple fiber coupling enables a delivery system to have the same or larger cutting area as that of a large single fiber but with much greater flexibility. Cutting area is proportional to the square of the fiber diameter, whereas stiffness is proportional to the fourth power of the fiber diameter.[41] Thus, if a system is designed for a single fiber of 200-μm diameter, four fibers of 100-μm diameter could be substituted and give the same cutting area at the distal tip. However, the flexibility of the four 100-μm fibers would be four times greater than that of a single 200-μm fiber.

Coupling multiple fiber delivery systems to a laser requires stable and consistent performance from that laser. Wasted space at the input of a multiple fiber delivery system requires that the lasers have high energy output. Most multiple fiber inputs would consist of a circular bundle. It is difficult, however, to group these individual fibers together without having air gaps between them. The portion of the laser beam that passes between the fiber input surfaces is not coupled to any fibers. Thus, a substantially greater input energy is required to achieve a high output density when a multiple fiber delivery system is used. Furthermore, for a multiple fiber system to operate safely, similar energy densities must be exiting from each fiber. If the energy density from each fiber is not the same, some of the fibers may be below ablation threshold. It follows that since each input of a multiple fiber bundle occupies a different portion of the laser beam, the beam must have uniform energy density.

Another technique for creating a more flexible delivery system is to expand the beam at the distal tip. If the beam of a 200-μm fiber is allowed to expand to 400 μm outside of the fiber, it will cut a 400-μm hole, providing that the energy density is sufficient. Expanding the diameter by a factor of two, however, quadruples the energy required for an unexpanded beam. For instance, transmitting an energy fluence of 200 mJ/sq m through a fiber allowed to expand to twice its diameter would result in an energy density of 50 mJ/sq m at the ablation site. Therefore, tip expansion requires that high energy densities must be transmitted through the fiber. This high energy density transmission may be achieved by using tapered fibers at the input end of the delivery system in order to "funnel" more energy into the fibers without causing input surface damage.[24, 42]

A means by which to expand the beam at the output tip can also be complicated. For the ultraviolet and infrared lasers, in particular, beam expansion can be difficult because blood is opaque to these frequencies.[17] One method to eliminate blood is to block the vessel with a balloon and flush with saline. The resultant free beam expansion in the vessel creates a large cutting area with a flexible system, but it may be difficult to control.[43] Another method utilizes funnel-like tapered fibers at the output tip.[24] In this case, high energies are transmitted through small flexible fibers and then allowed to expand in the tapers at the distal output.

CATHETER DESIGN

Early research in laser angioplasty revealed two significant safety issues: laser perforation and mechanical trauma.[44, 45] Fluorescence emission spectroscopy is one of the most recent technologies being experimented with to prevent arterial wall perforation.[26, 27] This technique delivers low-energy light to the tissue and records the subsequent emission.

The emission spectra are then analyzed to determine whether this tissue is plaque or healthy arterial wall. However, the use of spectroscopy for catheter guidance has some fundamental limitations. If spectroscopic feedback is obtained from one fiber of a multiple fiber system, the remaining fibers may cut into healthy tissue while the feedback fiber is in contact with diseased tissue. A small, single fiber delivery system could eliminate this problem. However, a small fiber would produce a small channel that has minimal clinical significance. These problems could be solved by implementing a large cutting multiple fiber delivery system that obtains feedback from each fiber. Each fiber of the delivery system could be selected for transmission after determining that it is in contact with a lesion.[46, 47] This type of system, though scientifically possible, is cumbersome and complex and would be difficult to operate. Thus, although fluorescence emission spectroscopy may prove to be a valuable tool in the future for the guidance of laser angioplasty delivery systems, it has not been fully developed for present use.

A more practical and proved technology uses a guidewire to maintain safety in the vessel. The guidewire is advanced into the distal portion of the artery and provides a track over which the laser catheter may be advanced. The excimer laser catheter functions as a contact cutting system because blood is opaque to excimer laser energy. A laser catheter that cuts in a forward direction and remains colinear with the vessel wall ensures that the laser energy is not directed at the vessel wall.

The second significant safety issue in laser angioplasty is mechanical trauma, which at worst case results in vessel perforation. Mechanical trauma to the interior of the vessel wall can be avoided by blunting the distal tip of the fiberoptic delivery system. Colinear orientation and flexibility are features of a delivery system that minimize the risk of mechanical perforation. Thus, design modifications made in the fiberoptic delivery systems were dedicated to these issues: flexible and atraumatic tips, colinear orientation.

At present, two types of laser delivery systems are being evaluated in the excimer clinical trials. The system used for total occlusions has an optical fiber centrally located within a specially constructed balloon angioplasty catheter. A mechanically modified fiberoptic tip creates a blunt edge on the working surface to avoid abrasion and mechanical perforation. The modification of the fiberoptic tip also allows expansion of the cutting area. The specially designed balloon angioplasty catheter has a large lumen and a short, squared-off balloon for coaxial positioning. On the proximal end of the balloon catheter, a Y adaptor allows for fiberoptic insertion and periodic injection of radiopaque contrast material. The balloon catheter is advanced over a standard guidewire to the lesion, and the guidewire is then removed. The fiberoptic catheter is then advanced to the tip of the balloon catheter. Radiopaque markers are present on both the fiberoptic catheter and the balloon catheter to allow alignment. The balloon is inflated with a 50:50 mixture of contrast media and saline. While the balloon is dilated, the fiberoptic catheter is advanced into the lesion under fluoroscopic control while contrast medium is injected periodically. The balloon catheter is then deflated and advanced over the fiberoptic catheter. The fiberoptic catheter thus acts as a guidewire. This process is continued until the entire length of the occlusion is recanalized. When the procedure is terminated, the balloon catheter has been advanced completely through the occlusion and the fiberoptic catheter is withdrawn. If necessary, balloon angioplasty can then be performed. This laser angioplasty system is unique in that a 7 F balloon angioplasty catheter is used to provide coaxial orientation and intermittent contrast injection.

The second system, for treatment of stenotic lesions, incorporates several small, flexible optical fibers concentrically arranged around the guidewire lumen within a catheter. Flexibility of the tip is fundamental to this ''over-the-wire'' system in order to ensure that the catheter follows the guidewire to avoid the laser energy from coming in contact with the vessel wall. Figure 4–6 illustrates such a multifiber over-the-wire delivery system.

CLINICAL RESULTS OF EXCIMER ANGIOPLASTY USING THE PROTOTYPE DELIVERY SYSTEMS

Percutaneous excimer laser angioplasty has been performed at Cedars-Sinai Medical Center in Los Angeles. The first 25 patients had superficial femoropopliteal laser angioplasties using a 308-nm excimer laser-balloon system. The laser had a pulse width of 140 nsec at a pulse frequency of 20 Hz. Eighteen patients had total occlusions and seven had stenoses. A single fiber within a 7 F catheter treated the occluded vessels and a 5 F over-the-wire delivery system treated the stenotic lesions.

Of the 18 patients with total occlusions who were treated, 3 had occlusions less than 5 cm; 5 had occlusions between 5 and 10 cm; 8 had occlusions between 10 and 20 cm, and 2 had occlusions greater than 20 cm. Acute success for both total occlusions and stenoses was 80%. Fifteen of 18 (83%) total occlusions were successfully recanalized. Two of the three failures were occlusions longer than 20 cm. Five of the seven stenoses (71%) were successfully treated.

A fiberoptic delivery system comprised of 12 200-μm fibers has been used in the coronary arteries of ten pigs. Negotiating two or three coronary arteries in each heart and lasing up to 10,000 pulses, it was demonstrated that the delivery system tracked the guidewire even through tortuous segments without perforation, dissection, or spasm. With FDA approval the coronary trial of excimer laser angioplasty began in October 1988. The multifiber system was used to recanalize a vein graft in an 85-year-old woman. The patient had previously undergone two coronary artery bypass graft (CABG) surgeries and three PTCA procedures. The vein graft was 95% occluded with no collateral flow. The laser made three passes and operated for a total of 26 seconds. The delivery system created a 1.5-mm channel. After subsequent balloon angioplasty, 5% of the stenosis remained.

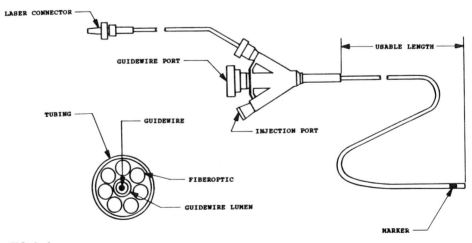

FIG 4–6.
Multifiber laser catheter.

SUMMARY

Laser angioplasty has now been successfully performed both intraoperatively and by percutaneous intervention of fiberoptic delivery systems. The fiberoptic delivery system is a critical component of the laser system and has three essential characteristics. First, it must be sufficiently flexible so that it can negotiate tortuous arteries without causing mechanical trauma. Thus, both flexibility and bluntness of the tip are essential. Second, it must avoid laser perforation of the vessel wall. In most cases, this will necessitate use of a central guidewire. Third, the delivery catheter must be small enough to traverse distal arteries while remaining capable of producing clinically efficacious channels. As a result of the achievement of these design criteria, a simple, safe, and reliable laser angioplasty system is a valuable tool for intravascular treatment.

Acknowledgments

The authors wish to thank Dr. James S. Forrester, Dr. Warren S. Grundfest, and Dr. Frank Litvack for their helpful input and comments and Melinda Madigan and Larry Wainblat for their assistance. Sam Shaolian, Brian Packard, and Al Diaz were instrumental in designing the laser angioplasty delivery catheters discussed in this chapter. We thank Hugh Narciso and Theresa Newton for coordinating the clinical trials.

REFERENCES

1. Miller S, Chynoweth A: *Optical Fiber Communications.* Orlando, Fla, Academic Press Inc, 1979.
2. Lawson KR, Cutler OR: UV cured coatings for optical fibers. *J Radiat Curing* 1982; 9:4–10.
3. Lawson KR, Ansel RE, Stanton JJ: Optical fiber buffer coatings cured with ultra-violet light. *Fiberoptic Communications* 80, San Francisco, September 1980.
4. McGinniss VD: Photo initiation of acrylate systems for UV curing, Association of Finishing Processes of the Society of Manufacturing Engineers technical paper FC, 760486, 1976, pp 476–486.
5. Ansel RE, Stanton JJ: Conference on physics of fiber optics. American Ceramic Society, April 1980.
6. Nevis EA: Alteration of the transmission characteristics of fused silica optical fibers by pulsed ultra-violet radiation. *Proc SPIE* 1985; 540:181–185.
7. Taylor RS, Leopold KE, Mihailov S, et al: Damage and transmission measurements of fused silica fibers using long optical pulse XeCl lasers. *Optics Commun* 1987; 63:26–31.
8. Goldenberg T, Anderson W: Internal communication, Advanced Interventional Systems, Irvine, Calif, 1988.
9. Beck WB, Hodge MH, Skutnik BJ, et al: Hard Clad Silica (HCS) fibers for data and power transmission. Proceedings of the European Fiberoptic Communications and Local Area Networks Exposition (EFOC/LAN) 85, 1985, pp 146–151.
10. Skutnick BJ, Hodge MH, Nath DK: High strength, reliable, Hard Clad Silica (HCS) fibers. EFOC/LAN, 85, 1985, Proc:232–236.
11. Skutnick BJ, Hille RE: Environmental effects on Hard Clad Silica optical fibers: Fiber optics in Adverse Environments II. *Proc SPIE* 1984; 506:184–188.
12. Taylor RS, Leopold KE, Brimacomb RK, et al: Fiberoptic delivery systems for the excimer laser recanalization of human coronary arteries in open heart surgery: Optical fibers in medicine II. *Proc SPIE* 1988; 906:225–235.

13. Tran D, Levin K: Zirconium fluoride fiber requirements for mid-infrared laser surgery applications: Optical Fibers in Medicine. *Proc SPIE* 1986; 713:36–37.
14. Bonner R, Smith P, Leon M: Quantification of tissue effects due to a pulsed Er:YAG laser at 2.9 μm with beam delivery in a wet field via zirconium fluoride fibers: Optical Fibers in Medicine II. *Proc SPIE* 1986; 713:2–5.
15. Linsker R, Srinivasan R, Wynne J, et al: Far ultra-violet laser ablation of atherosclerotic lesions. *Lasers Surg Med* 1984; 4:201–206.
16. Grundfest W, Litvack F, Goldenberg T, et al: Pulsed ultraviolet lasers and the potential for safe laser angioplasty. *Am J Surg* 1985; 150:220–226.
17. Chutorian DM, Selzer PM, Kosek J, et al: The interaction between excimer laser energy and vascular tissue. *Am Heart J* 1986; 112:739–745.
18. Grundfest W, Litvack F, Forrester J, et al: Laser ablation of human atherosclerotic plaque without adjacent tissue injury. *J Am Coll Cardiol* 1985; 5:929–933.
19. Goldenberg T, Litvack F, Grundfest W, et al: Design criteria for in vivo laser angioplasty: Optical fibers in medicine. *Proc SPIE* 1987; 713:53–55.
20. Isner J, Dov G, Steg G, et al: Percutaneous, in vivo excimer laser angioplasty: Results in two experimental animal models. *Lasers Surg Med* 1988; 8:223–232.
21. Srinivasan R: Ablation of polymers and biological tissue by ultra-violet lasers. *Science* 1986; 234:559–565.
22. Cumberland DC, Sanborn TA, Tayler DI, et al: Percutaneous laser thermal angioplasty: Initial clinical results with a laser probe in total peripheral artery occlusions. *Lancet* 1986; 1:1457–1459.
23. Abela G: Laser recanalization: Preliminary clinical experience. *Cardiovasc Dis Chest Pain* 1987; 3:3–8.
24. Singleton DL, Paraskevopoulos G, Taylor RS, et al: Excimer laser angioplasty: Tissue ablation, arterial response, and fiber optic delivery. *IEEE J Quant Elect* 1987; 23(10):1772–1782.
25. Abela GS, Normann SJ, Cohen DM, et al: Laser recanalization of occluded atherosclerotic arteries in vivo and in vitro. *Circulation* 1985; 71:403–411.
26. Prince M, Deutsch T, et al: Selective laser ablation of atheromas. *Circulation* 1985; 72(suppl 3):401.
27. Leon MB, Smith PD, Bonner RF: Laser angioplasty delivery system: Design considerations, in White RA, Grundfest WS (eds): *Lasers in Cardiovascular Disease.* Chicago, Year Book Medical Publishers Inc, 1987, p 52.
28. Laudenslager J: Physics of lasers with potential application in vascular diseases: Current state of the art and future prospects. JPL CIT.
29. Allison SW, Gillies GT, Magnuson DW, et al: Pulsed laser damage to optical fibers. *Appl Optics* 1985; 24(19):3140–3144.
30. Ready J: *Effects of High-Power Laser Radiation.* Orlando, Fla, Academic Press Inc, 1971.
31. Lowdermilk WH, Milam D: Review of ultra-violet damage threshold measurements at Lawrence Livermore National Laboratory: Excimer lasers, their applications, and new frontiers in lasers. *SPIE* 1984; 476:143–162.
32. Griscom D: Defect structure of glasses: Some outstanding questions in regard to vitreous silica. *J Noncrystalline Solids* 1985; 73:51–77.
33. Lowdermilk H, Milam D: Laser-induced surface and coating damage. *IEEE J Quantum Elect* 1981; 17(9):143–434.
34. Rainer F, Lowdermilk H, Milam D: Bulk and surface damage thresholds of crystals and glasses at 248nm. *Optical Eng* 1983; 22(4):431–434.
35. Goldenberg T: US Patent no. 4,641,912: 1987.
36. Goldenberg T: US Patent no. 4,732,448: 1988.
37. Geschwind H, Monhkolsmai D, Stern J, et al: Laser angioplasty with contact sapphire probe: Optical fibers in medicine. *Proc SPIE* 1986; 713:49–52.
38. Borst C: Percutaneous recanalization of arteries: Status and prospects of laser angioplasty with modified fiber tips. *Lasers Med Sci* 1987; 2:137.

39. Smith L, Bechtel J, Bloembergen N: Picosecond laser induced breakdown at 5321 and 3547 A: Observation of frequency dependent behavior. *Phys Rev B* 1987; 15:4039–4055.
40. Isner JM, Donaldson RF, Funai JT, et al: Factors contributing to perforations resulting from laser coronary angioplasty: Observations in an intact human postmortem preparation of intraoperative laser coronary angioplasty. *Coronary Artery Surg* 1985; 72(suppl 2):191–199.
41. Skutnik: High strength large core pure silica fiber for laser power transmission. Optical fibers in medicine III. *Proc SPIE* 1988; 906:204–250.
42. Harrison C: Tapered optical fibers. Technical overview. Presented at CLEO, San Francisco, June 1986.
43. Stiles S: Laser angioplasty's ingenious hardware. *Cardiology* 1988:45–52.
44. Abela GS, Seeger JM, Barbieri E, et al: Laser angioplasty with angioscopic guidance in humans. *J Am Coll Cardiol* 1986; 8:184–192.
45. Ginsburg R, Wexler L, et al: Percutaneous transluminal laser angioplasty for treatment of peripheral vascular disease. *Radiology* 1985; 156:619–624.
46. Richards-Kortum R, Kittrell C, Feld MS: Laser-induced spectral diagnosis of artherosclerosis. Presented at CLEO, San Francisco, June, 1986.
47. Feld MS: *An Optical Guidewire for Laser Angiosurgery Spectroscopy*. Santa Barbara, Calif, ACC, September 1988.

PART 2

Clinical Applications

Chapter 5

Overview of Laser Applications in the Treatment of Cardiovascular Disease

Thomas L. Robertson, M.D.

Empirical studies of the effects of laser energy on cardiovascular tissues have demonstrated the potential for a variety of therapeutic advances. These include angioplasty, endarterectomy, repair of aneurysms and arterial dissections, venous valvectomy, sealing of vascular anastomoses, transmyocardial neovascularization, myectomy, endocardiectomy, valvuloplasty, interruption of abnormally functioning conduction pathways, ablation of arrhythmogenic foci, and retardation or reversal of atherosclerosis.

The variety and precision of energetic interventions and observational capabilities evolving from laser technology have led to rapid expansion of knowledge in the physical sciences and appreciation of unusual potential in fundamental and applied biomedical research.[1] Lasers now available or in development can produce light energy across much of the electromagnetic spectrum from the far-infrared through the visible and ultraviolet ranges into the x-ray region, from microwatt to terawatt power levels, and from pulse transients of only a few femtoseconds to continuous irradiation.

The utility of lasers in fundamental cardiovascular research has been established. Berns et al.[2] at the University of California at Irvine, using an instrument that incorporates a fine and precise laser irradiating capability through a microscope with computer vision and control, have demonstrated the functional significance of subcellular organelles by sharply localized ablations. For example, ablation of the ribosomal gene area in the X chromosome of cultured cells results in reduced synthesis of ribosomal proteins. This functional deficit is transmitted to subsequent cell generations. In another laser technologic application, Lakatta et al.[3] have used backscattered, laser-induced fluorescence in beating hearts to study the role of calcium ions released from sarcoplasmic reticulum. This group is currently using this methodology to determine the role of calcium cycling in the generation of late systolic afterpotentials during ischemia and reperfusion.

Progress toward clinical applications has been impeded by technical difficulties and, importantly, by lack of specific information about laser energy interaction with cardiovascular tissues. It has become apparent that the effects of laser energy on tissue differ widely according to lasing parameters and the specific characteristics of the tissue and surrounding medium.[4] To evaluate adequately the potential uses of laser technology for treatment of cardiovascular disease, systematic studies are needed to observe short- and long-term tissue effects according to laser wavelength, energy level, and timing characteristics with consideration of the modulating effects of the surrounding medium.

NATURE OF LASER EFFECTS ON TISSUE

The physical properties of tissue and surrounding medium (blood, interstitial fluid, and irrigating solutions) determine focus, reflection, and scattering of laser energy as well as conduction of resultant thermal energy away from the site of laser-tissue interaction. Thus, the operating characteristics of the laser and optical and other properties of the tissue and surrounding medium interact to determine the depth of penetration, the volume of tissue affected, and the induced physical changes.

Whereas physical changes have been attributed usually to thermal effects (dehydration, coagulation, charring, and gasification), at high energy and short pulse duration, photochemical mechanisms may result in disruption of chemical bonds. Laser-induced, high-energy plasma formation can be used to disintegrate tissue in a controlled fashion. Also, tissue effects may be modulated by the presence of chromophores. At low power, clinically relevant differences in fluorescence may be induced, and this may prove to be useful diagnostically and as a guide to therapy. In addition, other therapeutically useful tissue effects may be mediated by other mechanisms.

VARIETY OF LASERS

Of the numerous lasers that are available from commercial suppliers, a number are being evaluated for cardiovascular applications. These include carbon dioxide (CO_2), erbium:yttrium-aluminum-garnet (Er:YAG), carbon monoxide, neodymium (Nd):YAG, alexandrite, argon ion, tunable dye, krypton ion, copper vapor, gold vapor, and excimer lasers. Other lasers are in development, such as the free-electron lasers, which will provide wavelengths not currently available with other lasers. Certain CO_2, Nd:YAG, and argon ion lasers have become available for ophthalmologic, dermatologic, or general surgical indications, and these have been evaluated most extensively for potential cardiovascular applications.[5-8] However, the lasing characteristics needed for specific cardiovascular applications may require developmental initiative. For example, Forrester et al.[9] have been able to ablate cardiovascular tissue in vivo in a reproducible, controlled fashion using pulsed ultraviolet laser energy from a specially constructed xenon chloride excimer laser, which is conducted through a proprietary optical fiber, whereas other investigative teams have had difficulty reproducing similar results with commercially available devices.

ANGIOPLASTY

Several approaches to percutaneous angioplasty have been investigated using a variety of laser energy sources and optical fibers to conduct the laser energy to obstructing arterial lesions. Several investigative teams have attempted to use argon ion or Nd:YAG laser energy conducted through an optical fiber, introduced through guiding catheters, to remove arterial obstructions. Ginsberg et al.[10] reported improvement in blood flow in peripheral arteries following penetration of obstructing atherosclerotic plaques, which could then be dilated with conventional balloon angioplasty technique. Because perforation of the arterial wall or thrombosis occurred in several patients, these investigators concluded that further laboratory investigation and laser-catheter system development were needed.

Optical Fibers

Commercially available optical fibers transmit the near-infrared and visible wavelengths with relatively little energy loss and have been used intravascularly with Nd:YAG and argon ion lasers in animal and clinical experimental studies, as noted above. With bare optical fibers, perforation of the arterial wall has been a problem attributed to both mechanical and thermal mechanisms; stiffness of some optical fibers appears to be a factor in mechanical perforation. Furthermore, clot and debris may accumulate on the fiber tip during intravascular laser irradiation. This may result in "burn back" (damage to the distal end of the fiber) or in bonding of the fiber to the arterial wall; the former interrupts transmission of laser energy from the distal end of the fiber, and the latter results in detachment of variable amounts of arterial intima and media when the fiber is withdrawn. Optical fibers are under development that meet flexibility and peak power requirements for transmission of pulsed ultraviolet and mid-infrared laser energy in vivo.

Thermal Probes

The problems with the distal ends of optical fibers have been approached in several ways. Two general types of metal caps have been attached to the ends of optical fibers and used as thermal probes to open arterial obstructions. One is solid and another is open at the end. Both are heated rapidly by laser energy conducted through the optical fibers and are operated in the 200 to 400°C range to vaporize or melt atheromatous arterial obstructions. Thermal probes with open tips provide egress of the laser beam to irradiate arterial obstruction distal to the catheter tip. These systems are being evaluated as means to create larger channels than result with the solid metal-tipped probes.[11]

Metal-tipped laser catheter systems have been used in over 200 peripheral arterial angioplasties and over a dozen coronary angioplasties; thermal probes have been used to penetrate tight stenoses or total occlusions, including cases with long occlusions. The resulting channels, though small, allow placement of conventional balloon angioplasty catheters, which are then used in the conventional way to dilate obstructions. Investigators evaluating thermal probes are attempting to determine the following: (1) success of angioplasty in cases with advanced disease not suitable for conventional balloon angioplasty, including frequency of improved perfusion, failure to penetrate obstructions, and perforation and thrombosis rates; (2) long-term results, including clinical outcome and frequency of continued patency and recurrent stenosis.

Preliminary results by Abela et al.[12] and Sanborn et al.[13] in the United States and by Cumberland et al.[14] in England suggest that thermal probes may offer advantages for some patients. There is inadequate information to evaluate the long-term outcome of thermal injury to the arterial wall. There are preliminary indications that successful opening and restenosis rates may favor thermal probe–initiated angioplasty over conventional balloon catheter–initiated angioplasty in patients with peripheral vascular disease.[15] It may be speculated that myointimal proliferation or recurrent atherosclerosis at the site of angioplasty may be retarded by thermal injury, but the potential for late scar formation or thrombosis requires further evaluation.

Other Contact Probes

Fourrier et al.[16] in France have developed a catheter system that uses an Nd:YAG laser coupled to an optical fiber, which in turn is coupled to a sapphire contact tip. With this experimental system, relatively long obstructions in peripheral arteries in a few patients have been recanalized. Other contact-tip laser-catheter systems are also under development.

An optical shield is under development by Cothren et al. at the Massachusetts Institute of Technology, and Kramer et al. at the Cleveland Clinic Foundation.[17] This approach may obviate some of the disadvantages encountered with bare optical fibers and with metal-tipped catheters. An optically clear glass cap is attached to the end of a catheter that incorporates an array of optical fibers, which are fixed in relation to the optical shield so that overlapping laser beams emitted from the fibers irradiate distally in a controlled fashion. This catheter system is being developed with the capability for machine discrimination of laser-induced fluorescence patterns to differentiate atheroma from normal arterial-wall tissue. In operation, the optical shield at the end of the catheter would be pressed against an obstructing atheroma. A low-power laser beam would be used to induce fluorescence, and a distinctive pattern typical of atheroma would trigger irradiation through the optical fibers that are aimed at the atheroma. Cessation of the typical fluorescence and/or sensing of normal arterial wall tissue would signal termination of irradiation through the relevant optical fibers. Optical fibers not focused on tissue producing the laser fluorescence signal typical of atheroma would not be energized. This *intelligent* catheter system may be adapted for use with a variety of laser fiberoptic configurations according to future developments.

Pulsed Laser Catheter Systems

To obviate thermal injury to arterial tissue, several investigative teams have evaluated pulsed lasers with operating parameters that result in little or no evidence of residual injury to the arterial wall.[18–20] Laboratory experiments with infrared, visible light, and ultraviolet laser energy delivered in 10 to 100-nsec pulses have been reported in which atherosclerotic plaque was ablated with minimal injury to the remaining tissue. Katzir et al.[21] and Sartori et al.[22] have investigated the use of pulsed Nd:YAG and excimer lasers to produce clean ablation. With appropriate operating parameters, comparable smooth ablation was obtained with minimal thermal injury to the remaining arterial wall. These experimental results indicate that pulsed laser energy at a variety of wavelengths may be used to remove pathologic cardiovascular tissue, including calcified atherosclerotic tissue, without significant residual tissue injury.

The mechanism responsible for clean ablation is disputed. The photoproducts resulting from such ablation have been described, on the one hand, as characteristic of thermal processes but, on the other hand, as characteristic of photochemical reactions. Calmettes and Berns[23] have published results indicating that, under certain conditions, multiphoton processes occur. Depending on the experimental conditions, the products of such ablation may include particles on the order of many microns in size.[24]

An impediment to the use of pulsed laser energy for percutaneous angioplasty is the need for optical fibers that can deliver pulsed laser energy sufficient for ablation without fiber breakdown in vivo. Forrester et al.[9] have reported progress in the development of an experimental optical fiber that conducts sufficient energy from a xenon chloride excimer laser for ablation of atherosclerotic plaque and other tissues. There is preliminary evidence of clean ablation using erbium:YAG laser energy in the mid-infrared region of the electromagnetic spectrum, which is conducted through a zirconium fluoride fiberoptic waveguide.[25]

ENDARTERECTOMY

Laser endarterectomy has been evaluated in experimental animals and, to a limited extent, in patients at open surgery. Eugene et al.[26-28] compared endarterectomy performed with CO_2, Nd:YAG, and argon ion lasers to remove atherosclerotic intima in experimental studies. Results with the argon laser were superior as to ease of performance, smoothness of the resulting luminal surfaces, adherence of remaining intima and media, damage to the arterial wall, and healing characteristics. Using a hand-held CO_2 laser, Livesay et al.,[29] in a preliminary report, indicated successful short-term results with distal endarterectomy in coronary artery revascularization procedures in a small series of patients.

ABLATION OF MYOCARDIUM

Myotomy, Myectomy, and Transmyocardial Neovascularization

Experimental studies and early clinical experiments have demonstrated the feasibility of removing or altering myocardial tissue for therapeutic objectives. Isner and Clarke[30] used an argon laser to perform myotomy and myectomy in a patient with asymmetric septal hypertrophy with resulting clinical improvement in left ventricular outlet obstruction. Preliminary work by Mirhoseini and Clayton[31] in the United States and investigators in Japan and the Soviet Union suggests that neovascularization of ischemic myocardial tissue may follow creation of channels by transmyocardial laser irradiation. Under certain conditions these new channels were reported to endothelialize and provide for the flow of blood directly from the left ventricle. These results have not been confirmed by other investigators in the United States.

Arrhythmia Control: Photoablation and Endocardiectomy

Several investigative teams have evaluated CO_2, Nd:YAG, and argon laser energy to ablate abnormally functioning cardiac conduction tissue or arrhythmogenic foci.[32-36] Experiments with both percutaneous and open surgical approaches suggest that laser ablation may be performed in a more precise manner than with conventional techniques. The potential for percutaneous approaches has generated interest among investigators, and the development of catheter systems that would incorporate electrophysiologic, angioscopic, and laser irradiating capabilities.

VALVULOPLASTY

In preliminary experimental work, Isner and Clarke[37] have found that calcific deposits on otherwise normal-appearing valves may be ablated without significant damage to the underlying valvular structures. Such an approach, if further developed, could provide an alternative to valve replacement in some patients. Ultimately, it may be possible to develop a system for safe percutaneous removal of atherosclerotic and calcific accretions from cardiac valves.

VASCULAR REPAIR

Construction of Anastomoses

Conventional surgical anastomoses may be complicated by bleeding or thrombosis and by late closure due to granuloma formation, scarring, myointimal hyperplasia, or atherosclerosis. To improve clinical outcome, several investigators have evaluated CO_2, Nd:YAG, and argon ion lasers for a variety of anastomoses.[38–41] Early results suggest that tissue sealing and fusion at anastomotic sites may be accomplished with disparate laser parameters. Arteriovenous anastomoses in experimental animals produced with the argon ion laser have compared favorably with conventional technique as to increased anastomotic strength, thrombogenicity, and healing characteristics. In addition to laser wavelength, results may depend also on the laser energy delivery system, the technical details of instrument and tissue manipulation, and the size and specific characteristics of the vessels to be fused and sealed.

Aneurysm Repair

Progress has been made in the development of approaches to repairing arterial aneurysms in experimental animals. In the animal model developed by O'Reilly et al.,[42] aneurysm cavities have been partially obliterated by inducing clot formation and local tissue injury, which was followed by fibrosis and reendothelialization of the luminal surface.

Arterial dissection occurs spontaneously in acute aortic dissection or iatrogenically following angioplasty. Animal experiments have demonstrated the feasibility of fusing dissected intima to the media by first reapproximating the dissected tissue planes with a special balloon angioplasty catheter and then irradiating through the balloon with an Nd:YAG laser.[43–45] This approach may compete with other percutaneous catheter techniques under development for placement of vascular stents in dissected segments of artery.

Chromophores

Following the work of Spears et al.[46] in which hematoporphyrin derivative was shown to have affinity for atherosclerotic tissue, considerable interest has focused on the use of dyes that are preferentially absorbed by atherosclerotic tissue and absorb light at wavelengths that are minimally absorbed by normal tissue. Tetracycline has been evaluated by several investigators because of its staining characteristics and absorption peaks at wavelengths generated by the argon laser. Abela et al.[47] reported selective ablation of atherosclerotic lesions in an animal model following tetracycline staining and argon laser irradiation. In this controlled study, evidence of regression was observed in both the control and tetracycline-treated groups, but the degree of regression was substantially greater in the tetracycline-stained vessels.

Prince et al.[48] reported the ablation of human atherosclerotic tissue with minimal injury to adjacent normal arterial intima when a tunable dye laser at low power was used at a wavelength that was preferentially absorbed by naturally occurring carotenoids that accumulate preferentially within atherosclerotic plaque. These encouraging experiments suggest that endogenous or exogenous chromophores that concentrate preferentially in atheroma may provide the means for selective ablation or for inducing regression of atherosclerotic tissue with minimal or no injury to normal arterial wall.

REGRESSION OF ATHEROSCLEROSIS

Gerrity et al.[49] observed rapid healing, intimal fibrous scarring, but no indication of accelerated atherosclerotic response at 8 weeks following low-energy CO_2 laser removal of atherosclerotic plaques in hyperlipemic swine. In hypercholesterolemic, atherosclerotic rhesus monkeys, Abela et al.[50] showed evidence consistent with regression of atherosclerotic plaque in areas adjacent to iliofemoral arterial sites that had been ablated 7 to 60 days earlier by argon ion laser irradiation delivered through an optical fiber. Thus, evidence of regression or reduced bulk of atherosclerotic tissue has followed subablative[49, 50] and low-power laser radiation as noted above.[47] The mechanism of these regressive changes is unclear. Regression following laser irradiation near ablative levels suggests a thermal effect; however, the low-power experiment suggests a mechanism other than response to thermal injury. If laser-induced regression or interruption of progression of atherosclerosis can be demonstrated as a long-term effect, important new therapeutic advantages may be realized with percutaneous angioplasty and for open surgical endarterectomy and anastomosis in revascularization procedures.

SUMMARY

Laboratory and preliminary clinical investigations have demonstrated that the use of lasers in the treatment of a number of cardiovascular problems is feasible. A variety of approaches is being studied with an increasing number of laser systems. Ideal operating parameters for specific applications are yet to be determined. Recent progress suggests that therapeutic advances will be realized in anastomotic sealing, endarterectomy, percutaneous removal of arterial obstruction, regression of atherosclerosis, open surgical percutaneous ablation of arrhythmogenic foci and abnormal conduction pathways, and other cardiovascular applications.

REFERENCES

1. Hochstrasser RM, Carey KJ: Lasers in biology. *Laser Focus/Electro-opt* 1985; 21:100–118.
2. Berns MW, Aist J, Edwards J, et al: Laser microsurgery in cell and developmental biology. *Science* 1981; 213:505–513.
3. Lakatta EG, Capogrossi C, Kort AA, et al: Spontaneous myocardial calcium oscillations: Overview with emphasis on ryanadine and caffeine. *Fed Proc* 1985; 2977–2983.
4. Regan JD, Parrish JA: *The Science of Photomedicine.* New York, Plenum Publishing Corp, 1982.
5. Abela GS, Normann S, Cohen D, et al: Effects of carbon dioxide, Nd:YAG, and argon laser radiation on coronary atheromatous plaques. *Am J Cardiol* 1982; 50:1199–1205.
6. Isner JM, Clarke RH: The current status of lasers in the treatment of cardiovascular disease. *IEEE J Quantum Electronics* 1984; 20:1406–1420.
7. Gerschwind HJ, Boussignac G, Teisseire B, et al: Conditions for effective Nd:YAG laser angioplasty. *Br Heart J* 1984; 52:484–489.
8. Macrue R, Martins JRM, Tupinamba AS: Possibilidades terapeuticas do raio laser em atromas. *Arq Bras Cardiol* 1980; 35:9–12.
9. Forrester JS, Litvack F, Grundfest WS: Laser angioplasty and cardiovascular disease. *Am J Cardiol* 1986; 57:990–992.
10. Ginsberg R, Wexler L, Mitchell RS, et al: Percutaneous transluminal laser angioplasty for treatment of peripheral vascular disease: Clinical experience with 16 patients. *Radiology* 1985; 156:619–624.

11. Abela GS, Barbieri E, Roxey T, et al: A method of quantitative plaque ablation using power-time matrix laser application, abstracted. *Circulation* 1986; 74(suppl 2):6.
12. Abela GS, Seeger JM, Barbieri E, et al: Laser recanalization under angioscopic guidance in humans. *J Am Coll Cardiol* 1986; 8:182–194.
13. Sanborn TA, Greenfield AJ, Guben JK, et al: Human percutaneous and intraoperative laser thermal angioplasty—Initial clinical results as an adjunct to balloon angioplasty. *J Vasc Surg* 1987; 5:183–190.
14. Cumberland DC, Sanborn TA, Taylor DI, et al: Percutaneous laser thermal angioplasty— Initial clinical results with a laserprobe in total peripheral artery occlusions. *Lancet* 1986; 1:1457–1459.
15. Sanborn TA, Faxon DP, Christian C, et al: Laser thermal angioplasty: Reduced restenosis compared to balloon angioplasty, abstracted. *Circulation* 1986; 74(suppl 2):6.
16. Fourrier JL, Marache P, Brunetaud J, et al: Laser recanalization of peripheral arteries by contact sapphire in man, abstracted. *Circulation* 1986; 74(suppl 2):204.
17. Cothren RM, Hayes GB, Cramer JR, et al: A multifiber catheter with an optical shield for laser angiosurgery. *Lasers Life Sci* 1987; 1:1–12.
18. Grundfest WS, Litvack F, Forrester JS, et al: Laser ablation of human atherosclerotic plaque without adjacent tissue injury. *J Am Coll Cardiol* 1985; 5:929–933.
19. Deckelbaum LI, Isner JM, Donaldson RF, et al: Use of pulsed energy delivery to minimize injury resulting from carbon dioxide laser irradiation of cardiovascular tissues. *J Am Coll Cardiol* 1986; 7:898–908.
20. Linsker R, Srinivasan R, Wynne JJ, et al: Far-ultraviolet laser ablation of atherosclerotic lesions. *Lasers Med Biol* 1984; 4:201–206.
21. Katzir A, Isner JM, Clarke RH, et al: Development of an infrared fiber radiometer for non-contact temperature monitoring during laser irradiation: Initial measurements regarding mechanism of ablation, abstracted. *Circulation* 1986; 74(suppl 2):497.
22. Sartori MP, Henry PD, Sauerbrey RA, et al: Tissue interaction and measurement of ablation rates with UV and visible lasers in canine and human arteries. *Lasers Surg Med* 1987; 7:300–306.
23. Calmettes PP, Berns MW: Laser induced multiphoton processes in living cells. *Proc Natl Acad Sci USA* 1983; 80:7197–7199.
24. DeJesus ST, Isner JM, Rongione AJ, et al: Embolic potential of cardiovascular laser irra-diation. *Proc Soc Photo-Opt Instr Engl* 1986; 713:47–49.
25. Bonner RF, Smith PD, Leon M, et al: A new erbium laser and infrared fiber system for laser angioplasty, abstracted. *Circulation* 1986; 74(suppl 2):361.
26. Eugene J, McColgan SJ, Pollock ME, et al: Experimental arteriosclerosis treated by con-ventional and laser endarterectomy. *J Surg Med* 1985; 39:31–38.
27. Eugene J, Pollock ME, McColgan SJ, et al: Fiber optic versus direct laser delivery for en-darterectomy of experimental atheromas. *Proc Int Soc Opt Eng* 1985; 576:55–58.
28. Eugene J, McColgan SJ, Pollock ME, et al: Experimental arteriosclerosis treated by argon ion and neodymium-YAG laser endarterectomy. *Circulation* 1985; 72(suppl 2):200–206.
29. Livesay JJ, Leachman DR, Hogan PJ, et al: Preliminary report on laser coronary endarter-ectomy in patients. *Circulation* 1985; 72(suppl 3):302.
30. Isner JM, Clarke RH: Laser myoplasty for hypertrophic cardiomyopathy: In vitro experience in human postmortem hearts and in vivo experience in a canine model (transarterial) and human patients (intraoperative). *Am J Cardiol* 1984; 53:1620–1625.
31. Mirhoseini M, Clayton MM: Revascularization of the heart by laser. *J Microsurg* 1981; 2:253–260.
32. Abela GS, Griffin JC, Hill JA, et al: Transvascular argon laser induced atrial ventricular conduction ablation in dogs, abstracted. *Circulation* 1983; 68(suppl 3):580.
33. Lee BI, Gottdiener JS, Fletcher RD, et al: Transcatheter ablation: Comparison between laser photoablation and electrode shock ablation in the dog. *Circulation* 1985; 71:579–586.
34. Isner JM, Estes NAM, Payne DD, et al: Laser assisted endocardiectomy for refractory ven-tricular tachyarrhythmias: Preliminary intraoperative experience. *Clin Cardiol* 1987; 10:201–204.

35. Svenson RH, Gallagher JJ, Selle JK, et al: Intraoperative laser photoablation of ventricular tachycardia, abstracted. *Circulation* 1986; 74(suppl 2):461.

36. Saksena S, Hussain SM, Gelchinsky I: Successful mapping-guided argon laser ablation of ventricular tachycardia in man. *Circulation* 1986; 74(suppl 2):186.

37. Isner JM, Clarke RH: Laser-assisted debridement of aortic valve calcium. *Am Heart J* 1985; 109:448–452.

38. Schober R, Ulrich F, Sander T, et al: Laser-induced alteration of collagen substructure allows microsurgical tissue welding. *Science* 1986; 232:1421–1422.

39. McCarthy WJ, Hartz RS, Yao JST, et al: Vascular anastomoses with laser energy. *J Vasc Surg* 1986; 3:32–41.

40. Frazier OH, Painvin GA, Morris JM, et al: Laser assisted microvascular anastomoses—Angiographic and anatomopathologic studies on growing microvascular anastomoses—Preliminary report. *Surgery* 1985; 97:585–590.

41. White RA: Technical frontiers for the vascular surgeon: Laser vascular anastomotic welding and angioscopy-assisted intraluminal instrumentation. *J Vasc Surg* 1987; 5:673–680.

42. O'Reilly GV, Forrest MD, Schoene WC, et al. Laser induced thermal coagulation of berry aneurysms: Preliminary experimental experience. Submitted for publication.

43. Hiehle JF Jr, Bourgelais DBC, Shapshay S, et al: Nd:YAG laser fusion of human atheromatous plaque-arterial wall separations in vitro. *Am J Cardiol* 1985; 56:953–957.

44. Serur JR, Sinclair IN, Spokojny AM, et al: Laser balloon angioplasty (LBA): Effect on the carotid lumen in the dog, abstracted. *Circulation* 1985; 72(suppl 3):457.

45. Sanborn TA, Sinclair IN, Serur JR, et al: In vivo laser thermal seal of neointimal dissection after balloon angioplasty in rabbit atherosclerosis, abstracted. *Circulation* 1985; 72(suppl 3):469.

46. Spears JR, Serur J, Shropshire D, et al: Fluorescence of experimental atheromatous plaques with hematoporphyrin derivative. *J Clin Invest* 1983; 71:395–397.

47. Abela GS, Barbieri E, Roxey T, et al: Laser enhanced plaque atherolysis with tetracycline, abstracted. *Circulation* 1986; 72(suppl 2):7.

48. Prince MR, Deutsch TF, Mathews-Roth MM, et al: Preferential light absorption in atheromas in vitro. *J Clin Invest* 1986; 78:295–302.

49. Gerrity RG, Coop FD, Golding AR, et al: Arterial response to laser operation for removal of atherosclerotic plaques. *J Thorac Cardiovasc Surg* 1983; 85:409–421.

50. Abela GS, Crea F, Seeger JE, et al: The healing process in normal canine arteries and in atherosclerotic monkey arteries after transluminal laser irradiation. *Am J Cardiol* 1985; 56:983–988.

Chapter 6

Percutaneous Laser Thermal Angioplasty

Timothy A. Sanborn, M.D.

By removing obstructing atheroma or thrombus through vaporization rather than by merely stretching or fracturing the plaque as in balloon angioplasty,[1] laser angioplasty or laser recanalization may be particularly useful as an adjunct or alternative to balloon angioplasty by (1) increasing the initial recanalization rate for lesions that are difficult or impossible to treat by conventional means or (2) decreasing the incidence of restenosis after angioplasty.

However, in initial experimental studies and early clinical trials, the technique has been limited by inadequate delivery systems, resulting in an unacceptably high perforation rate[2-6] and the creation of small recanalized channels that result in poor long-term patency.[5] The key limitation in these early trials of laser angioplasty was the lack of an adequate catheter-delivery system for safe and effective intravascular use. Modifications of the fiberoptic tips were the first approaches to improve upon these results with bare fiberoptics. The first, but certainly not the last, modified laser delivery system to demonstrate a high incidence of successful laser recanalization with a low incidence of vessel perforation is an argon laser heated metallic-capped fiberoptic device (Laserprobe-PLR, Trimidyne Inc., Santa Ana, Calif).

LASER PROBE PROPERTIES

The laser probe is a fiberoptic delivery system[7] that allows transmission of argon laser energy from the laser generator to the desired target and conversion of this light energy into controlled thermal energy at the distal end of the probe (Fig 6–1). In the first 2 seconds of argon laser energy delivery, the temperature on the surfaces of the probe rises sooner and higher at the probe tip and decreases toward the neck of the probe, but by 5 seconds the temperature distribution of the probe is nearly uniform.[8] When brought in contact with atherosclerotic tissue, the laser probe conducts this heat to the tissue and vaporization of the tissue occurs. As expected, increased laser energy resulted in greater depth of ablation. Interestingly, in this study increasing the force applied by the laser-heated device also resulted in more efficient ablation of tissue.[8] While this greater tissue

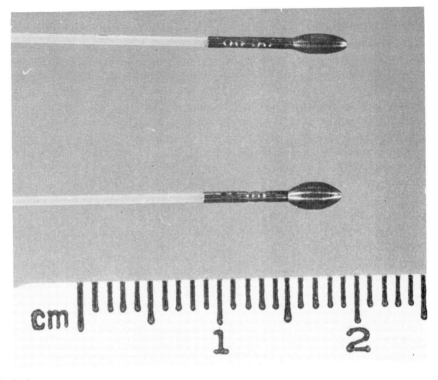

FIG 6–1.
1.5-mm laser probe (*top*); 2.0-mm laser probe (*bottom*). (From Sanborn TA, et al: Human percutaneous and intraoperative laser thermal angioplasty: Initial clinical results as an adjunct to balloon angioplasty. *J Vasc Surg* 1987; 5:83–90. Used by permission.)

ablation may simply be because of less thermal resistance from improved contact of the probe with the tissue, another possibility is that vacuolated tissue is compressed by the rounded probe. In a comparative study in this same report, irradiation of aortic tissue with bare argon optical fibers was found to result in a split, fragmented appearance on the surface of the aortic tissue and extensive dissection of the subintima, while the injury resulting from the laser probe was more controlled without evidence of vessel dissection. In this study, the laser-heated probe was also more effective in ablating fibrofatty plaque than nonatherosclerotic aorta. It can be speculated that this difference in thermal properties could explain the clinical observation that the laser probe preferentially vaporizes obstructive atheroma and thrombus during laser recanalization rather than the vessel wall and that this explains why the incidence of vessel perforation is reduced.

EXPERIMENTAL IN VIVO RESULTS

Three in vivo experimental studies have now been published that demonstrate not only improved safety and efficacy of this laser-heated probe compared to bare fiberoptics[2, 9] but also indicate an incidence of less restenosis than occurs with conventional balloon angioplasty.[10] First, in a series of atherosclerotic rabbit iliac artery stenoses,[2] angiography revealed greater widening of luminal stenoses in animals treated with the laser probe device as compared to those treated with the standard fiberoptic system. More important, while perforation of the vessel wall occurred frequently with the fiberoptic fiber, only one mechanical perforation occurred in 12 animals treated with the laser probe.

Histology revealed striking differences with these two fiberoptic systems. With direct laser radiation from the bare fiberoptic, a deep localized laser "crater" was noted along one side of the vessel wall, with charring and considerable thrombus formation (Fig 6–2,A). On histologic cross sections of eccentric lesions, the major portion of the atherosclerotic lesion was often "missed" by the narrow laser beam. In contrast, those vessels treated with the laser-heated metallic probe showed histologic evidence of thermal injury distributed evenly around the entire luminal circumference with minimal charring and thinner, flatter thrombus formation (Fig 6–2,B). These histologic data suggest that circumferential rather than localized distribution of energy is a factor in these improved results.

These results were confirmed in a series of postmortem human coronary arterial

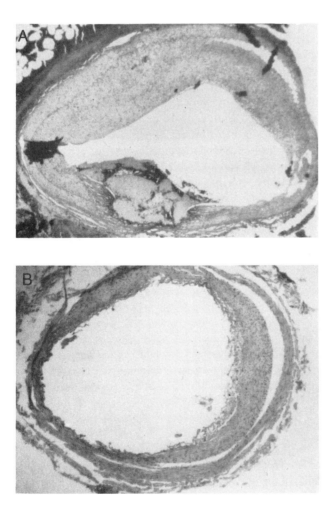

FIG 6–2.

Histologic specimens of iliac artery. A, example of direct argon-laser radiation resulting in a localized laser defect along one side of the vessel wall that extends through the neointima into the media. A gradient of thermal injury characterized by cell swelling and tissue edema is also noted. In addition, considerable thrombus that fills the newly formed laser defect is present. B, example of laser probe thermal injury distributed evenly around the entire luminal circumference. Hematoxylin-eosin, × 80. (From Sanborn TA, et al: Experimental angioplasty: Circumferential distribution of laser thermal energy with a laser probe. *J Am Coll Cardiol* 1985; 5:934–938. Used by permission.)

xenographs transplanted into canine femoral arteries.[9] Angiography demonstrated recanalization in all five arteries treated with a laser-heated probe, compared to three of five arteries treated with a bare fiberoptic. There was also less vessel perforation with the metallic-capped fiber compared to the bare fiberoptic.

Recent follow-up angiographic and histologic studies in the rabbit model demonstrated good long-term patency with laser thermal angioplasty in comparison to conventional balloon angioplasty.[10] While the immediate enlargement of the angiographic luminal diameter was similar for both procedures, the vessels treated with 1.5- to 2.0-mm laser probe devices had less angiographic restenosis and a significantly larger mean luminal diameter than those treated with balloon angioplasty. On histology, 4 weeks after the laser procedure, there was a larger lumen, minimal thrombosis or smooth muscle cell proliferation, and a thin neointima covered with a fibrous cap (Fig 6–3,A). In contrast, those vessels treated with balloon angioplasty demonstrated evidence of prior fracture and dissection of the vessel wall, with more of a fibrocellular proliferative response and ongoing thrombus formation (Fig 6–3,B). Morphometric analysis of these histologic cross sections confirmed a significantly larger luminal area after laser thermal angioplasty compared with balloon angioplasty. Thus, laser thermal angioplasty was associated with less restenosis and produced a significantly larger mean luminal diameter and mean luminal area than conventional balloon angioplasty. The differences in the pathophysiology of these techniques is probably responsible for these observations. That is, with laser recanalization of these high-grade stenotic lesions there is (1) partial laser vaporization or removal of atherosclerotic material and (2) perhaps more importantly, a smoother, less thrombogenic surface is left behind compared to that seen with balloon angioplasty. Whether there is an additional thermal effect on the arterial wall that inhibits platelet accumulation and/or smooth muscle cell proliferation is another intriguing concept.

LASER-THERMAL ANGIOPLASTY IN PERIPHERAL VESSELS

After the safety and efficacy of this device was demonstrated in experimental animals, a clinical trial was initiated to investigate its role in performing percutaneous laser thermal angioplasty as an adjunct to balloon angioplasty in patients with severe peripheral vascular disease.[11, 12] The initial aims were twofold: (1) to demonstrate the safety of this laser device and (2) to determine whether this procedure could add to conventional balloon angioplasty by increasing the initial success rate in peripheral artery total occlusions and recanalizing occlusions in which balloon and guidewire techniques had failed.

Use in Total Occlusions

In an initial report, laser recanalization was achieved in 50 of 56 (89%) femoropopliteal and iliac artery occlusions.[11] From a previous assessment of the angiogram and/or gentle probing of the proximal origin of the occlusion with a guidewire, the lesions were subjectively classified as "easy" (17) or "difficult" (21) to cross by conventional angioplasty methods. Eighteen occlusions were classified as "impossible" either because previous angioplasty attempts had failed (11) or because they were considered unsuitable for conventional angioplasty (7). All 17 easy, 19 of 21 difficult, and 14 of 18 impossible occlusions were successfully recanalized. Since there were two acute reocclusions in the first 24 hours, the overall initial clinical success rate was 86%. These results compare

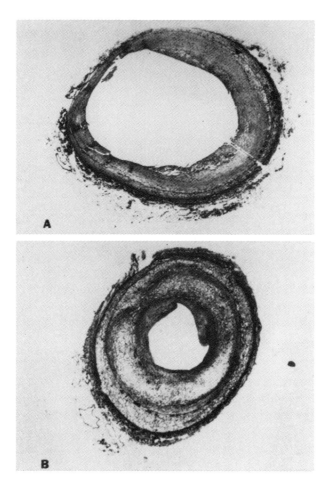

FIG 6–3.
A, cross-section of the patent rabbit iliac vessel 4 weeks after laser thermal angioplasty, demonstrating minimal fibrocellular proliferative response and a thin, condensed fibrous cap. B, histologic section 4 weeks after balloon angioplasty, revealing moderate fibrocellular proliferation caused by the dilation that partially filled the lumen and obliterated the prior dissection planes between the neointima and the media. (Verhoeff-van Geison elastin strains; × 26). (From Sanborn TA, et al: Angiographic and histologic consequences of laser thermal angioplasty: Comparison with balloon angioplasty. *Circulation* 1987; 75:1281–1286. Used by permission.)

favorably to recent clinical success rates of 72% to 78% for conventional balloon angioplasty.[13, 14]

In this initial series, the perforation rate was less than 2%, and the one perforation was attributed to excess mechanical pressure within a hard calcified occlusion rather than a thermal perforation. There were no clinical sequelae as a result of this perforation. Angiographic examples of laser-assisted balloon angioplasty of total occlusions are shown in Figures 6–4 and 6–5.

MULTICENTER EXPERIENCE

This initial clinical experience with laser thermal angioplasty in peripheral arteries[11, 12] suggests that this technique is a safe and effective adjunct to balloon angioplasty in that

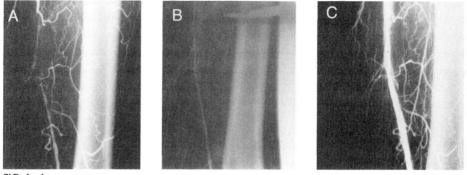

FIG 6–4.
Angiograms of a 4-cm total occlusion of the superficial femoral artery (**A**) that was recanalized with three pulses of 12 W of argon laser energy delivered to the laser probe for 10 seconds' duration each (**B**). This was followed by balloon angioplasty to yield a good angiographic result (**C**). (From Sanborn TA, et al: Human percutaneous and intraoperative laser thermal angioplasty: Initial clinical results as an adjunct to balloon angioplasty. *J Vasc Surg* 1987; 5:83–90. Used by permission.)

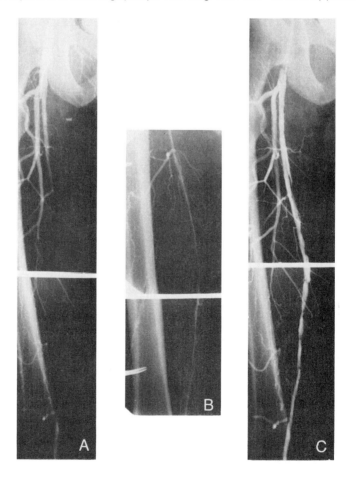

FIG 6–5.
Angiograms of a 15-cm right superficial femoral artery occlusion. **A**, before treatment. **B**, after recanalization with 6 pulses (5 seconds' duration) of 12 W of argon laser energy delivered to a 2.5-mm laser probe. **C**, after dilation with a 6-mm balloon catheter. (From Sanborn TA, et al: Peripheral laser-assisted balloon angioplasty: Initial multi-center experience in 219 peripheral arteries. *Arch Surg*, in press. Used by permission.)

it can recanalize lesions that previously could not be treated by conventional means.[11] However, these initial results were obtained at two centers with extensive experimental[2, 10] and prior clinical experience with argon laser angioplasty.[6] One question that needed to be answered was whether this new technique could be easily learned and used safely and effectively by physicians experienced in conventional peripheral balloon angioplasty techniques. The following is a summary of the clinical experience with the laser probe at ten centers.[15]

Physician Training

Physician training was key in the development of this initial experience in as safe a manner as possible. After the technique had been developed in over 40 patients at two centers, eight additional investigators with extensive experience in peripheral balloon angioplasty were trained through a combination of the following: (1) obtaining knowledge of laser safety, laser physics, and laser tissue interaction; (2) gaining "hand-on" experience in atherosclerotic rabbits or postmortem specimens; (3) observing videotapes and/ or actual "live" cases; and finally (4) clinical participation in several laser cases with one of the established investigators.

Today, more than 3 years after this initial experience, cardiovascular laser training remains a significant concern. Unfortunately, in some institutions, significant debate and in a few cases "turf battles" have developed over which physicians are best qualified to perform these procedures. In some instances, for political reasons, laser credentials have actually been denied to individuals who may be the best qualified. The cardiovascular area should not be any different from other areas of medicine and surgery in which lasers are used and standards of practice have been developed according to the guidelines as established by the American Society of Laser Medicine and Surgery.

More important than attending a laser course or watching a few cases, however, is the need to be skilled in conventional peripheral balloon angioplasty and interventional radiology techniques. It has often been said that laser recanalization of a lesion is sometimes the easiest part of the angioplasty procedure. The antegrade puncture as well as the choice and handling of various guidewires and balloon catheters requires considerable experience that is unique to a vascular radiologist. Despite my own training in cardiac catheterization and coronary angioplasty, I have always performed our laser-assisted balloon angioplasty procedures in collaboration with one of my colleagues in Radiology. This cooperation is key in order to obtain the best result with the lowest risk of complications for the patient. Most other successful cardiovascular laser centers have also developed similar types of collaborative approach to laser angioplasty, whether it be a cardiologist and a vascular radiologist working together with surgical consultation or a vascular surgeon teamed up with an interventional radiologist. The free exchange of different techniques and methods adds significantly to the overall likelihood of success.

Initial Investigators and Lesion Classification

Between April 1985 and November 1986, laser-assisted balloon angioplasty was performed in 219 peripheral arteries in 204 patients at ten medical centers. These centers and their principal investigators are as follows: Boston University Medical Center, Boston: Timothy A. Sanborn, M.D., and Alan J. Greenfield, M.D.; Johns Hopkins Medical Center, Baltimore: Robert I. White, M.D., and Robert R. Murray, M.D.; Northern General Hospital, Sheffield, England: David C. Cumberland, M.D., and Christopher L.

TABLE 6–1.
Initial Angiographic and Clinical Results

Angioplasty Category	N	Mean Lesion Length (cm)	Angiographic Success*		Clinical Success*	
Possible	149	6.8	128	(86)	116	(78)
Stenosis	41		40	(98)	39	(95)
Occlusions	108		88	(81)	77	(71)
Impossible	70	11.7	44	(63)	39	(56)
Stenosis	4		4	(100)	4	(100)
Occlusions	66		44	(67)	53	(79)
Total	219	8.3	172	(79)	155	(71)

*Number in parentheses represents percent success in each group.

Welch, M.D.; Seton Medical Center, Daly City, Calif: Richard K. Myler, M.D.; Stanford Medical Center, Palo Alto, Calif: Robert Ginsberg, M.D.; St. Anne's Hospital, Chicago: Amir Motarjeme, M.D.; St. Joseph's Hospital, Wichita, Kan: Daniel Tapati, M.D.; St. Vincent's Hospital, Indianapolis: Donald E. Schwarten, M.D.; Texas Heart Institute, Houston: D. Richard Leachmann, M.D.; and University of Arkansas Health Sciences Center, Little Rock: Ernest J. Ferris, M.D., and Timothy C. McCowan, M.D.

In this initial series, the indications for angioplasty were severe claudication that was unresponsive to exercise therapy and pentoxifylline in 96 (44%) lesions and rest pain, nonhealing ulcer, or gangrene in 123 (56%) lesions. Nine straight iliac arteries and 210 femoropopliteal arteries were treated. There were 166 (76%) occlusions and 53 (24%) stenoses. From previous assessment of the angiogram and/or by gentle probing at the proximal end of an occlusion with a guidewire (without an attempt to cross the lesion), all lesions were classified by the clinical investigator as to the probability of success by conventional peripheral balloon angioplasty (i.e., possible or impossible) as previously reported.[11] Prior failed attempts with conventional balloon angioplasty were considered in the impossible category. Altogether, 149 (68%) of these lesions were considered possible to treat by conventional balloon angioplasty, while almost one third (70) of these lesions were impossible to treat by conventional balloon angioplasty (Table 6–1).

Acute Angiographic and Clinical Results

The overall initial angiographic and clinical success for all 219 lesions was 71%, with the likelihood of angioplasty success (possible or impossible) influencing immediate technical and clinical success (see Table 6–1). For lesions considered possible to treat by conventional balloon angioplasty, the clinical success rate of 78% is equal to or better than that reported in the literature for conventional balloon angioplasty.[14, 16] In this series, clinical success was achieved in 39 of 41 (95%) stenoses and 77 of 108 (71%) total occlusions in this "possible" category.

Potentially, one of the most important benefits of laser thermal angioplasty is the ability to quickly and safely recanalize lesions that are impossible to treat by conventional means. In particular, over one half (56%) of those lesions that were not amenable to balloon angioplasty alone were successfully treated with laser-assisted balloon angioplasty.

Complications

In this initial multicenter series, which represented an expansion from two initial clinical centers to a total of ten, the complications that arose from laser-assisted balloon angioplasty were minimal (Table 6–2). Most notable, the perforation rate with this laser device was only 4.1%, and there was no requirement for emergency bypass surgery. This perforation rate was only 2.1% in those lesions considered possible to treat by balloon angioplasty alone. In a trial that represents not only the clinical development stage of a new device but also early operator learning experience, it is important to note that the incidence of various complications is no greater than that noted in two recent reports[17, 18] of conventional balloon angioplasty (see Table 6–2). One early concern with laser angioplasty was the incidence of perforation, which complicated early clinical trials.[4, 6] In the present series, the 4.1% incidence of vessel perforation with no significant clinical sequelae is much lower than that of previous clinical series using bare argon laser fiberoptics for peripheral laser angioplasty, in which vessel perforation was noted in 2 of 15 (13%)[4] and 3 of 16 (19%)[6] vessels.

The decreased incidence of vessel perforation with this device is probably multifactorial. From a design standpoint, the rounded but tapered tip provides a blunt object that is less likely to perforate the artery mechanically compared to sharp, pointed fiberoptics.[2] Secondly, the metal probe has been shown to disperse thermal energy uniformly around the tip so as not to focus all laser energy in one spot.[8] Histologic analysis after the use of this device indicates a thermal effect around the entire luminal circumference of a diseased vessel.[2] Thus, dispersion and circumferential distribution of thermal energy rather than attempting to aim a narrow laser beam could also contribute to reduce perforation. Finally, vaporization of fibrofatty plaque with this laser probe device was possible at lower temperatures than for normal (elastic and collagen) tissue[8]; this may also contribute to reduce perforation.

Probe Detachment

Early in this clinical trial, probe tip detachment from the fiberoptic occurred in four patients; all but one of these probes could be retrieved and removed. Subsequent to this early experience, a 0.014-in. safety (anchor) wire was incorporated into the device to add stability to the union between the fiberoptic and the metal tip and to prevent further probe detachment. This wire runs along the entire intravascular length of the fiberoptics

TABLE 6–2.
Incidence of Complications in 219 Arteries

Complications	Probe Related %	Probe Related No.	Procedure Related %	Procedure Related No.	Incidence With Conventional Balloon Angioplasty, % Gardiner et al.[17]	Incidence With Conventional Balloon Angioplasty, % Sos et al.[18]
Death	0	(0)*	0	(0)	0.3	0
Emergency surgery	0	(0)	0	(0)	3.0	—
Embolization	0	(0)	2.7	(6)	1.5	5
Probe detachment	1.8	(4)	—	—	—	—
Groin hematoma	0	(0)	3.2	(7)	4	2
Infection	0	(0)	0	(0)	—	—
Perforation	4.1	(9)	4.6	(10)	—	0–3
Rupture	0	(0)	0	(0)	0.4	0–1
Spasm	0	(0)	1.8	(4)	—	0–5
Subintimal dissection	5.0	(11)	5.0	(11)	4	1

*Number in parentheses represents number of complications in 219 patients.

TABLE 6–3.
Learning Curve of Success and Complications

Clinical Center	N	Clinical Success	Intimal Dissection	Perforation
Boston University	19	16 (84)*	0	0
Northern General Hospital	105	73 (70)	4 (3.8)	3 (2.9)
Other 8 centers (avg-12 per site)	95	66 (69)	7 (7.4)	7 (7.4)

*Number in parentheses represents percent of total attempts.

so that, if tip detachment should occur, the probe could be retrieved. In addition, by keeping the probe moving constantly during laser delivery and the cooling period, it was found that adherence to the vessel wall, one of the potential causes of probe detachment, was significantly reduced.

Learning Curve of Success and Complications

In this multicenter clinical trial, clinical success and incidence of complications improved considerably as the operator gained experience with the laser probe device (Table 6–3). In terms of complications, the lowest incidence of perforations (0%) occurred at Boston University where extensive experiments and a "tactile" sense for the device had been gained from prior experimental studies in atherosclerotic rabbits and postmortem specimens. However, clinical centers could also learn this technique and gain experience with the device quite rapidly without a high incidence of complications. For example, at Northern General Hospital the incidence of perforation decreased from 1 in 14 patients (7%) to 2 in the first 40 patients (5%), and then 1 in the last 65 patients (1.5%).

Thus, this multicenter series of 219 peripheral artery laser-assisted balloon angioplasty procedures indicates that there is evidence that the process of laser thermal angioplasty with an argon-laser–heated metallic-capped fiberoptic allows for nonsurgical treatment of lesions difficult or impossible to treat by conventional means. Furthermore, the technique can be easily learned by those experienced in peripheral angioplasty. It can also be performed without added risk compared to conventional balloon angioplasty.

FOLLOW-UP RESULTS

While recanalization with laser devices may be a useful adjunct to improve the initial chance of a successful angioplasty in peripheral artery total occlusions, the real challenge will be to determine whether laser angioplasty by whatever pathophysiologic mechanism (vaporization, thermal compression, sealing) can actually improve long-term clinical patency and reduce recurrence. At present, the laser probe is the only laser catheter with adequate clinical experience for assessment of long-term results; 1-year cumulative results were recently reported and compared to results of recently published series for conventional balloon angioplasty.[19] Angiographic examples of laser-assisted balloon angioplasty with follow-up angiography are shown in Figures 6–6 and 6–7.

When long-term results of peripheral angioplasty are examined, recurrence rates varied considerably depending on the type of lesion (stenosis vs. occlusions), lesion length, and the definition of recurrence. With subgroup analysis of this initial series, a potential benefit of combined laser recanalization and balloon angioplasty was suggested in femoropopliteal arteries (Table 6–4). For example, the 1-year cumulative recurrence

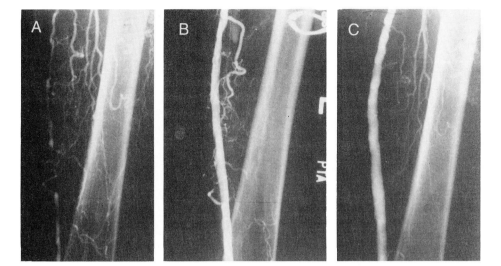

FIG 6–6.
Angiography of a 4-cm superficial femoral artery occlusion with a tortuous 8-cm stenosis proximal to the occlusion. **A,** image obtained before angioplasty. **B,** image obtained immediately after laser-assisted balloon angioplasty. Traversing the tortuous proximal stenosis required shaping a curve in the 0.014-in. guidewire attached to the laser probe. With the curved guidewire, it was possible to torque the laser probe through the stenosis. After the occlusion had been crossed with the laser-heated probe, the probe was slowly withdrawn through the occlusion and the stenosis with continuous laser-pulse delivery to further enlarge the entire lumen before balloon angioplasty. **C,** image obtained at repeat angiography 2 months later, at the time of angioplasty of the opposite leg. (From Sanborn TA, et al: Percutaneous laser thermal angioplasty: Initial results and 1-year follow-up in 129 femoropopliteal lesions. *Radiology* 1988; 168:121–125. Used by permission.)

rates for stenoses and short occlusions (1 to 3 cm in length) were only 5% and 7% respectively.[19] These results were considerably better than recent balloon angioplasty series in which 1-year recurrence rates of 20% to 30% or more were reported for short occlusions.[14, 16, 20] The definition of clinical patency is important in comparing these results as a 12% to 20% redilation rate was not considered a recurrence in two of these recent series.[14, 16] For longer occlusions treated with laser-assisted balloon angioplasty, a 1-year recurrence rate of 24% for 4- to 7-cm occlusion and 42% for occlusion > 7 cm is also better than a recurrence rate of 50% for occlusion > 3 cm reported in one series.[20]

On one hand, these results are influenced by operator learning and experience and the initial development stage of a device; clinical success and patency should improve with more catheter and device modifications. On the other hand, these results could be influenced by other patient demographic factors such as case selection, diabetes, smoking, distal vessel run-off, and medications. Obviously these results have to be confirmed and a multicenter randomized trial should be considered. These initial results do serve as a useful reference for future laser or mechanical devices.

Possible explanations for these lower recurrence rates after laser recanalization and balloon angioplasty are that the technique partially vaporizes or thermally compresses the atherosclerotic lesion and leaves behind a smoother, less thrombogenic arterial surface. Obviously, for longer occlusions, more atherosclerotic material will have to be removed. Larger probes may be beneficial in removing more material or leaving behind a smoother surface with a larger lumen so that balloon angioplasty may not be required at all. Preliminary clinical experience with a "second generation" of larger 2.5-mm devices

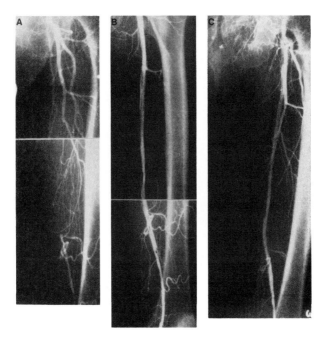

FIG 6–7.
Angiography of an 18-cm left superficial femoral artery occlusion (**A**) that was recanalized first with a 2.0-mm Laserprobe-PLR-Plus using eight sequential pulses (5 to 10 seconds each) of 10 W of argon laser energy delivered to the probe tip. The lesion was then dilated along the entire length of the lesion with a 6-mm by 10-mm balloon catheter (**B**). One year later, the patient was asymptomatic in his left leg but had developed symptoms in his right leg. On diagnostic arteriogram the left superficial femoral artery was still patent (**C**), and the right superficial femoral artery had a short lesion that could be treated successfully with conventional balloon angioplasty. The 1-year follow-up arteriogram courtesy of Dr. Gerald L. Honick, M.D., Oklahoma City. (From Sanborn TA: *Laser Med Surg News and Advances* 1988; 6:26–35. Used by permission.)

capable of being passed over guidewires indicates that this may be possible; this has been noted by Sanborn et al.[21] The recent study in the smaller (1- to 2-mm) rabbit iliac arteries discussed earlier suggests that laser recanalization with the laser probe device alone may cause less restenosis than conventional balloon angioplasty.[2]

TABLE 6–4.
Comparison of 1-Year Cumulative Patency Rates*

Technique	Stenoses	Occlusions		
		<3 cm	4–7 cm	>7 cm
Laser-assisted balloon angioplasty	95	93	76	58
Balloon angioplasty alone				
Hewes et al.	81[†]	67[†]	82[†]	68[†]
Murray et al.	72[†]	86[‡]		
Krepel et al.	80	93	50 (>3 cm)	

*Note values are expressed as percentages. From Sanborn TA, Cumberland DC, Green-field AJ, et al: Percutaneous laser thermal angioplasty: Initial results and 1-year follow-up in 129 femoropopliteal lesions. *Radiology* 1988; 168:121–125. Used by permission.
[†]Redilation rate of 12% to 20% was not considered recurrence.
[‡]Value for all occlusions.

Percutaneous Coronary Laser Feasibility

Based on this experience in peripheral vessels, clinical trials of percutaneous coronary use of lasers were recently initiated using specially designed coronary laser-heated probes.[22, 23] These preliminary studies indicated that a coronary laser catheter can be used percutaneously to reduce coronary stenoses angiographically (Fig 6–8); however, laser recanalization of the stenoses was limited by the inflexible, prototype nature of the device.[22] In addition, a high incidence of myocardial infarction in one study[23] raised concerns about the thrombogenicity or vasospastic nature of these early prototype devices. Currently, laser probe catheters with improved flexibility, trackability, profile, a central lumen design, and temperature feedback are being investigated and appear promising.

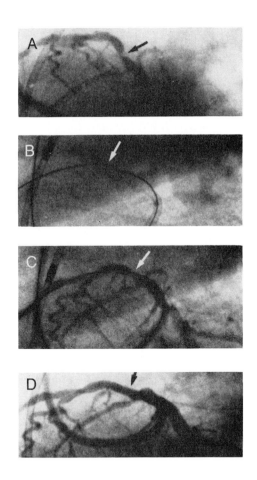

FIG 6–8.
The 60-degree left anterior oblique, 10-degree caudal views of a 90% eccentric left anterior descending artery lesion *(arrows)* before treatment (**A**), after laser thermal angioplasty results with the laser probe through the lesion and the angiographic results of laser thermal angioplasty (**B** and **C**), and after balloon angioplasty (**D**). (From Sanborn TA, et al: Percutaneous coronary laser thermal angioplasty. *J Am Coll Cardiol* 1986; 8:1437. Used by permission.)

CONCLUSIONS

We are definitely entering a new era of interventional techniques. There is already evidence that at least one laser device can supplement the vascular radiologists' complement of balloons and wires for recanalizing lesions that previously could not be treated.[11] Perhaps more exciting is the suggestion that long-term results for femoropopliteal angioplasty may be improved with laser techniques.[19] We have learned that bare fiberoptics are unsafe and provide inadequate recanalized channels. A second generation of modified fiberoptic tips offers significant improvements in safety and efficacy compared to bare fiberoptics. The improved results are attributed to self-centering rounded tips, circumferential vaporization, thermal compression by the "contact" devices, and a residual luminal surface that has less fracture, dissection, and restenosis than balloon angioplasty. Experimental research as well as randomized comparative clinical trials are greatly needed to determine which laser devices can improve upon the two major limitations of balloon angioplasty: recanalization of chronic total occlusions and restenosis.

REFERENCES

1. Sanborn TA, Faxon DP, Haudenschild CC, et al: The mechanism of transluminal angioplasty: Evidence for formation of aneurysms in experimental atherosclerosis. *Circulation* 1983; 68:1136–1140.
2. Sanborn TA, Faxon DP, Haudenschild CC, et al: Experimental angioplasty: Circumferential distribution of laser thermal energy with a laser probe. *J Am Coll Cardiol* 1985; 5:934–938.
3. Abela GS, Normann SJ, Cohen DM, et al: Laser recanalization of occluded atherosclerotic arteries in vivo and in vitro. *Circulation* 1985; 71:403–411.
4. Ginsburg RL, Wexler L, Mitchell RS, et al: Percutaneous transluminal laser angioplasty for treatment of peripheral vascular disease: Clinical experience with 16 patients. *Radiology* 1985; 156:619–624.
5. Choy DSF, Stertzer SH, Myler RK, et al: Human coronary laser recanalization. *Clin Cardiol* 1984; 7:377–381.
6. Cumberland DC, Taylor DI, Procter AE: Laser-assisted percutaneous angioplasty: Initial clinical experience in peripheral arteries. *Clin Radiol* 1986; 37:423–428.
7. Hussein H: A novel fiberoptic laser probe for treatment of occlusive vessel disease. *Optical Laser Technol Med* 1986; 605:59–66.
8. Welsh AJ, Bradley AB, Torres JH, et al: Laser probe ablation of normal and atherosclerotic human aortic in vitro: A first thermographic and histologic analysis. *Circulation* 1987; 76:1353–1363.
9. Abela GS, Fenech A, Crea F, et al: "Hot tip": Another method of laser vascular recanalization: *Lasers Surg Med* 1985; 5:327–335.
10. Sanborn TA, Faxon DP, Garber GR, et al: Angiographic and histologic consequences of laser thermal angioplasty: Comparison with balloon angioplasty. *Circulation* 1987; 75:1281–1286.
11. Cumberland DC, Sanborn TA, Tayler DI, et al: Percutaneous laser thermal angioplasty: Initial clinical results with a laser probe in total peripheral artery occlusions. *Lancet* 1986; 1:1457–1459.
12. Sanborn TA, Greenfield AJ, Guben JK, et al: Human percutaneous and intraoperative laser thermal angioplasty: Initial clinical results as an adjunct to balloon angioplasty. *J Vasc Surg* 1987; 5:83–90.
13. Zeitler E, Richter EI, Seyferth W: Femoropopliteal arteries, in Dotter CT, et al (eds): *Percutaneous Transluminal Angioplasty*. Berlin, Springer-Verlag, 1983, pp 105–114.
14. Hewes RC, White RI, Murray RR, et al: Long-term results in superficial femoral artery angioplasty. *Am J Radiol* 1986; 146:1025–1029.

15. Sanborn TA, Cumberland DC, Greenfield AJ, et al: Peripheral laser-assisted balloon angioplasty: Initial multi-center experience in 219 peripheral arteries. *Arch Surg,* in press.

16. Murray RR, Hewes RC, White RI, et al: Long segment femoropopliteal stenoses: Is angioplasty a boon or a bust? *Radiology* 1987; 162:473–476.

17. Gardiner GA, Myerovitz MF, Stokes KR, et al: Complications of transluminal angioplasty. *Radiology* 1986; 159:201–208.

18. Sos TA, Sniderman KW: Percutaneous transluminal angioplasty. *Semin Roentgenol* 1981; XVI:26–41.

19. Sanborn TA, Cumberland DC, Greenfield AJ, et al: Percutaneous laser thermal angioplasty: Initial results and 1-year follow-up in 129 femoropopliteal lesions. *Radiology* 1988; 168:121–125.

20. Krepel VM, van Andel GJ, van Erp WFM, et al: Percutaneous transluminal angioplasty of the femoropopliteal artery: Initial and long-term results. *Radiology* 1985; 156:325–328.

21. Sanborn TA, Mitty HA,Train JS, et al: Sole laser thermal angioplasty for infrapopliteal and below knee popliteal lesions: Preliminary results in 10 patients. *Radiology,* in press.

22. Sanborn TA, Faxon DP, Kellett MA, et al: Percutaneous coronary laser thermal angioplasty. *J Am Coll Cardiol* 1986; 8:1437–1440.

23. Cumberland DC, Starkey IR, Oakley GDG, et al: Percutaneous laser-assisted coronary angioplasty. *Lancet* 1986; 2:214.

Chapter 7

Intraoperative Laser Thermal Angioplasty

Edward B. Diethrich, M.D.

Nonsurgical vascular interventionalists have worked for decades to devise tools that could successfully obliterate arterial blockages, once the province of the vascular surgeon. Their percutaneous experience, angiographic skills, and ingenuity led to the development of the balloon catheter, a milestone in the treatment of vascular occlusive disease. It was only natural, therefore, that they should continue the search for alternative devices that could be attached to catheters for convenient percutaneous introduction. Their creativity has spawned several useful techniques in the last few years, not the least of which is their adaptation of laser technology to intravascular recanalization.[1-15]

In the late 1970s, when angioplastic techniques were introduced, vascular surgeons by and large did not display a great deal of interest, preferring to concentrate on the classical surgical approaches to revascularize the peripheral arterial circulation.[16] This was not surprising, inasmuch as most surgeons had long ago abdicated the role of arteriographer to the diagnostic radiologist or cardiologist. Hence, few surgeons had any significant experience with guidewires and catheters, save the occasional vascular surgeon who was trained in translumbar techniques. So while the leading vascular surgical specialists were busy studying graft patency, endothelial seeding, and strategies to manage vascular infections, they were referring patients to interventionalists for angioplastic procedures, standing by in case an adverse event demanded emergency surgery.

This did not change for nearly 10 years. Vascular surgeons continued to operate, as their nonsurgical counterparts worked to overcome the deficiencies in balloon angioplasty. Recognizing that displacing the plaque by compression created a blood interface ripe for thrombogenesis and restenosis, the interventionalists sought a means to ablate effectively the majority of atherosclerotic plaque, either to establish a sufficient conduit or to reduce the volume of material to be compressed by the balloon. While some investigated techniques for mechanical ablation, notably atherectomy devices, others pursued the application of laser energy in the hopes that complete ablation would be possible.

The potential for vascular laser therapy was rapidly appreciated by the interventionalists as a natural progression in their disciplines. At the Harbor-UCLA laser training course I attended in late 1986, only a handful of surgeons were among the 50 participants, despite the fact that the program was created by an academic vascular surgeon, Dr.

Rodney White. At the conclusion of this course, it occurred to me that there were areas that should be addressed by specialists trained in vascular surgical techniques. Certainly, some cases of peripheral occlusive disease would present access problems for the percutaneous approach. What about the totally occluded proximal superficial femoral artery (SFA) or the patient with common femoral, profunda femoris, and SFA disease? Would not a surgical approach, combining laser angioplasty with classical endarterectomy techniques, be worth exploring? Furthermore, would not the surgeon, when faced with a laser angioplasty failure or a complication, be superbly qualified to use alternate techniques to offer the patient satisfactory revascularization? It was with these thoughts in mind that I established a protocol at the Arizona Heart Institute, in February 1987, to determine the safety and efficacy of laser and laser-assisted angioplasty in the treatment of atherosclerotic occlusive disease.

Designed for the surgeon who wishes to become proficient in vascular laser techniques, this chapter outlines the instrumentation and devices needed to properly equip an operating room for laser therapy. Further, it explains the thermal lasing techniques using today's most popular closed beam laser delivery systems and newer hybrid probe designs, and it explores various other areas of importance, including patient selection, limitations of the procedure, anticipated results, complications, and some thoughts regarding the future applications for laser therapy in the intraoperative setting.

THE OPERATING THEATER

Of all the factors that could adversely affect the technical performance of a surgeon about to undertake vascular laser recanalization, poor quality or inadequate intraoperative fluoroscopic imaging may well be the most significant. Interventionalists pride themselves on their ability to localize obstructing lesions properly, thereby facilitating a successful angioplasty. This task is made easier by the high resolution radiographic equipment available in radiologic and cardiac catheterization laboratories. Operating suites are not normally thus equipped.

In order to match the arteriographic capabilities of the interventionalists, the surgeon must have access to this specialized imaging equipment. The Arizona Heart Institute's operating theaters at Humana Hospital-Phoenix were specially designed to accommodate the state-of-the-art vascular laser instrumentation; however, any standard operating suite can be successfully upgraded for these procedures.

The primary components of the vascular laser operating theater center around intraoperative arteriography. The surgical C-arm roentgenographic unit (Diagnost OP-C, International Surgical Systems) with image enhancer is integrated with a 3/4-in. videotape recorder and monitor for contrast injection visualization. A second monitor with an Eigen disk is also used to provide still images of selected arteriographic segments, facilitating "road mapping" or real-time subtraction, a tool essential to complex laser angioplasty procedures. For hard-copy documentation, Polaroid film packs with adaptors may be integrated with the radiographic equipment.

Standard monitoring equipment must also be available for electrocardiography and systemic arterial pressure measurements and differentials. For contrast studies, we use Omnipaque 300 (Winthrop Laboratories), which gives excellent imaging quality with minimal side effects.

To optimize the usefulness of the radiographic equipment in vascular laser procedures, a new nonmetallic, carbon fiber surgical table (model 205, International Surgical Systems)

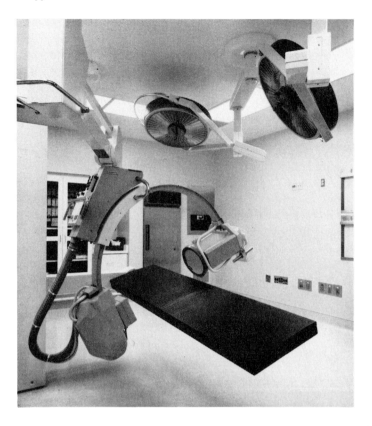

FIG 7–1.
Nonmetallic carbon fiber surgical table developed especially for vascular laser procedures has complete clearance beneath for intraoperative arteriography.

(Fig 7–1) has been developed especially for these techniques. The table, supported by a pedestal at one end, provides complete clearance beneath and allows 15 degree side-to-side roll with 20 degree Trendelenburg tilt (standard and reverse). A metric ruler (USA XRAY) is used to quantify and designate lesions. Placed on the table beneath the patient's pelvis, it is calibrated from the level of the umbilicus to provide these reference measurements.

Laser Sources and Delivery Systems

Laser energy is provided in our operating theater by a neodymium:yttrium-aluminum-garnet (Nd:YAG) source (Optilase 1,000 or MBB 4,000, Trimedyne, Inc.) capable of producing up to 60 W of pulsed or continuous wave energy. This has replaced the argon system in our facility because the broader performance characteristics of the Nd:YAG are compatible with probes up to 5.0 mm in diameter. However, the argon produces equally satisfactory results with probes up to 2.5 mm.[17] (Newer versions of argon lasers with incrementally sized probes are undergoing clinical trials.)

As I mentioned, we have used primarily the closed beam laser delivery systems operated in the continuous mode for our intraoperative protocol. A variety of these fiberoptic probes (Fig 7–2) are available for vascular use. The most common peripheral model we use is the 2.5-mm metal-tipped probe (Laserprobe-SLR, Trimedyne, Inc.) with a 600-μm fiber that achieves a temperature of 1004°C in air but approximately 450°C intraluminally when heated by 14 W of laser energy.

A comparably sized probe has a channel placed eccentrically on the probe's tip (Laserprobe-PLR Flex, Trimedyne, Inc.) for passage over a 0.035-in. guidewire. This probe is employed whenever a wire is used to cross the lesion initially, allowing lasing to be accomplished over the wire. Smaller 2.0-mm versions of these models are also available. Other probes are being studied, including a 2.5-mm laser catheter (Laser Catheter PLR, model 525, Trimedyne, Inc.) that tracks coaxially over the 0.035-in. guidewire.

A newer addition to the family of probes is the 2.5-mm Spectraprobe (Trimedyne, Inc.); this has a spear-headed sapphire tip with a 2-μm central window that emits 10% to 20% direct laser light. This probe's partial open beam preceding the metal tip appears promising in dealing with calcified lesions resistant to the closed beam delivery system.

Needles, Sheaths, Wires, and Balloons

This equipment is usually foreign to the surgeon who does not perform catheterization and contrast studies. However, the safe and efficient manipulation of these devices must be learned, particularly if the percutaneous route is to be used in the peripheral vessels, the route we prefer to use because of its simplicity and freedom from incision-related complications.

For percutaneous access, we begin with an 18-gauge Potts-Cournard needle with obturator (USCI-Bard). This acts as a guide through which a wire is passed for introduction

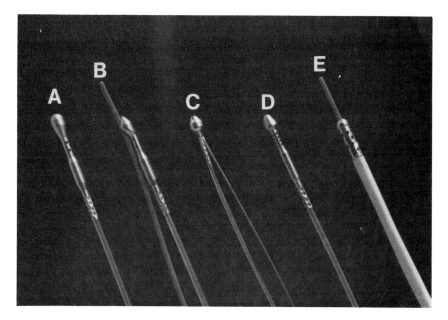

FIG 7–2.
A variety of probes are currently available for peripheral angioplasty. **A,** the commonly used 2.5-mm surgical recanalization probe (SLR). **B,** the 2.5-cm eccentric probe (PLR-Flex) over a guidewire. **C,** the 2.5-cm eccentric probe with anchor wire (PLR-Plus). **D,** the 2.5-mm Spectraprobe. **E,** the experimental 2.5-mm laser catheter (PLR-525) over a coaxial guidewire.

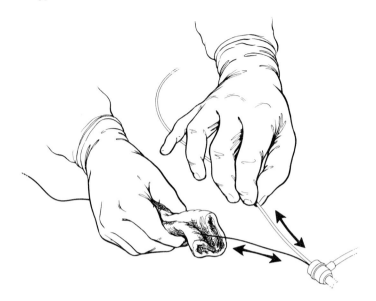

FIG 7–3.
Using a moistened gauze to hold the "eel" guidewire assists in the delivery of this extremely slippery wire.

of the commonly used 8 or 9 F introducers with sheaths (Cordis) (larger arteries may require the 11 or 12 F introducers for use with the 3.5-mm probes). Sheaths are used in cases of surgical access as well in order to control introduction of the laser probe, guidewire, or balloon.

Intravascular guidance is a critical factor in safely navigating the probe to and through a lesion so as to apply the thermal energy appropriately without injuring the arterial wall. There are various types of guidewires available, among them the standard 0.035-in. J-wire (Medrad) and the 0.014 in. Veriflex (USCI-Bard). However, our preference is for a new hydrophilic wire that becomes uncommonly slippery when wet (hence its nickname: the "eel"). This 145-cm, 0.035-in. guidewire (Glidewire, Medi-tech, Inc.) is easier to handle with a moistened gauze (Fig 7–3).[18] Despite some initial difficulty the operator may have adjusting to this wire, it is this lubricity that makes this guidance mechanism extremely effective in negotiating even the most severely stenosed lesions and tortuous arteries.

One precaution should be taken with this wire because of its potential heat lability. The manufacturer does not recommend its use with a heated probe, but we have averted any difficulty by simultaneously moving the probe and wire independently so that the metal tip is not in contact with any one point of the wire for a prolonged period of time.

For post-lasing dilatation (essential except in the few instances in which the large probes may adequately open the artery), a variety of balloon catheters are employed, depending on the nature of the lesions. In the superficial femoral artery (SFA) and popliteal arteries, the most frequently used balloons range from 4 to 6 mm in diameter by 4 to 10 cm in length (Medi-tech, Inc.); the iliac arteries require the 8 or 10 mm by 8 cm models (Fig 7–4). Dilatation is performed in 30- to 60-second intervals at atmospheric pressures ranging from 6 to 17, depending on the balloon characteristics and nature of the lesion.

Inflation of these balloons is facilitated with a syringe-like device for instilling the heparinized saline solution into the balloon (Indeflator Plus, ACS). A dial on the device calibrates the atmospheres of pressure being applied by the balloon. While this is not mandatory, I have found it adds a recordable dimension to the procedure that may be valuable in long-term follow-up.

PROTOCOL DESIGN AND PREOPERATIVE ASSESSMENT/PREPARATION

It is appropriate here to digress a moment to expound on the rationale for the protocol that has helped guide and refine our intraoperative laser techniques. First, it is important to note that our major goal was to establish a large group of laser-treated patients in whom periodic, objective reevaluation would provide longitudinal data to support or refute the efficacy of laser therapy in atherosclerotic occlusive disease. There was no intent to compare laser angioplasty to vein or prosthetic bypass grafting, so the study was in no way randomized.

Hence, the protocol offered laser angioplasty to every patient as an initial intervention, reserving classic revascularization procedures for cases that failed to respond to laser treatment or in combination with laser therapy when necessary. Even lesions amenable to standard balloon angioplasty (e.g., subtotal occlusions) were lased primarily. Balloon dilatation was used routinely following laser treatment in this protocol (this would allow us to observe the laser's influence, if any, on patency rates of the balloon procedure) except in isolated cases in which sole laser therapy created an adequate arterial lumen.

The substantiation for our "unlimited" application of the laser was based on the vascular surgeon's ability to gain entry to any artery, even in the presence of extensive occlusive disease, circumventing the access limitation of the nonsurgical specialists. Further, the surgeon was qualified to convert a failed laser angioplasty procedure to a classical revascularization operation, culminating in a successful outcome for the patient.

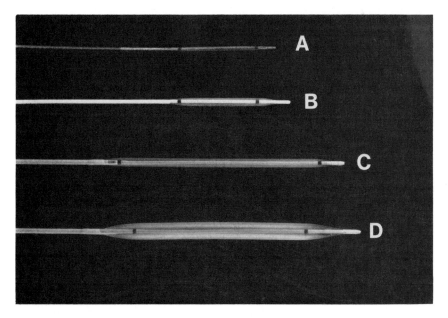

FIG 7–4.
An assortment of balloon catheters (Medi-tech) can be used for post-laser dilatation. **A,** SV 2 mm × 4 cm. **B,** ultra-thin 4 mm × 4 cm. **C,** Blue-max 4 mm × 10 cm. **D,** DC 8 mm × 8 cm.

Thus, by testing laser angioplasty under the broadest possible array of vascular pathologies in an unrestricted population, we would discern both the applicability and limitations of the procedure rapidly, while being able to refine lasing techniques and optimize instrumentation in a clinical environment presenting unlimited variations of atherosclerotic disease.

To this end, all patients seen in our clinic with symptoms of lower limb arterial insufficiency (hip, thigh, or calf claudication; rest pain; ulceration; or threatened limb loss) are considered candidates for laser angioplasty. They undergo a thorough cardio-vascularly oriented examination to identify their risk factors, characterize their peripheral pathology, and detect any concomitant atherosclerotic disease in need of treatment.

An arterial Doppler examination (preferably with exercise if symptoms and physical examination permit) is made to establish a baseline ankle/brachial systolic pressure index (ABI) for use in evaluating long-term patency. Documentation of the lower extremity arterial system is accomplished using translumbar, retrograde, or antegrade arteriography, depending on the location of the lesions; translumbar aortography and antegrade studies are used if both iliac arteries are totally occluded or both common femoral arteries are severely diseased.

Although the treatment plan in these patients is to use laser-assisted angioplasty rather than conventional surgical procedures, all patients electing laser angioplasty are informed that a bypass procedure or endarterectomy may be performed when necessary and if possible if the laser technique fails to establish an open vessel with satisfactory distal circulation.

Of course, certain categories of patients are scheduled for combined laser and surgical revascularization from the onset due to the nature of their lesions. For example, in the case of common femoral and profunda femoris lesions with disease in the superficial femoral artery, the procedures used would be common femoral angioplasty (CFA) and profunda endarterectomies, profundaplasty, and SFA laser angioplasty.

Patients electing laser angioplasty are started on 325 mg/day of aspirin and 75 mg dipyridamole, three times per day, 48 hours before surgery. Inasmuch as the majority of these patients are scheduled for same-day admission, the standard preoperative workup required for hospitalization is done in advance at the Institute.

PATIENT PREPARATION AND APPROACH SELECTION

Epidural block is our preferred form of anesthesia for laser-assisted procedures re-gardless of the entry technique. This mode of anesthesia has several advantages over local or general methods. The patient is conscious and can observe the procedure while experiencing no discomfort from the laser probe, balloon catheter, or contrast material. More importantly, though, the epidural block produces a profound sympathetic response that eliminates to a great extent the vasospasm observed with local anesthesia. If epidural block is contraindicated (patients with previous spinal operations or in whom a throm-bolytic agent will be used), local or, more rarely, general anesthesia may be employed.

Initially in our experience, bilateral SFA angioplasties were performed simultane-ously. However, these procedures are now staged; the procedure on each limb is performed on successive days, with the epidural catheter left in place while the patient stays in the Intensive Care Unit for circulatory observation. Patients with both iliac and SFA lesions are treated similarly, with the upper segment done initially followed by the lower lesions on successive days.

The operative approach is determined by the location of the lesions and the necessity for exposure of the common femoral artery. In general, the open technique is required for approach to the iliac, common femoral, profunda femoris, and superficial femoral arteries in instances of: (1) complete occlusion of the common or external iliac artery (with absent femoral pulse) if percutaneous needle insertion is not possible; (2) common femoral or profunda femoris lesions in conjunction with SFA occlusion and stenoses; (3) extensive atherosclerotic disease preventing introduction of the sheath at the site of percutaneous entry; or (4) situations requiring femoral-femoral bypass grafting (i.e., one iliac artery can be successfully lased, but the occluded contralateral artery is resistant to laser/balloon dilatation). Popliteal and tibial branch lesions need open access only when the route of approach through the proximal SFA is occluded.

OPERATIVE PROCEDURE

Inasmuch as the details of percutaneous access for peripheral laser-assisted angioplasty appear elsewhere (see Chapter 6), I will concentrate now on the surgical approach that is used in slightly less than half of our cases.

With the patient's groin prepped in the standard manner and covered with a steri-drape without any metal clips around the extremity, the open approach begins with a vertical incision exposing the CFA from the inguinal ligament distally to its bifurcation into the origin of the profunda femoris artery and the proximal SFA. Heparin, 1,500 to 2,500 units, depending on the patient's size, is given intravenously prior to clamping the common femoral and profunda femoris arteries. In the open technique, there is often no need to clamp the SFA since it is generally occluded at its origin.

With the arteries cross-clamped, an arteriotomy is made in the CFA for introduction of the sheath and laser probe. The incision is extended approximately 3 mm into the SFA. If a significant obstruction exists in either the profunda femoris or common femoral arteries, a classic endarterectomy is performed, intentionally terminating near the origin of the SFA.

If the SFA is obstructed at the incision site, the probe is introduced into the atherosclerotic plaque and passed distally to create a 2- to 4-cm channel in the SFA. The catheter sheath is then inserted through the arteriotomy; a small bolus of contrast material is injected through the sheath to confirm its location and identify any potential pathway for the probe through the distal arterial obstruction.

With the entry site thus prepared, the hydrophilic guidewire is passed down the artery to test the proximal obstruction (iliac lesions will be discussed separately). If the wire does not pass the lesion, the 2.5-mm SLR probe is used initially. However, if the wire traverses the lesion, the eccentrically channeled PLR probe is selected. Before use, all probes are tested by submersion in saline to confirm the presence of energy at the tip (bubbles).

With the laser turned off, the probe is passed through the sheath to the proximal lesion. Lasing begins at 12 W, with the probe constantly moving in a to-and-fro motion (this keeps the probe from sticking to the vessel wall and accumulating charred debris on the tip). If the wire is used, the probe is also spun around the wire's entire circumference as it is advanced to increase surface contact with the lesion, thereby ablating more plaque. If a wire is not used, contrast material is injected continuously throughout lasing to monitor the probe's movement in relation to the artery, helping to avoid perforation or an aberrant pathway.

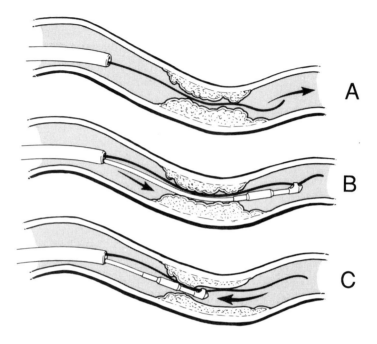

FIG 7–5.
A, the reverse lasing technique begins with a guidewire passed through the lesion over which is threaded the eccentric probe **(B). C,** with the wire in place, the probe is activated and pulled retrograde through the plaque.

Lasing continues until the probe either creates an open channel in a total obstruction or "debulks" a tight stenosis. If long occlusions or multiple stenotic segments are found in tandem, treatment continues in stepwise fashion until all lesions have been treated. The probe is withdrawn under continuous activation so that the tip exits the sheath clean without carbon particles. When the artery has been opened, retrograde blood flow can be observed through the sheath's side tubing.

In cases of very resistant plaque, the closed beam probe may not traverse the lesion. For these lesions, the new partial open beam Spectraprobe is passed to the recalcitrant obstruction and activated in the continuous mode at an energy setting of 12 W in order to open the artery with the combined efforts of the heated tip and active laser light.

In some instances the preceding laser light of the Spectraprobe opens only a small channel through the lesion without actual penetration by the tip. Forcing this nonguided probe into a lesion may cause deviation and perforation; therefore, a technique for reverse direction lasing is used (Fig 7–5). In this procedure, the eccentric probe is passed through the narrow channel over a guidewire to the distal aspect of the obstruction. The probe is activated and pulled retrograde through the lesion to open the artery further.

Lesions in the iliac arteries require a few alterations in the technique that bear mention. These larger bore arteries, when treated with the 2.5-mm probe, retain a greater proportion of plaque for the balloon to displace. Theoretically, more aggressive ablation of tissue should result in greater long-term patency. To achieve this, serially sized experimental probes up to 5.0 mm are now being studied in the iliac and large superficial femoral arteries.

Furthermore, from an intraoperative assessment standpoint, we have determined that arteriography alone cannot reliably document a successful recanalization in the iliac system. To provide a positive definition for procedural success in these arteries, pressure gradients are now routinely measured. By attaching a pressure line to the side port of the sheath, the pressure gradient across the lesion can be monitored (Fig 7–6). Only when the gradient has been obliterated can the arterial segment be considered adequately recanalized.

Elimination of the pressure gradient is the single most important determinant of a successful procedure in the aortoiliac arterial segment, but even then restenosis cannot be ruled out. In our experience, if a gradient of more than 15 mm Hg persists or if the arterial segment appears diffusely diseased or irregular after laser-assisted angioplasty, an intravascular stent is inserted over a balloon. The results of this technique to date have been very gratifying.

Because the largest sized probes available at this time cannot completely recanalize an artery in most cases, balloon dilatation is necessary to expand the vessel fully. A balloon catheter compatible with the size of the artery is introduced over the guidewire

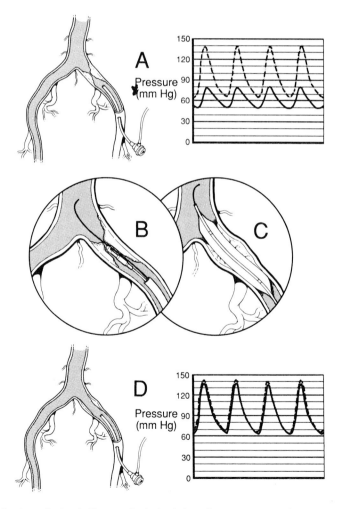

FIG 7–6.
Pressure gradient monitoring in iliac angioplasty. **A,** baseline measurement is taken. **B,** lasing opens a channel, but the gradient persists due to residual plaque. **C,** the segment is dilated until the gradient is abolished **(D).**

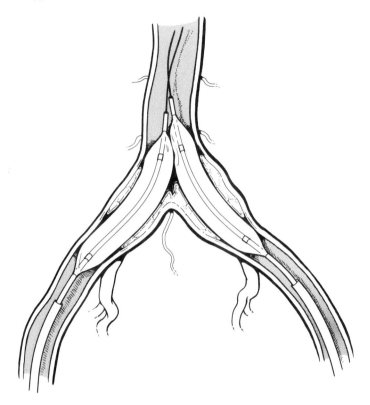

FIG 7–7.
The "kissing balloon" technique uses two wires and two balloons positioned at the bifurcation. Simultaneously inflating the balloons stabilizes the bifurcation and eliminates the shifting of atherosclerotic material from one side to the other.

and inflated for 30- to 60-second intervals up to 17 atmospheres in serial fashion at each stenotic segment. If the inflation characteristics of the balloon indicate substantial residual plaque, the compromised segment is relased as it is in the SFA area.

A useful dilatation method for treating bifurcation disease is the "kissing balloon" technique commonly used by radiologists. For bilateral disease, identical procedures are performed on both vessels. After each artery is successfully dilated, a guidewire is threaded through each into the aorta (Fig 7–7). Two balloons, inserted so as to lie at the bifurcation, are dilated simultaneously. This places more consistent pressure on the atherosclerotic plaque and stabilizes the bifurcation, eliminating the shifting of material from one side to the other. The kissing balloon technique is likewise applicable to the popliteal trifurcation but with the simultaneous dilatations over dual wires performed sequentially at each branching.

Following successful dilatation, a final control arteriogram is taken before the treated arteries are released to smooth the intima. This "glazing," performed at 5 W, presumably benefits long-term patency by reducing surface irregularities to give a more satisfactory blood-intimal interface. (We are indebted to Dr. Richard Myler for coining this phrase following his early morning visit to a doughnut shop, where he noticed the glazed doughnuts had the smooth, unblemished surface he wanted to achieve intra-arterially for unrestricted blood flow.)

Once all lesions are treated, the arteriotomy in the CFA is closed with a knitted

Dacron patch. If a profunda endarterectomy has been performed, the patch on the CFA is extended to the profunda femoris artery as well.

It is important to note here that a flap of atherosclerotic plaque is usually created by the probe at the proximal aspect of significant SFA lesions. When opening the severely diseased SFA, the probe has a tendency to deviate posteriorly from the coaxial plane, leaving residual plaque on the anterior wall at the site of the incision (Fig 7–8). If this flap is left untreated, the reestablished blood flow will dissect this area, causing the proximal artery to reocclude.

To prevent this problem, a new procedure has been devised, named the boat-dock technique (Fig 7–9). A small piece of knitted Dacron graft material (Sauvage) is cut the length of the arteriotomy. Each end of the patch is trimmed to a point resembling the bow of a boat. The residual atherosclerotic plaque at the proximal SFA is secured anteriorly against the artery wall with 5–0 Prolene suture. The Dacron patch is then sutured to the secured plaque as if a boat were being moored into dock. When completed, the atherosclerotic plaque, like a pennant on the bow, is fixed in position. Just prior to completing the suture line, the clamp in the SFA is relased and retrograde flow from the newly created posterior channel can be observed. Attention to these details is extremely important to assure success in treating disease at the origin of the SFA.

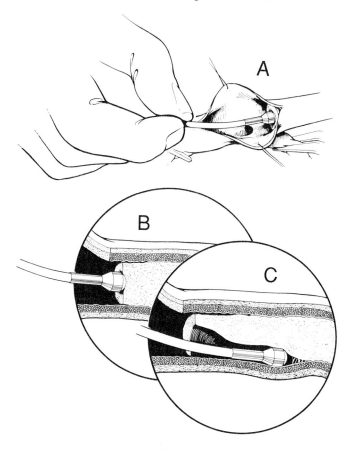

FIG 7–8.
A and B, in the open approach to severe SFA lesions, the probe encounters the plaque in the coaxial plane. C, however, posterior deviation of the probe creates an anterior atherosclerotic flap that, if unrepaired, can compromise circulation and cause restenosis.

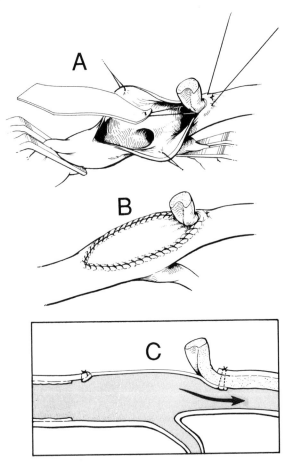

FIG 7–9.
The "boat-dock" technique for anterior flap repair. **A,** the flap is secured anteriorly against the artery wall with 5-0 Prolene suture. A knitted Dacron patch sized to fit the arteriotomy is trimmed to a point on either end, resembling the bow of a boat. It is moved into position over the arteriotomy as if a boat were being moored into dock. **B,** the graft is sutured in place, leaving the atherosclerotic flap exteriorized, dangling like a pennant on the boat. **C,** the cross-sectional view of the unobstructed channel provided by the boat-dock technique with the flap fixed in position.

With the procedure now complete, heparinization is not reversed; a Jackson-Pratt drain is placed along the base of the incision, and the patient is transferred to the recovery room.

POSTOPERATIVE CARE

Patients are observed in the intensive care unit (ICU) overnight for signs of bleeding or a change in pulse status. Heparin administration (approximately 1,000 units/hour, intravenous drip) is begun upon arrival in ICU (one hour after sheath removal for percutaneous cases) to maintain the activated coagulation time (ACT) above 200 seconds for 48 hours. This anticoagulation regimen has helped to lessen early thrombosis; however, careful observation is necessary due to the potential for hematoma formation at the wound site.

Ambulation is begun within 12 hours after the procedure, provided there are no contraindications and the recovery from anesthesia is complete. In addition, the aspirin (325 mg/day) and dipyridamole (75 mg, three times per day, orally) therapy begun prior to operation is reinstituted as soon as oral intake is tolerated. Discharge from the hospital usually takes place 12 hours after discontinuation of the heparin therapy.

Postoperative evaluation and exercise arterial Doppler examination are performed within 10 days. Doppler studies and selective arteriography are scheduled at 6-month intervals for documentation of long-term results. Either return of symptoms or failure to improve after operation is an indication for earlier arteriographic studies.

DISEASE CATEGORIZATION AND DETERMINATION OF LASER SUCCESS

During the evolution of our techniques, it became obvious that outcome was related to the location, nature, and extent of the atherosclerotic disease process. Because any one limb may have several sites of atheromatous accumulation of varying degrees of severity, we consider each diseased arterial segment in a limb a separate lesion for comparison of postoperative and long-term success rates. The categorization of the distribution and severity of the 1,100 arterial lesions we have treated in 555 patients over the first 18 months of our experience (Table 7–1) reflects this association of disease pathology with its level of occurrence.

Success of a laser procedure is assessed in the immediate postoperative period by the surgeon based on arteriographic evidence of a satisfactory lumen and presence of palpable pulses. Within 10 days following the procedure, the patient is interviewed and evaluated hemodynamically. For the procedure to remain classified as a success, the

TABLE 7–1.
Lesion Categorization for Laser-Assisted Angioplasty According to Location and Severity

Category	No. of Lesions	Access Surgical	Access Percutaneous Angioplasty	Postoperative Laser Success
I. (Iliac)	175 (16%)	50 (29%)	125	119 (68%)
A. Occlusion	90	33	57	58 (64%)
B. Stenosis	85	17	68	61 (72%)
II. (SFA)	595 (54%)	324 (54%)	271	460 (77%)
A. Occlusion				
Proximal	297	240	57	216 (73%)
Mid	77	25	52	68 (88%)
B. Occlusion/no runoff*	26	20	6	11 (42%)
C. Stenosis	195	39	156	165 (85%)
III. (Popliteal)	211 (19%)	75 (36%)	136	164 (78%)
A. Occlusion	106	41	65	83 (78%)
B. Occlusion/no runoff	23	13	10	12 (52%)
C. Stenosis	82	21	61	69 (84%)
IV. (Tibial/peroneal)	91 (8%)	23 (25%)	68	53 (58%)
A. Occlusion	22	6	16	12 (55%)
B. Occlusion/no runoff	21	5	16	5 (24%)
C. Stenosis	48	12	36	36 (75%)
Grafts	28 (3%)	27 (96%)	1	19 (68%)
A. Vein	12	12	—	5 (42%)
B. Prosthetic	16	15	1	14 (88%)
TOTAL	1,100 (100%)	499 (45%)	601	815 (74%)

*No runoff refers to the absence of observed pretreatment visualization of the tibial vessels.

TABLE 7–2.
One-Year Follow-up of Laser-Assisted Angioplasty in 124
Patients

Category	No. of Lesions	Success*
I. (Iliac)	30	26 (87%)
A. Occlusion	20	17 (85%)
B. Stenosis	10	9 (90%)
II. (SFA)	100	88 (88%)
A. Occlusion		
Proximal	42	38 (90%)
Mid	27	24 (89%)
B. Occlusion/no runoff†	3	0 —
C. Stenosis	28	26 (93%)
III. (Popliteal)	13	9 (69%)
A. Occlusion	8	5 (63%)
B. Occlusion/no runoff	2	0 —
C. Stenosis	5	4 (80%)
IV. (Tibial/peroneal)	15	9 (60%)
A. Occlusion	4	2 (50%)
B. Occlusion/no runoff	1	0 —
C. Stenosis	10	7 (70%)
Grafts	8	6 (75%)
A. Vein	3	2 (67%)
B. Prosthetic	5	4 (80%)
TOTAL	**168**	**138 (82%)**

*As determined by continued absence of symptoms and
maintenance of a >0.5 improvement in the ABI over the
preoperative value.
†No runoff refers to the absence of observed pretreatment
visualization of the tibial vessels.

patient must be free of symptoms and demonstrate a >0.15 improvement in the ABI over the preoperative baseline value.[19]

According to the postoperative success data in our population, the best results were seen in the SFA segment, surprisingly with slightly better outcome in the occluded vessels at the midartery level. Results in the popliteal segment were comparable to the SFA for both stenoses and occlusions. Tibial/peroneal occlusions and segments with no runoff (no observed pretreatment visualization of the tibial vessels) fared worst of all. Stenotic lesions in all segments responded uniformly better than occlusion, but not always to a significant degree. Laser treatment of grafts was moderately successful.

Acute failure of the tandem laser/balloon procedure was due primarily to inability to cross refractory calcified lesions (14%, 154 procedures). The remainder of the postoperative failures were associated with poor distal runoff or slow flow (6%, 66), an inability to create an adequate channel (4%, 44), or collapsible lesions (2%, 22).

The longitudinal follow-up studies are continuing, with data being accumulated beyond 1 year. While the preliminary 1-year follow-up population is too small to support any conclusions, the statistics provide some clear direction for the future.

Examining the arterial categories (Table 7–2), it is clear that the best results persist in the SFA and iliac arteries, while the infrapopliteal arteries, once thought to be an ideal system for laser treatment, suffer more restenosis.

LIMITATIONS AND COMPLICATIONS

As our experience with laser-assisted angioplasty grew, certain events and observations seemed to exert an influence on the procedure and its results. Some of these events had obvious effects on the technique's performance and produced immediate failure; others were clinical impressions whose impact might eventually surface in the form of late failures. We appropriately developed seven categories for these occurrences and added their documentation to our protocol in the hopes of finding correlations to outcome (Table 7–3).

Among those events that acutely affected the procedure are mechanical failures. These are problems relative to instrumentation and unrelated to the laser-tissue interaction. Malfunction of the laser delivery system, breakage of the fiber, separation of the probe tip, defects in the sheath, access problems, and dissection or perforation due to the guidewires or balloon catheters fall into this category.

Another more common cause of acute failure is the inability of the probe to cross a lesion. Usually this is due to the presence of recalcitrant calcified plaque. Even the energy of the new partial open beam probe with its preceding raw laser light is sometimes ineffective if the plaque is heavily impregnated with calcium.

The misdirection of the probe is also a potential source of failure. It is not uncommon to find lesions situated at a junction with large collateral branches. An unguided probe, in seeking the least resistant path, chooses the unobstructed collateral rather than the desired direction across the lesion. Continuous injection of contrast material is crucial here to monitor the probe's direction.

The path of the probe after entering the lesion is subject to difficulty with another form of deviation, dissection of a false lumen. In order to establish an acceptable arterial channel, a probe not only has to pass through an obstruction, but also it has to exit the lesion in the true lumen beyond. The inability of the probe to reenter the correct arterial channel creates a neolumen that can lead to at least partial failure. (In a few cases, we observed this intraoperatively and expected absent pulses, only to find the pulses present; however, long-term failure is more common.)

Associated hemodynamic variables also influence outcome. As with any revascularization procedure, success ultimately depends upon the integrity of the distal circulation. In diabetic patients, for example, small vessel disease is common, and their lack of arterial runoff makes recanalization much less successful. Laser therapy is, therefore, as ineffective as conventional revascularization procedures in patients with inadequate runoff.

Another hemodynamic factor impacting laser success is reduced flow proximal to a successfully lased segment. In actuality, the presence of a proximal lesion impeding flow should never occur; proximal lesions are always treated primarily according to standard vascular surgical principles. On two occasions in our experience, however, the severity of an identified proximal lesion was underestimated, resulting in inadequate pressure to

TABLE 7–3.
Intraoperative Failure Codes for Laser-assisted Angioplasty

Category	Description
Mechanical	Due to sheath, wire, balloon, probe,* fiber, delivery system, access route
Failure to cross	Due primarily to calcification
No reentry	Due to inability to reenter the proper distal lumen
No runoff	Due to severe obstruction of distal arterial circulation
Proximal lesion	Due to undetected or underestimated lesion proximal to lased segment
Slow flow	Due to hemodynamic and physical conditions hampering flow to distal vessels (e.g., small arteries, iatrogenic incisional flaps, extensive dissection planes, etc.)
Collapsible lesion	Due to lesion's return to pretreatment or near pretreatment configuration

*Does not include mechanical injury, i.e., perforation or dissection.

sustain the patency of a treated distal segment. This prompted us to be more vigilant in assessing proximal stenoses with direct pressure measurements, ultimately leading to more aggressive treatment of what appeared to be subcritical stenoses.

In our experience, preoperative arteriograms sometimes fail to demonstrate the infrapopliteal arteries (poor timing, slow flow due to severe proximal stenosis, etc.). At times, this caused us to assume preoperatively a lack of arterial runoff only to find that, when the proximal arterial segment was opened, the trifurcation vessels could be visualized and were patent. Clinical assessment of laser recanalization success must take into account true vs. perceived absence of distal runoff in order to avoid overstating the value or ability of the laser probe to negotiate total obstructions in the smaller arteries.

A final hemodynamic factor is classified as "slow flow," and it includes several factors that would account for lack of flow sufficient to maintain distal arterial integrity. Among these are small arteries, extensive dissection planes, and iatrogenic intimal flaps at the incision site. Identification of the latter prompted our development of the boat-dock patch angioplasty technique.

Another not uncommon cause of eventual failure is related to the composition of atherosclerotic plaques. Many lesions have a significant fibrotic component. Although these lesions are easily lased and dilated by the balloon, the fibrous "elastic memory" returns the artery to its pretreatment or near pretreatment state. This happens both acutely on the operating table or over weeks, leading to subsequent reocclusion or restenosis.

Although many of these "failure codes," as they are known, represent some of the limitations of laser-assisted angioplasty, we have gained sufficient experience to identify three primary roadblocks to a successful laser recanalization.

First is calcification. With today's commercially available technology, many calcified lesions will remain untreatable. However, new laser configurations being studied are showing great promise in dealing with this problem.

Another limitation that precipitates acute failure is the lack of adequate distal circulation. Again, our current technique is limiting in terms of opening occluded distal arterial beds. New laser wires and experimental delivery systems may hold some promise for the future.

Finally, the ability to control restenosis/reocclusion is vital to arterial patency. The use of longitudinal studies such as ours to follow the course of patients over years will be instrumental in uncovering the causes of reclosure and dealing with them effectively. At present, we have been alerted in our follow-up studies to a strong tendency toward restenosis and accelerated arteriographic defects at sites of treated subcritical stenoses. It may well be that thermal injury plays a great part in this, as I will discuss further on.

Mechanical injury in the form of perforation can also be a major cause of failure in laser angioplasty.[1, 2, 9, 14, 20–22] In the beginning of our study, we observed five different types of arterial injury related to the probe; however, not all the injuries were clinically relevant. To correlate probe deviation with clinical outcome more accurately, we composed three categories of perforation, with injuries ranging from the simplest form of dissection to the most deleterious type of adventitial rupture.

Class I.—This category encompasses dissections that do not penetrate the adventitia. In the first scenario, the laser probe leaves the true lumen or the intended plane of dissection, deviating into an aberrant pathway. It may shear an arterial side branch, but it eventually relocates distally in the correct, open arterial channel. There is no adverse reaction to this dissection and, in most cases, the situation goes unnoticed.

A more consequential event is the laser probe deviating into the atherosclerotic plaque, usually when it encounters calcium deposits. Unlike the clinically satisfactory situation above, however, the probe does not reenter the true distal lumen or create a satisfactory dissection plane that can restore arterial continuity. Under these circumstances, the procedure is usually abandoned with no untoward consequences.

Class II.—In this situation there is true arterial wall penetration through the adventitia with two possible outcomes. In the first, contrast material is seen outside the arterial wall but without active bleeding. Here, in the more common situation, the probe has penetrated the artery in an area of dense atherosclerotic material, so little if any blood is flowing through that segment.

Occasionally, such an injury is attended by leakage of blood from the artery. Because of the severe disease, the blood flow is under very low pressure, so clot formation seals the penetration site. No operative intervention is required.

Class III.—This is the same type of damage as in Class II, but the active bleeding continues through the perforation site and surgical intervention is necessary to control the hemorrhage. Because we have not encountered any Class III perforations, our 7% rate of mechanical arterial injury has been fairly evenly distributed between Classes I and II (3.8% and 3.2%, respectively).

Another area of concern is the incidence of thrombosis. As a complication, thrombosis is rare (4% in our series) and usually easy to treat with thrombolytic therapy (urokinase or streptokinase) or mechanical thrombectomy and relasing. However, dealing with the cause of this problem has not proved as simple.

In most of these patients, the anticoagulation therapy had been limited to use of antiplatelet drugs preoperatively and postoperatively and intraoperative heparinization. However, in an effort to reduce early thrombosis and restenosis, the therapy was enhanced to include a 1,000 unit/hour heparin drip initiated postoperatively and adjusted to maintain the activated coagulation time above 200 seconds for 48 hours. This has diminished the incidence of acute postoperative thrombosis, but it will be some time before its impact on restenosis is determined.

DISCUSSION

A question I am often asked at meetings is, "Who should be doing laser angioplasty?" Looking at the figures in our experience, despite our preference for the percutaneous route, 45% of the procedures have required an open surgical approach. Further, we have often found it necessary to perform additional classical vascular surgical procedures, ranging from endarterectomy to graft placement, in order to revascularize the limb completely. This underscores one of the major points regarding the philosophical dichotomy between surgeons and interventionalists on the question of angioplasty.

Angioplasty, and particularly percutaneous transluminal coronary angioplasty, has created a phenomenon foreign to the surgical mentality: incomplete revascularization. The surgeon's philosophy has always been to reconstruct the vascular area, whatever the damage, as completely as possible. In the femoral popliteal system that would mean achieving restoration of pulses; in the coronary vasculature, it would entail one or several bypasses of multiple lesions to restore adequate circulation to the myocardium.

However, the interventionalists now speak of the "target" lesion, the one responsible for the symptoms or event. Treatment of this isolated "symptomatic" obstruction, therefore, often results in less than complete revascularization.

The surgical view clearly seems more acceptable in terms of total benefits to the patient. In this new technological field, the surgeon therefore provides an opportunity for unlimited rather than restricted restoration of circulation. Of course, this assumes that the surgeon has learned from his interventional colleagues the skills, both technical and judgmental, requisite to the efficacious performance of angioplasty itself. Adding the laser component is new to all of us, so in that regard, surgeons, radiologists, and cardiologists are all at an equivalent starting position.

Another point to consider is morbidity. Complications are bound to occur regardless of the type of specialist performing the procedure; however, only the surgeon can draw on the full array of surgical and nonsurgical remedies available for expedient correction of an untoward event. A linear tear created by balloon dilatation of an iliac artery resulting in acute hemorrhage demands immediate operative intervention.

Adding all these factors, it seems that surgeons are especially well qualified to adopt laser angioplasty for use with their existing revascularization techniques. The potential for percutaneous entry offers a dimension unfamiliar to the surgeon, but one that should be welcomed as an added patient benefit.

Of course, none of this precludes the option that is always available: forming a team on which the surgeon and radiologist or cardiologist work together. I have seen this concept at some centers, and it can function well.

The final answer to this question will depend, at least for now, on the individual departmental ground rules at local hospitals. Unilateral exclusion obviously cannot be tolerated; however, the surgeon's role as he or she achieves proficiency in angioplastic techniques should become more significant.

The second most common question I hear is, "Why use a potentially dangerous laser probe in stenoses that can be traversed by a wire or dilated by a balloon?" We know that the balloon causes significant damage to the architecture of the plaque. This factor has been identified as the cause for the high rate of restenosis seen with the balloon.[22] The object of either thermally or photochemically "debulking" the lesion prior to balloon dilatation is to lessen the amount of atherosclerotic material to be compressed. Theoretically, it is hoped this will reduce the intraluminal thrombogenic surface area. Preliminary results in a small patient series do seem to point to enhanced patency with the tandem procedure,[24] but it will be some time before significant clinical studies can validate this hypothesis.

It should be remembered that the original attraction to laser therapy was its anticipated ability to completely ablate atheroma, obviating the need for balloon dilatation. Many of my earlier articles called for larger diameter probes to accomplish this goal. In concept, this still remains viable; however, I have made some interesting observations that may impact this avenue of technological development.

First, larger probes definitely are associated with more debris, i.e., carbonization on the tip. This is not unexpected; however, it does increase the potential for embolization. Further, the larger probes may not create as smooth and well defined a channel as the smaller probes. Disruption of greater volumes of tissue with the larger probes may leave a markedly irregular surface, thereby setting the stage for acute occlusion or restenosis.

Second, and more important, there is the issue of thermal damage to the adjacent normal tissue. Experimental studies have provided some facts from which we may extrapolate the following points for consideration. Tissue damage is directly related to energy dosage: the product of the probe's wattage and the length of time (in seconds) of

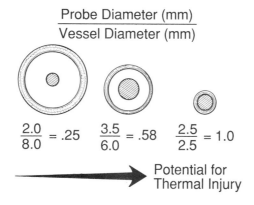

Probe Diameter (mm)
Vessel Diameter (mm)

$$\frac{2.0}{8.0} = .25 \quad \frac{3.5}{6.0} = .58 \quad \frac{2.5}{2.5} = 1.0$$

Potential for
Thermal Injury

FIG 7–10.
The potential for thermal injury from a hot-tip laser probe is likely to be a relationship between the diameters of the probe and vessel. In this relationship, as the ratio of the probe's size to that of the artery approaches 1, the potential increases.

its tissue contact. Measured in joules, this amount of energy can be further tailored to express the amount of energy delivered to a square millimeter of tissue (the energy fluence).[25, 26] Because these measurements were derived from direct laser irradiation, it might be better to depict the concept graphically for the closed beam as a ratio of the diameter of the probe to that of the vessel (Fig 7–10), so that as the ratio approaches 1, the potential for thermal injury increases.

Also influencing this concept would be the insulating qualities of plaque. Our experiments have shown that the temperature of a thermal probe drops from 450°C in the open artery by one half or more during plaque penetration, rising only slightly until the lesion is traversed. This dissipated heat is absorbed by the plaque, which acts as a protective barrier for the surrounding arterial wall. It is obvious, therefore, that a probe whose diameter closely approximates that of the vessel, in removing a greater portion of the plaque, might obliterate this damping factor, causing significant thermal injury. I would like to emphasize that these are merely observations and impressions from our experience; however, I am convinced that the entire concept of thermal injury deserves further investigation.

Another controversial issue related to the thermal injury quandary is the use of post-dilatation glazing to smooth the disrupted plaque. Theoretically again, this is a valid concept, inasmuch as an ideal angioplastic procedure should produce a blood interface as near normal structurally and functionally as possible. Unfortunately, current dilatation techniques do not meet this goal. No one has yet found a way to minimize the disruption of the endothelium and reduce thrombogenicity, hence the use of heparin and antiplatelet therapies.

From the onset of our protocol, we ended each angioplasty with glazing. Originally, we set the probe to 5 W regardless of artery diameter, lesion location, or the original treatment energy. A few months into the study, it was proposed that we glaze at the treatment wattage, which we did for a time.

The results of our high temperature glazing became apparent rather quickly, as patients thus treated began to appear with advanced, lengthy restenotic segments (Fig 7–11).

From our thermistor studies, we had determined that the probe maintained the temperature of 450°C during glazing in the freshly dilated vessel. Further, the reduced plaque density produced by the tandem procedure nearly eliminated the thermal protective barrier, increasing the likelihood of thermal damage.

Other researchers have now established that 95 to 140°C is the ideal temperature for "fusing" the disrupted atherosclerotic lining of the vessel.[27-29] This temperature can be achieved with 5 W of energy delivered to a 2.5-mm probe, and we have returned to that level.

These events caused us to reexamine the initial energy dosage of other cases of restenosis we were seeing. Not surprisingly, our investigation substantiated the vessel/probe ratio theory, because the greater proportion of restenoses were appearing in the smaller arteries.

In the beginning, we had been so enthusiastic about the laser probe's potential for recanalizing all diseased segments that we used it in the distal popliteal, anterior, and posterior tibial arteries and the tibial peroneal trunk branches. These are small arteries, and even using the 2.0-mm probe, the vessel/probe ratio can come very close to unity.

In the operating room, we saw excellent angioplasty results with reestablished flow, only to observe an acute thrombosis, sometimes within hours, particularly if there was inadequate distal runoff.

Disappointed, we modified our protocol such that subtotal occlusions of the tibial arteries are *not* lased, a significant deviation from our original concept. However, if a guidewire will not cross a total tibial occlusion, the laser probe is used in an attempt to create an open channel. The newly developed 1-mm laser wire, having shown initial success in England, may help to modify our procedures in these vessels.

In summary, our protocol has remained flexible, adjusting to the changing technology and applying newly disclosed information in an effort to optimize the technique. We have returned to our original glazing temperature, but we may dispense with it altogether if later studies disprove its purported benefits.

Although we thought the laser probe a panacea for distal arterial occlusions, we have had to cease laser treatment in these smaller subtotally occluded arteries due to significant thermal damage.

We approach lengthy lesions knowing that they may contain significant calcium deposits that will interfere with successful probe passage, even the partial open beam model. We have had to accept the fact that some lesions resistant to even the increased energy outlay of this hybrid probe are best treated with bypass grafting.

On the positive side, the laser success we have observed has given us confidence to offer laser angioplasty to patients at an earlier stage in their disease process than would be done for surgical treatment. The uncomplicated arterial access needed and short recovery time make this an ideal therapy for the less symptomatic patients. They can be free of claudication before it becomes too debilitating, and even if restenosis precipitates symptoms further on, retreatment is relatively simple. We have performed "re-do" procedures on a small group of our patients with excellent results.

Of course, to the prudent mind this brings the following question. "Does early intervention with the current technique influence the atherosclerotic process, either favorably or not?" If we are creating arterial lesions beyond those that the procedure aimed to treat (e.g., subcritical stenoses progressing to occlusion due to thermal injury or balloon-induced damage, which we cannot disregard), then we are doing no service to the patient.

On the other hand, we know that atherosclerosis is progressive, so incomplete lesions naturally advance to occlusions, often times with significant thrombosis beyond the obstruction. Does the laser offer an opportunity to prevent that clinical course by earlier intervention with a simple procedure? My guess is yes, but until data can support it, this remains an hypothesis.

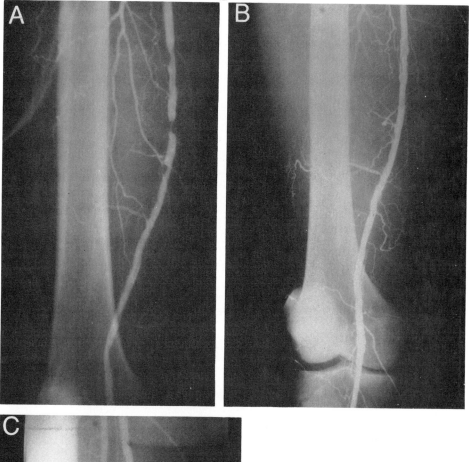

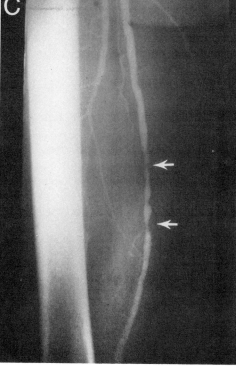

FIG 7–11.
A, a 56-year-old patient with one near total occlusion of the superficial femoral artery and two subcritical stenoses. **B,** the post-operative arteriogram following treatment of all lesions with laser/balloon angioplasty. **C,** an arteriogram of the same artery 6 months later when the patient's symptoms recurred. Note the increased stenotic changes at the proximal and distal lesions *(arrows)* indicative of thermal injury.

I strongly believe, however, that early or earlier treatment with the laser in contrast to femoral-popliteal bypass is clearly justified. I have not found restenosis or reocclusion following laser therapy to be anatomically or pathologically worse than the original condition (provided there was no thermal damage). With the femoral-popliteal bypass, failure often is attended by interruption of collateral vessels and more extensive thrombosis than was present with the initial lesion. In the iliac arterial system, it is clear that laser-assisted angioplasty is the treatment of choice over classic surgical procedures for short obstructive lesions.

As for other recommendations on patient selection, we have seen that total occlusions appear to do better in the SFA than in the iliacs, but, in general, stenoses respond somewhat more favorably in all segments.

In terms of length, short, discrete lesions are more amenable to lasing than long occluded segments. In the lengthy blockages, the probe is more likely to produce multiple false lumens that ultimately create an inadequate central channel.

Lastly, larger vessels and the proximal arteries are more suitable to lasing. Here, the greater diameter ratio of probe to artery lessens the potential for thermal injury, although it leaves more plaque in need of displacement by the balloon.

FUTURE PROSPECTS FOR INTRAOPERATIVE LASER THERAPY

I sincerely doubt that the closed beam probe will remain the standard it is today. The logic that created it initially was spawned by impatience with the slow progress of open beam technology. Now, research in this area is bearing fruit; new laser sources with selectable wavelengths are on the way with more sophisticated imaging and feedback circuitry to monitor ablation. Laser absorption characteristics are being defined for atheroma and normal intimal tissue so that this selectivity can be prudently applied. Additionally, sophisticated guidance systems, most notably direct intra-arterial ultrasound imaging, may open yet unexplored laser angioplasty potentials.

Moreover, the pulsed beam systems potentially offer substantial improvement to the technique. They use very high energy beams that successfully vaporize plaque, but the rapid, pulsatile nature of the energy bursts significantly reduces the potential for thermal injury to adjacent tissue.

If the open beam probes continue to progress toward their original conceptualization, that of a precisely controllable surgical ''knife'' to ablate plaque selectively and safely, then the closed beam probe will become a relic. Until then, I am confident that we now have the capability to offer significant benefits to the patient with our current delivery system. With a keen eye to patterns of difficulty, their characterization, and their resolution through altered technique, we can safely provide laser angioplasty as an effective alternative to bypass grafting, though its replacement of surgical intervention is still in the future.

Indeed, if this conclusion is correct, it is then incumbent upon surgical specialists to prepare adequately for this new therapeutic modality. To do less will ultimately doom the surgeon to the role of ''backup'' for a failed procedure or emergent situation.

REFERENCES

1. Abela GS, Norman SJ, Cohen D, et al: Laser recanalization of occluded atherosclerotic arteries: An in vivo and in vitro study. *Circulation* 1985; 71:403–411.
2. Abela GS, Seege JM, Barbieri E, et al: Laser angioplasty with angioscopic guidance in humans. *J Am Coll Cardiol* 1986; 8:184–192.
3. Choy DJ, Sterter SH, Myles RK, et al: Human coronary laser recanalization. *Clin Cardiol* 1984; 7:377–381.
4. Crea F, Davies G, McKenna W, et al: Percutaneous laser recanalization of coronary arteries, letter. *Lancet* 1986; 2:214.
5. Cumberland DC, Sanborn T, Taylor DI, et al: Percutaneous laser thermal angioplasty: Clinical experience in peripheral artery occlusions. *J Am Coll Cardiol* 1986; 2:211A.
6. Cumberland DC, Sanborn TA, Taylor DI, et al: Percutaneous laser thermal angioplasty: Initial clinical results with a laser probe in total peripheral artery occlusions. *Lancet* 1986; 1:1457–1459.
7. Cumberland DC, Taylor DI, Proctor AE: Laser-assisted percutaneous angioplasty: Initial clinical experience in peripheral arteries. *Clin Radiol* 1986; 37:423–428.
8. Dries DJ, Lawrence PF, Syverud J, et al: Response of atherosclerotic aorta to argon laser. *Lasers Surg Med* 1985; 5:321–326.
9. Ginsberg R, Wexler L, Mitchell RS, et al: Percutaneous transluminal laser angioplasty for treatment of peripheral vascular disease: Clinical experience with sixteen patients. *Radiology* 1985; 156:619–624.
10. Grundfest WS, Litvak F, Forrester JS, et al: Laser ablation of human atherosclerotic plaque without adjacent tissue injury. *J Am Coll Cardiol* 1985; 5:929–933.
11. Grundfest WS, Litvak F, Hickey A: The current status of angioscopy and laser angioplasty. *J Vasc Surg* 1987; 5:667–673.
12. Kaplan MD, Case RB, Choy DS: Vascular recanalization with argon laser: Role of blood in transmission of laser energy. *Lasers Surg Med* 1985; 5:275–279.
13. Sanborn TA, Faxon DP, Kellett MA, et al: Percutaneous coronary laser thermal angioplasty. *J Am Coll Cardiol* 1986; 8:1437–1440.
14. Sanborn TA, Greenfield AJ, Guben JK, et al: Human percutaneous and intraoperative laser thermal angioplasty: Initial clinical results as an adjunct to balloon angioplasty. *J Vasc Surg* 1987; 5:83–90.
15. Selzer DM, Murphy-Chutporan D, Ginsburg R, et al: Optimizing strategies for laser angioplasty. *Invest Radiol* 1985; 20:860–866.
16. Diethrich EB, Rozaci J, Timbadia E, et al: Laser angioplasty: A surgical perspective. *Medicamundi* 1987; 32:127–132.
17. Diethrich EB, Rozaci J, Timbadia E, et al: Argon laser-assisted peripheral angioplasty. *Vasc Surg* 1988; 22:77–87.
18. Diethrich EB, Timbadia E, Bahadir I: Hydrophilic guidewire for laser-assisted angioplasty, letter. *J Vasc Surg* 1988; 8:201–202.
19. Hewes RC, White RI, Murray RR, et al: Long-term results of superficial femoral artery angioplasty. *AJR* 1986; 146:1025–1029.
20. Sanborn TA, Faxon DP, Haudenschild C, et al: Experimental angioplasty: Circumferential distribution of laser thermal energy with a laser probe. *J Am Coll Cardiol* 1985; 5:934–945.
21. Sanborn TA, Haudenschild CC, Garber GR, et al: Angiographic and histologic consequences of laser thermal angioplasty: Comparison with balloon angioplasty. *Circulation* 1987; 75:1281–1286.
22. Diethrich EB, Bahadir I: Complications of laser-assisted angioplasty: Recognition, classification, and treatment. *Vasc Surg* (in press).
23. Sanborn TA, Haudenschild CC, Garber GR, et al: Angiographic and histologic consequences of laser thermal angioplasty: Comparison with balloon angioplasty. *Circulation* 1987; 75:1281–1286.

24. Sanborn TA, Cumberland DA, Greenfield AJ, et al: Percutaneous laser thermal angioplasty: Initial results and 1-year follow-up in 129 femoropopliteal lesions. *Radiology* 1988; 168:121–125.
25. Welch AJ, Bradley AB, Torres JH, et al: Laser probe ablation of normal and atherosclerotic human aorta in vitro: A first thermographic and histologic analysis. *Circulation* 1987; 5:1353–1363.
26. Strikwerda S, Bott-Silverman C, Ratliff NB, et al: Effects of varying argon ion laser intensity and exposure time on ablation of atherosclerotic plaque. *Lasers Surg Med* 1988; 8:66–71.
27. Jenkins RD, Sinclair IN, Anand R, et al: Laser balloon angioplasty: Effect of tissue temperature on weld strength of human postmortem intima-media separations. *Lasers Surg Med* 1988; 8:30–39.
28. Anand RK, Sinclair IN, Jenkins RD, et al: Laser balloon angioplasty: Effect of constant temperature versus constant power on tissue weld strength. *Lasers Surg Med* 1988; 8:40–44.
29. Jenkins RD, Sinclair IN, Anand RK, et al: Laser balloon angioplasty: Effect of exposure duration on shear strength of welded layers of postmortem human aorta. *Lasers Surg Med* 1988; 8:392–396.

Chapter 8

Cardiovascular Application of Continuous Wave Laser Systems

Takanobu Tomaru, M.D.

George S. Abela, M.D.

James M. Seeger, M.D.

A laser beam has certain characteristics different from those of light generated from conventional sources. A laser device can generate a highly directional beam of monochromatic light and can produce intense power densities on a target tissue, which may result in vaporization and resection of tissue. Because of these properties, laser energy is appropriate for the treatment of certain types of cardiovascular disease. The wavelengths of lasers currently used in the medical field range from ultraviolet to infrared. Popular lasers used in the treatment of cardiovascular disease include neodymium:yttrium-aluminum-garnet (Nd:YAG), argon ion, carbon dioxide (CO_2), tunable dye, and excimer. Laser energy is delivered as continuous or short pulsed energy and, except for excimer laser, these lasers are continuous wave lasers.

Enthusiasm for laser angioplasty is based on the ability of lasers to deliver energy through small, flexible optical fibers and the ability of lasers to vaporize and resect tissue. In addition, the potential for selective absorption of laser energy by different tissues means that tissue removal could be very specific. Fiberoptic transmission of laser energy means that laser angioplasty can be adapted to standard catheterization techniques. Although balloon angioplasty and bypass surgery are widely used and accepted procedures, they do not accomplish the actual physical removal of the atherosclerotic plaque. This means that in some patients coronary or peripheral revascularization cannot be accomplished. In these patients, laser angioplasty may provide an alternative approach for successful arterial recanalization. In this chapter, we describe the progress and status of continuous wave (CW) laser technology in the cardiovascular area and also discuss the future directions.

TABLE 8–1.
Laser Characteristics

Laser	Carbon Dioxide	Nd:YAG	Argon
Type	Gas (molecules)	Crystal	Ion gas
Wavelength	10,600 nm	1,064 nm	488, 514 nm
Color	Far infrared	Near infrared	Blue-green
Power	0–100 W	0–120 W	0–20 W
Pulsed mode	Possible	Possible	Impossible
Absorption	Water	Tissue protein	Hemoglobin Melanin
Transmission through fluid	Poor	Fair	Good
Delivery	Silver halide	Silica fiber	Silica fiber
Tissue penetration	Poor	Good	Moderate

LASER SYSTEM FOR CARDIOVASCULAR AREA

The basic laser system used in the cardiovascular area includes a laser source and a catheter-based delivery device. Currently, there are three types of CW laser that have been used for vaporizing atheromatous plaque: (1) argon ion laser, which emits radiation with predominant wavelengths of 488 to 514 nm (blue-green), operates on a CW basis or in a mechanically chopped mode, and is capable of average powers up to approximately 20 W; (2) Nd:YAG laser, which emits radiation with a wavelength of 1,064 nm (in the near infrared), can be run either in CW or pulsed mode, and is capable of operating at high average powers (>100 W); and (3) CO_2 laser, which emits radiation with a wavelength of 10,600 nm (far infrared), can operate either in CW or pulsed mode, and is capable of powers up to 100 W (Table 8–1). Argon light is well absorbed by chromophores, such as hemoglobin, and has good tissue penetration.[1, 2] The Nd:YAG laser beam transmits readily through water and has deep penetration into tissue causing heat generation. Carbon dioxide laser energy is strongly absorbed by water and has limited tissue penetration with only local superficial heating. In addition to these three lasers, the dye pump laser, whose wavelength is tunable, is currently in use with spectroscopic analysis for selective plaque ablation.

The laser delivery system contains a flexible thin optical fiber through which laser energy can be transmitted in densities that will vaporize plaque and not damage the fiber. Currently available fibers to transmit laser energies are made of quartz silica. Silica fibers can transmit argon, Nd:YAG, and portions of ultraviolet, but not CO_2 wavelength. Silver halide optical fibers may transmit CO_2 wavelength but are not clinically available because of high energy loss and toxicity.

Laser energy emitted from a bare optical fiber directly to the target tissue often results in perforation of the vessel, even at low energy levels (Fig 8–1,A).[3–5] Thus fiber modification has been necessary to produce a clinically useful laser delivery system. Modified optical fiber tips with microlens[6] or sapphire lens at the fiber tips[7] emit laser beam directly but appear to be more useful for clinical purposes because the round fiber tip reduces mechanical vessel perforation. A fiberoptic delivery system that transmits laser energies to a metal cap attached to its distal end has also been developed.[8, 9] The metal tip, heated by laser energy, can vaporize atheromatous plaque and the histology of recanalized vessels is very similar to that seen after bare fiber recanalization. Finally, a "hybrid" probe has been developed to deliver laser energy through both a heated metal cap and microlens at the tip of the probe (Fig 8–1,B).[10] In this probe, a 300- or 600-μm core optical fiber is connected to one of the elliptical metal caps (either 1, 2, or 2.5 mm in diameter) at the tip. A 250-μm diameter window with a microlens in the metal cap, focuses an argon laser beam as it exits from the tip at a 15-degree angle.

EFFECTS OF LASER IRRADIATION ON VESSEL AND THROMBUS

When a laser beam is directed on a target tissue, at least three types of laser-tissue interactions occur. These include a physical process of "photoplasma explosion," a thermal process, and a photochemical process. Continuous wave lasers vaporize tissue mainly by a thermal process.[1, 3] The rapidity and degree of tissue heating depend on competing effects of tissue absorption of the laser energy resulting in heat accumulation and thermal diffusion and convection properties, which result in heat loss to the sur-

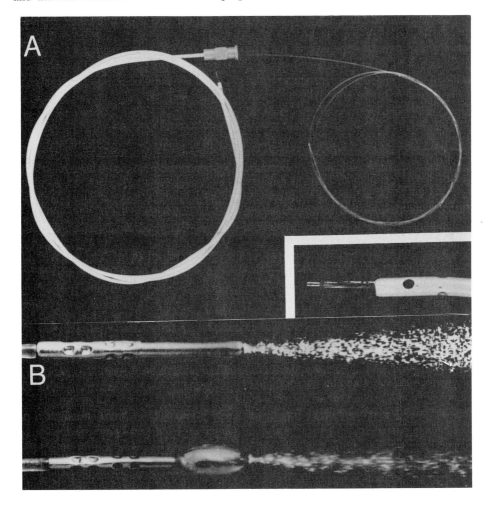

FIG 8–1.
A, a 0.2-mm core silica optical fiber with a metal-tipped marker emerging from the end of a 5 F catheter (magnified in *inset*). **B,** a 300-μm core optical fiber with a 1-mm *(top)* or 2-mm *(bottom)* elliptical metal cap at the tip. A 250-μm diameter window with a microlens focuses the argon beam as it exits from the tip at a 15-degree angle. (From Abela GS, Seeger JM, Barbieri E, et al: Laser angioplasty with angioscopic guidance in humans. *J Am Coll Cardiol* 1986; 8:182–194. Used by permission.)

rounding environment. Thermal diffusion is determined by the tissue absorption characteristic of light. Lipid or fibrous tissue is readily vaporized by CW laser energy, but heavily calcified tissue is resistant to laser ablation.

When CW laser light is absorbed by a target tissue, it is converted into heat, and tissue changes occur. As the target tissue temperature proceeds above 50°C, protein denaturation occurs. At temperatures above 60°C, collagen denaturation is observed on histology. As heating proceeds beyond 100°C, tissue water begins to boil and vaporize, resulting in tissue necrosis and carbonization. It has been demonstrated that CW laser irradiation can create controlled thermal injury to normal or atherosclerotic vessels.[1] Total energies or average powers necessary for penetration of vascular tissue vary with the laser system. However, a power threshold exists, below which successful tissue penetration does not occur even with prolonged lasing.

The argon laser has several advantages over other lasers. These include: (1) efficient conductivity through conventional flexible silica fibers; (2) effective tissue vaporization in blood medium; (3) moderate tissue penetration; and (4) the blue-green light is visible and a system failure is readily detectable. In saline, more CO_2 laser energy than argon laser energy is needed to obtain comparable tissue vaporization. This is probably due to the argon laser beam being more concentrated and thus penetrating deeper into the tissue. Blood enhances the absorption of argon and Nd:YAG laser, and less energy is required to produce equivalent plaque damage than when lasing is done in saline.

By-products of laser radiation have been evaluated in vitro and in vivo. These by-products include light chain hydrocarbons, CO_2, CO, and water vapor.[11] The amount of solid debris formed after lasing is reported to be minimal, as detected following laser recanalization of human peripheral arteries. The particle weight ranged from 0.2 to 1.8 mg.[10] These particles consisted primarily of charred and fused elements of denatured cellular elements.

Effects of laser irradiation on arterial thrombus are not well defined. An in vitro study has indicated that argon laser is well absorbed by clot, resulting in vaporization.[12] The Nd:YAG laser has also been shown to vaporize thrombus in vitro.[5] In vivo, 1-cm long thrombi in canine femoral arteries are completely vaporized using argon laser energy.[13] However, these thrombi were produced by thrombin injection and were rich in red blood cells, thus resulting in high absorption of the argon laser beam. Human arterial thrombi usually consist of platelet aggregates, fibrin, and blood cells, and they are significantly different from these artificial thrombi. Clinical data suggest that fresh thrombotic occlusion of human femoral arteries is not readily vaporized by argon lasing.[10]

To further investigate the effects of laser radiation on thrombus, we have conducted studies using a thrombus model that simulates clinical situations. The thrombus was produced by endothelial denudation and partial arterial constriction. Thrombotic obstructions were evaluated by angioscopy to provide a topographic cross-sectional view of the vascular lumen. Occlusive thrombi (1 to 2 cm long) were recanalized by argon lasing, but considerable amounts of residual thrombus remained, even after 30 laser exposures. Further study is needed to elucidate the laser-thrombus interaction using various powers and wavelengths.

Through histologic analysis the effects of CW laser radiation on normal or atherosclerotic arteries have been studied extensively. Abela et al. described that 1 to 5 joules (J) of CO_2 laser irradiation on atherosclerotic coronary arteries resulted in three zones of tissue injury when lasing was done in air. Zone one consisted of a crater that was the result of tissue vaporization, while zone two consisted of a region of thermal-induced necrosis and coagulation, and zone three comprised a distal and diffuse acoustic or shock

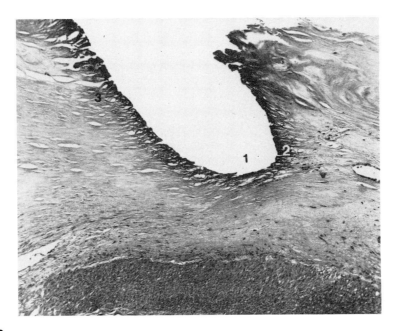

FIG 8–2.
Photomicrograph of a laser injury to a fibrous atherosclerotic plaque. The vessel was exposed to 2 joules of laser energy from a CO_2 laser source under dry conditions. This section shows a zone of tissue vaporization in the path of the laser *(1)*, a zone of adjacent tissue burn *(2)*, and a zone of acoustic shock and injury that begins at the tissue burn edge and fades gradually into normal tissue structure *(3)*. Hematoxylin-eosin; × 112. (From Abela GS, Normann S, Cohen D, et al: Effects of carbon dioxide, Nd:YAG, and argon laser radiation on coronary atheromatous plaques. *Am J Cardiol* 1982; 50:1199–1205. Used by permission.)

injury (Fig 8–2).[1] Under saline solution, laser radiation of atherosclerotic coronary arteries, using CO_2, argon, or Nd:YAG laser, resulted in little to no charring along the edge of the laser crater (zone 2) (Fig 8–3). Although many investigators have reported thermal injury after CW lasing, including collagen coagulation, necrosis, and charring, this varies with laser sources and energy parameters.[1, 14, 15] Argon energy is better absorbed by atherosclerotic tissue than Nd:YAG and can vaporize tissue, leaving a smooth surface.[1, 15] Elastic lamina of artery appears relatively resistant to laser injury because it is transparent to the argon laser beam and may act as an optical window (Fig 8–4).[10] In contrast, excimer, pulsed laser energy, which ablates atherosclerotic plaque with minimal thermal damage, may leave an irregular surface at the edge of the laser crater and may cause an increased amount of large-sized debris.[16, 17]

Healing process in normal or atherosclerotic arteries after direct laser irradiation has been studied using experimental animals (Fig 8–5).[18, 19] Two to four days after argon laser irradiation, a fibrin-platelet plug over the crater surface was noted. At 1 week, a low-grade cellular infiltration by smooth muscle cells and fibroblasts was seen in the crater site. Endothelial cell proliferation was observed weeks following lasing. Reendothelialization was complete by 1 to 2 months. Healing after lasing using a metal-capped fiber was similar.[20] Thus complete reendothelialization occurs after CW laser injury, regardless of the type of delivery system used.

EXPERIMENTAL LASER ANGIOPLASTY

In Vitro Studies

Preliminary investigations of the use of CW laser radiation to vaporize arterial tissue were done using direct beam lasing or a focusing lens.[14, 21] However, it was not until flexible, optical fibers were used to transmit laser energy that intraluminal laser angioplasty was considered to be feasible.[1, 3] The CW laser energy can be readily transmitted via flexible thin silica optical fibers. Optical fibers allow transmission of intense laser light to a target tissue at some distance from the laser source. In vitro studies showed that laser angioplasty using a flexible optical fiber could successfully recanalize obstructed human coronary arterial segments from argon or Nd:YAG energy sources.[4, 5] In addition, the effects of laser beam divergence and energy decay on the size of the recanalized channel were determined.[3] With the fiber tip in a fixed position, argon lasing at 3 W (30 to 90 joules) via an optical fiber could not recanalize or perforate totally occluded atherosclerotic rabbit arteries. However, recanalization was achieved as the fiber tip was advanced through the obstruction. The depth and diameter of the new channel were related to duration of exposure (Fig 8–6). Although these studies demonstrated that laser irradiation could recanalize atherosclerotic obstruction, arterial perforation remained a major limitation to human application.

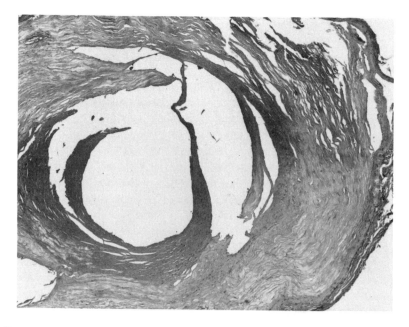

FIG 8–3.
Photomicrograph of a new lumen by exposure to Nd:YAG laser radiation in a totally occluded coronary artery immersed in saline solution. This artery was stained with Sudan black and then exposed to 25 J of laser energy. Note the incomplete vaporization of the plaque, with the injury in concentric fashion sparing deep layers; ×84. (From Abela GS, Normann S, Cohen D, et al: Effects of carbon dioxide, Nd:YAG, and argon laser radiation on coronary atheromatous plaques. *Am J Cardiol* 1982; 50:1199–1205. Used by permission.)

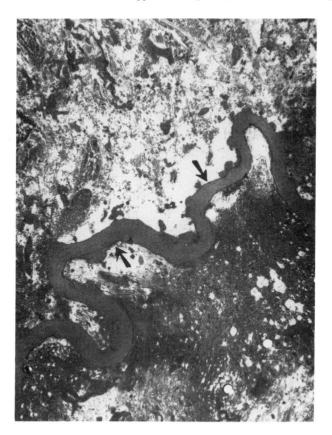

FIG 8–4.
Transmission electron micrograph of femoral artery from a laser-treated patient showing an intact elastic lamina *(arrows)*. The atheroma on the luminal side of the vessel above the lamina and the muscular layer below the elastic lamina show intense thermal necrosis; ×4,427. (From Abela GS, Seeger JM, Barbieri E, et al: Laser angioplasty with angioscopic guidance in humans. *J Am Coll Cardiol* 1986; 8:184–192. Used by permission.)

In Vivo Studies

Several preliminary animal studies were conducted using various laser systems. Lee et al.[22] demonstrated the feasibility of conducting laser energy into blood vessels of normal dogs. In addition, these investigators studied the acute and chronic response of in vivo laser exposure in atherosclerotic rabbits.[19] Argon lasing with power intensities of 1 to 2 W for 3 seconds produced a vaporized crater within an atherosclerotic plaque. However, excessive thermal damage to the vessel wall was seen when in vivo lasing was done without visualizing specific plaque targets. Finally, carbon dioxide laser energy transmitted through a silver halide optical fiber has also been shown to ablate atherosclerotic plaques in rabbit arteries with limited damage to the vessel wall.[23]

Abela et al.[3] reported on the use of laser irradiation to recanalize arterial obstructions in rabbits with atherosclerotic arteries. In 15 hypercholesterolemic rabbits, a catheter was positioned in the distal aorta using fluoroscopic guidance. An optical fiber with a metal ring at the tip was then advanced via the catheter and positioned against the plaque. Both Nd:YAG and argon lasing were done with varying power and pulse duration, and these

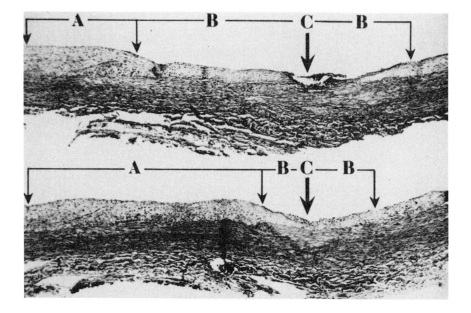

FIG 8–5.
Photomicrographs of hypercholesterolemic monkey aortas sacrified at 7 days *(top)* and 30 days *(bottom)* after lasing (2.5 W for 1 second). Zone A is the surrounding nonlased plaque; zone B is the plaque bordering the crater; zone C is the crater made by lasing. *Top,* the crater at 7 days is clearly visible with charred edges and a lumen filled with a coagulum of cellular debris. The bordering zone B is characterized by thinning of the intima, whereas the surrounding zone A shows the intimal thickening typical of this atherosclerotic model. Hematoxylin-eosin; × 25. *Bottom,* the crater at 1 month is reendothelialized and hypercellular. The reformed arterial intima at the crater site as well as the adjacent zone B is thinner than that in zone A. Hematoxylin-eosin; × 25. (From Abela GS, Crea F, Seeger JM, et al: The healing process in normal canine arteries and in atherosclerotic monkey arteries after transluminal laser radiation. *Am J Cardiol* 1985; 56:983–988. Used by permission.)

laser sources were effective in arterial recanalization (Fig 8–7). The severity of iliofemoral stenoses decreased from 78 ± 18 to 32 ± 11% in eight animals, and perforation occurred in seven animals with both laser sources. A deeper penetration into tissue by the Nd:YAG wavelength as compared with the argon wavelength was seen. Successfully recanalized arteries demonstrated centrally located channels without residual debris, suggesting that atheroma was vaporized (Fig 8–8). The intimal surface showed a thin zone of charring. As many investigations suggested, vascular perforations are frequent with bare or ring-tipped optical fibers. This may be related to the sharp configuration of the fiber tip as well as to beam divergence and scattering from the tip.

As previously noted, several modified fiber devices have been developed to reduce perforation. These include optical fibers with a metal marker at the tip for fluoroscopic guidance, microlens-tipped fibers,[6] sapphire-lens–tipped catheter systems,[7] and encapsulation of the fiber tip with a metal probe. The encapsulated fiber has been widely used for experimental and clinical laser angioplasty. A completely encapsulated optical fiber appears to be less traumatic to the artery than a bare fiber.[8, 9] This device (the "hot-tip" probe or laser probe) is usable only with a CW laser system. In this device, laser radiation is converted to heat by the metal cap. Pathophysiologic mechanisms of laser angioplasty using this device are mainly attributable to thermal vaporization of target tissue as well as mechanical compression. A recent thermographic study revealed that the laser thermal

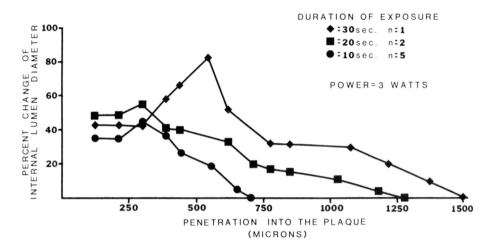

FIG 8–6.

The graph summarizing in vitro experiments in totally occluded arteries with the optical fiber tip fixed. Increasing duration of exposure to laser beam at constant power (3 W) led to a larger internal lumen diameter and deeper penetration into the atheromatous plaques. The size of the new channel created by laser radiation was expressed as the percent change in lumen diameter as compared with the size of the original occluding atheroma (vertical axis), and the depth of penetration is shown on the horizontal axis. Average changes in lumen diameter at selected depths of penetration are shown for exposures of 30-, 20-, and 10-second durations. (From Abela GS, Normann S, Cohen DM, et al: Laser recanalization of occluded atherosclerotic arteries in vivo and in vitro. *Circulation* 1985; 71:403–411.)

probe was more effective in ablating fibrofatty plaque than normal aorta.[24]

Theis et al. showed that atheromatous plaques in the iliac artery of monkeys could be vaporized using a metal-capped probe.[20] Lasing with 3 to 6 J tangentially produced a superficial lesion that extended into the intima, while lasing at 9 J tangentially produced a burn into media. In another experiment, Abela et al. attempted recanalization of occluded human atherosclerotic coronary xenografts transplanted into dog femoral arteries.[8] Lasing was done using an argon laser. Recanalization was achieved in all five arteries treated with a "hot-tip" probe and in three (60%) of five treated with a bare-ended fiber. Perforation occurred in one artery with the hot-tip probe and in three with a bare-ended fiber. In a similar study, Sanborn et al. compared the hot-tip probe with a bare fiber for dissolution of atherosclerotic obstruction in the aorta and iliac arteries of rabbits.[9] Widening of stenosed vessels was achieved in 2 (17%) of 12 using a bare fiberoptic system, compared with 8 (67%) of 12 using a hot-tip probe. Perforation of the vessel wall occurred more frequently with the bare optical fiber (9 of 12) as compared with the hot-tip probe (1 of 12). Microscopic examination of the vessel recanalized by either technique showed similar charring (Fig 8–9). However, a difference in pattern of thermal injury between these two systems was seen with a localized laser defect being noted with the bare optical fiber, while evenly distributed thermal injury resulted from the laser probe.[9] Thus, a metal-capped thermal probe was found to widen luminal stenosis with less vessel perforation than a bare fiberoptic catheter system. However, complete attenuation of the laser beam seemed to reduce the efficiency of tissue ablation, and the hot-tip probe required high temperature and good tissue contact for effective recanalization.

Coronary laser angioplasty in normal and thrombosed coronary arteries in live normal dogs has also been evaluated by our group.[25–27] Via a percutaneous approach, an 8 F catheter was introduced and a 300-μm core open-ended fiber was guided into the left anterior descending artery or left circumflex artery. Lasing was done using 1 to 2 W. This resulted in perforation in all dogs.[25] In ten animals with thrombosed coronary arteries, only one artery was recanalized without perforation (Fig 8–10).[26] These studies strongly suggested that open-ended fibers were not safe for coronary recanalization. The hot-tip probe was also tested in the coronary arteries of live dogs,[27] and the temperature of the probe tip was measured during lasing. Probe temperature greater than 350°C was associated with probe sticking and thrombotic occlusion of the vessels, while safe lasing in coronary circulation was possible at lower probe temperatures. This suggested that excessive thermal damage is responsible for complications and that probe temperature monitoring could provide safe approach to laser energy delivery.

Long-term vessel responses to laser recanalization potentially leading to thrombosis, restenosis, or aneurysms in normal or atherosclerotic arteries have been evaluated.[18] Most studies have shown minimal adverse changes at the lased sites.[19, 20, 28] Sanborn et al.[28] also examined the angiographic and histologic consequences of laser thermal angioplasty using a hot-tip laser probe and compared these findings to those with balloon angioplasty. In atherosclerotic rabbit arteries, the immediate enlargement of the arterial lumen diameter was similar for both procedures. However, 4 weeks after angioplasty, the vessels treated

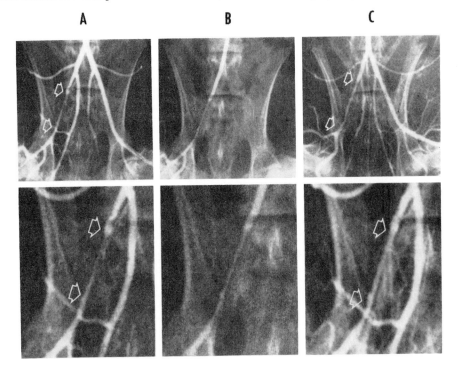

A   **B**   **C**

FIG 8–7.
A–C, *top panels* show low-power view of the lower abdominal aorta and both right and left femoroiliac circulations. A, the right external iliac artery was severely stenosed *(arrows)*. Magnified views (bottom panels) of the right internal and external iliac arteries show the stenosed external iliac artery in more detail. B, passage of the optical fiber across the stenotic segment resulted in mechanical recanalization with a small decrease in the percentage of stenosis. C, after application of laser energy (15 J), further decrease in the percentage of stenosis occurred *(arrows)*. (From Abela GS, Normann SJ, Cohen DM, et al: Laser recanalization of occluded atherosclerotic arteries in vivo and in vitro. *Circulation* 1985; 71:430–411. Used by permission.)

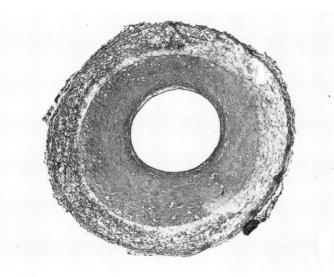

FIG 8–8.
Tissue section of an atherosclerotic femoral arterial stenosis recanalized by an argon laser. This vessel was severely stenosed before laser radiation. Intimal smooth muscle and foam cell proliferation occluded the vessel, and laser radiation has cleanly vaporized a portion of this tissue. A thin darkened zone of charring was seen at the edge of lumen. The luminal surface of the recanalized channel was very smooth (hematoxylin-eosin; ×68). (From Abela GS, Normann SJ, Cohen DM, et al: Laser recanalization of occluded atherosclerotic arteries in vivo and in vitro. *Circulation* 1985; 71:403–411.)

with a hot-top laser probe had less restenosis and a significantly larger lumen than those treated with conventional balloon angioplasty. Only one report in an atherosclerotic rabbit model has demonstrated aneurysmal formation in lased aorta.[19] This may be attributable to lasing with a larger and stiffer fiber without fluoroscopic guidance.

In our study using atherosclerotic monkeys, thermal damage was observed at the site of lasing, but thrombus formation was infrequent and was seen only in 10% of 20 lased arteries. No aneurysm was noted. In addition, intimal thickening at the site of lasing was limited compared to untreated sites 3 months after the procedure.

Laser balloon angioplasty has been developed by Spears et al.[29] for the treatment of coronary occlusive disease. The Nd:YAG laser irradiation is delivered to the arterial wall from a diffusing tip within a prototype balloon during angioplasty. The laser energy fuses disrupted elements of arterial wall, which are seen following balloon angioplasty, and may prevent abrupt reclosure or thrombosis. Preliminary results in canine coronary arteries suggest a persistent dilatation of the irradiated segment on 1-year follow-up. This irradiated area was also resistant to vasospasm induced by ergonovine.

Photosensitizing Studies

Atheromatous plaque may be sensitized by chromophore dyes, so that certain wavelengths of laser energy can be selectively absorbed into sensitized plaque, sparing the normal vessel. Sudan black stain of atherosclerotic aorta enhances tissue absorption of Nd:YAG laser energy and allows tissue penetration of the laser beam at lower energy levels.[1] Hematoporphyrin derivative localizes in plaque of rabbits, monkey, and human cadaver aorta, but the absorption peak of plaque containing hematoporphyrin was at 630 nm, and this did not seem to alter the plaque ablation or regression significantly.[30] In contrast, tetracycline, which also accumulates in plaque, absorbs the ultraviolet wavelength at 355 nm and effectively enhances plaque vaporization by a frequency-tripled Nd:YAG laser in vitro.[31] In addition, tetracycline enhances the thermal effects of the argon wavelength.[32] Finally, hemoglobin in blood may act as a potential chromophore and enhance argon and Nd:YAG laser effects.[1] Thus, photosensitizing may be useful for selective ablation of atheromatous tissue while sparing normal vessel wall. However, possible adverse effects including vascular reaction and toxicity are not well defined in clinical situations.

LASER ANGIOPLASTY IN HUMANS

Numerous clinical trials of laser angioplasty using CW laser systems in peripheral arteries have been done, and trials of coronary laser angioplasty using CW lasers have been recently initiated. In this chapter, we describe the reported studies on laser angioplasty in addition to our clinical experience.

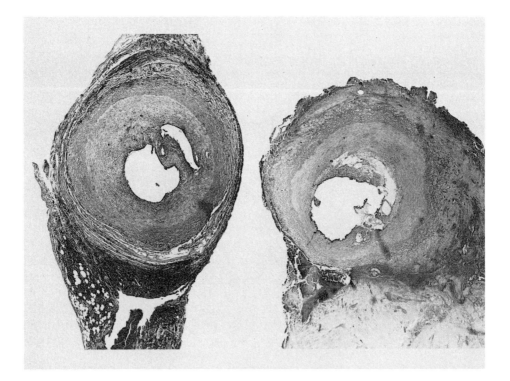

FIG 8–9.
Cross sections showing new vascular channels in two previously totally occluded arterial transplants. The left cross section shows a new centrally located vascular channel made by using a 0.8-mm hot-tip probe (hematoxylin-eosin; ×23). The right cross section shows a vascular channel made by a bare optical fiber. A total of 25 J was used. Hematoxylin-eosin; ×23. Both channels have the characteristic charred lining and are comparable in size. (From Abela GS, Fenech A, Crea F, et al: "Hot-Tip": Another method of laser vascular recanalization. *Lasers Surg Med* 1985; 5:327–335.)

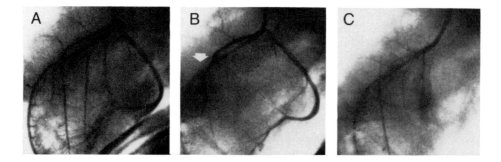

FIG 8–10.
Successful laser recanalization of the left anterior descending artery of a dog. **A,** control angiogram. **B,** angiogram after thrombus formation. An irregular filling defect of the proximal left anterior artery with distal occlusion *(arrow)* is seen; the diagonal branches are not opacified. **C,** angiogram after argon lasing (7 J). The left anterior descending artery is recanalized although the proximal filling defect is still present; the diagonal branches are seen. (From Crea F, Fenech A, Smith W, et al: Laser recanalization of acutely thrombosed coronary arteries in live dogs: Early results. *J Am Coll Cardiol* 1985; 6:934–938. Used by permission.)

Laser Angioplasty in Peripheral Arteries

As with balloon angioplasty, laser angioplasty was first attempted in peripheral arteries to investigate the safety and efficacy of the technique. Preliminary studies of CW laser recanalization of obstructed vessels were done using both Nd:YAG and argon laser systems to recanalize stenosed or occluded peripheral arteries. Geschwind et al.[33] reported successful percutaneous laser angioplasty using the Nd:YAG laser system in three arteries (two totally occluded and one stenosed). The laser beam was delivered through a 400-μm optical fiber, using a special catheter system to maintain a coaxial position. Ginsburg et al.[34] recanalized 8 of 17 obstructed arteries, including 5 of 9 totally occluded ones, using a bare optical fiber and argon lasing at 8.3 to 15.2 W. Heavily calcified lesions were resistant to laser recanalization using these systems. Complications included spasm in four cases, pain in seven, and perforation in three.

In the first trial of peripheral laser angioplasty approved by the United States Food and Drug Administration, the feasibility of laser angioplasty with angioscopic guidance in human peripheral arteries was demonstrated at the University of Florida.[10] During peripheral bypass operations, argon lasing at 1 to 8 W was done using a special optical fiber probe in 11 patients with totally occluded superficial femoral arteries. Seven (78%) of nine arteries were recanalized using a 2-mm "hybrid" probe, but perforation occurred in two. The recanalized channel size ranged between 2 and 3.5 mm in diameter. Although both organized thrombus and atheromatous occlusion were readily recanalized, fresh thrombus was not readily removed. Histologic cross section of the recanalized artery illustrated a relatively smooth-walled central lumen with minimal charring and thermal injury (Fig 8–11).

Subsequent clinical studies of laser angioplasty in the treatment of peripheral vascular disease have been reported (Table 8–2). Fourrier et al.,[35] using a 2.2-mm sapphire-lens–tipped fiber and Nd:YAG laser energy at 15 W recanalized 12 (75%) of 16 atherosclerotic occlusions in peripheral arteries. Three perforations occurred. Balloon angioplasty was performed in nine recanalized arteries, and eight of these were patent at 8 months after lasing. In contrast, all three arteries treated with laser angioplasty alone reoccluded.

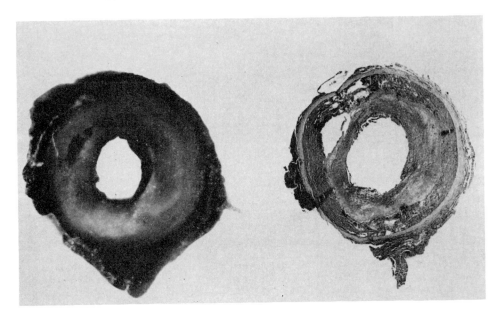

FIG 8–11.
Recanalized human artery. *Left*, fresh segment of superficial femoral artery after laser re-canalization. The central channel was made using a 2-mm probe. The original lumen appears in the 11 o'clock position. *Right*, histologic cross section of the recanalized artery illustrating relatively smooth-walled central lumen with minimal charring and thermal injury made with argon laser. The left upper quadrant shows original vascular lumen. Hematoxylin-eosin; × 12. (From Abela GS, Seeger JM, Barbieri E, et al: Laser angioplasty with angioscopic guidance in humans. *J Am Coll Cardiol* 1986; 8:184–192. Used by permission.)

Nordstrom et al.[36] reported the results of direct laser exposure for recanalization of peripheral arteries using a special balloon catheter to position the fiber so that the laser beam was delivered in a coaxial alignment. Argon lasing at 10 W (2- to 10-second pulses) resulted in recanalization of 33 (92%) of 36 arteries, including 10 (100%) of 10 stenosed arteries and 23 (88%) of 26 totally occluded arteries. Clinical improvement was observed in 23 (70%) of 33 patients. Two emboli and one perforation occurred. Sanborn et al.[37] reported the results of laser thermal angioplasty in 129 arteries. Argon lasing using a

TABLE 8–2.
Technical and Clinical Success of Percutaneous Laser Angioplasty

	Lesion*	n	Technical Success No.	Technical Success %	Clinical Success No.	Clinical Success %	Follow-up % Patency
Nordstrom et al.[36] (n = 36)	S O	10 26	10 23	100 88	— —	— —	— 50
Fourrier et al.[35] (n = 16)	O	16	12	75	12	75	67
Myler et al.[38] (n = 54)	O	54	31	57	—	—	73
Abela et al.[68] (n = 52)	O	52	40	77	34	66	—
Sanborn et al.[37] (n = 129)	S O	22 107	22 91	100 85	21 78	95 73	} 77

*S = stenosis; O = total occlusion.

laser thermal probe at 8 to 13 W resulted in recanalization of all 22 stenosed arteries and 91 (85%) of 107 occluded arteries. Clinical success was achieved in 99 patients using balloon angioplasty to increase the lumen size. There was a 4% frequency of perforation, but surgical reconstruction was not required in any patients. The 1-year cumulative clinical patency was 77% for the 99 lesions with an initial clinical success. However, another study of laser thermal angioplasty showed a lower recanalization rate of 57% in totally occluded arteries.[38] By February 1989, laser thermal angioplasty using laser probe was done in 227 patients and resulted in 73% technical and clinical success.

At the University of Florida, we have evaluated the short-term and long-term effects of laser recanalization of totally occluded peripheral arteries, including iliac and femoropopliteal lesions (2 to 30 cm in length). For laser recanalization we used a 2- or 2.5-mm hybrid probe on a 300- or 600-μm core optical fiber, respectively (Spectra probe, Trimedyne, Santa Ana, Calif). These probes have a side channel in the metal cap through which a 0.018-in. guidewire can be passed to allow some directional control of the probe. The entire system was preloaded in a 7 F thin-walled catheter (Cook, Bloomington, Ind.) prior to insertion of the optical fiber. The focused laser beam emitted from a microlens at the tip of the optical fiber creates a small internal channel through areas of total occlusion that the bullet-shaped tip follows. Argon lasing of 1-second pulses and 0.2-second intervals was used. Lasing was started at 5 W and increased to 16 W as needed to penetrate and cross the obstruction.

From March 1986 to March 1989, 52 percutaneous procedures were done using this technique. Recanalization was achieved in 40 (77%), and clinical success as determined by improvement of symptoms and increased ankle/brachial systolic pressure ratios (ABI) was seen in 34 patients (66%).[68] This is similar to the report of Myler et al.[38] of initial clinical success of 50% recanalization of total arterial occlusions. In most of the recanalized arteries, residual stenosis of >50% was seen, and immediate balloon angioplasty to increase the luminal size was done. This was considered necessary for adequate vessel recanalization. However, seven patients with <50% residual stenosis did not require balloon dilatation. Mean residual stenosis following laser angioplasty was 49.4% ± 14.1%, and this improved after balloon angioplasty to 31.3% ± 16.5% (Fig 8–12). Thermal monitoring of laser probe temperature during the procedure in patients indicated an average recanalization temperature of 136 ± 29°C. This is lower than that reported during vessel recanalization using a hot-tip probe. High temperatures were observed only when recanalization of calcific plaque was attempted.

Ankle/brachial pressure indices recorded in 18 patients who had successful recanalization were 0.54 ± 0.14 before treatment, 0.76 ± 0.22 after laser recanalization and balloon angioplasty. Two patients had acute thrombosis, and six perforations occurred. However, perforation was not a major complication and did not require either blood transfusion or emergency by-pass operation. Probe sticking to vessel wall occasionally occurred, but it was easily disengaged while activating the laser and pulling back. Arterial dissections were noted by angiography following balloon angioplasty but not with the laser.

On follow-up, symptom relief was maintained in 66% of patients. Percent stenosis on follow-up angiography after 6 to 12 months was 69.1% ± 27.8%. These studies indicated that laser angioplasty can recanalize long occlusive arterial segments (1 to 30 cm in length), with clinical success varying from 66% to 75%. In contrast, recent studies of balloon angioplasty alone have shown clinical success rates varying from 57% to 77% for treatment of arterial occlusions and 26% to 78% for treatment of occlusions greater than 3 cm in length (Table 8–3).[39–41] Thus the laser angioplasty appears to be an effective

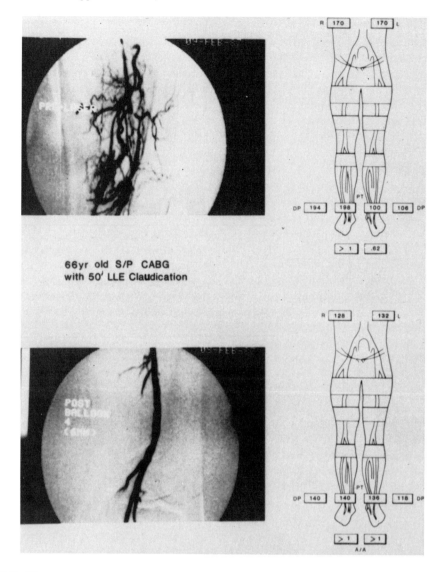

FIG 8–12.
Angiograms of laser balloon angioplasty. *Top left,* prelaser angiogram showing total occlusion of a left superficial femoral artery. Collaterals are seen filling the distal vessel. The patient had severe claudication at 50 ft. *Top right,* pretreatment arterial pressures obtained by Doppler measurement. The left ABI is 0.62. *Bottom left,* angiogram after laser-assisted balloon angioplasty showing successful recanalization with minimal residual stenosis. Collateral vessels disappeared. *Bottom right,* following laser balloon angioplasty, arterial pressures obtained by Doppler measurement. The left ABI is >1.

treatment for recanalization of totally occluded peripheral arteries. However, balloon angioplasty is required to enlarge lumen size in most cases to achieve clinical success.

Sanborn et al.[37] also reported that the 1-year cumulative clinical patency rate in 17 short occlusions was 93%. In contrast, clinical success in the longer occlusions (4 to 7 cm and greater than 7 cm) was 76% and 58%, respectively. Follow-up patency rates of laser angioplasty appear to be better than the patency rate of 50% for occlusions longer than 3 cm treated by balloon angioplasty alone.[39] The lower recurrence rate after laser

TABLE 8–3.
Technical and Clinical Success of Balloon Angioplasty

	Lesion*	No.	Technical Success No.	Technical Success %	Clinical Success No.	Clinical Success %	1-yr Cumulative % Patency <3 cm†	1-yr Cumulative % Patency 4–7 cm†	1-yr Cumulative % Patency >7 cm†
Krepel et al.[39]	S	127 ⎫	150	91	117	92			
(n = 164)	O	137 ⎭			21	57	93	50	...
Hewes et al.[40]	S	78	74	95	67	86			
(n = 130)	O	52	42	81	40	77	67	80	65
Murray et al.[41]	S	116	111	96	100	86			
(n = 193)	O	77	60	78	57	74	86	...	...

*S = stenosis; O = total occlusion.
†Indicates length of total occlusion (cm).

angioplasty may be explained by partial removal of atherosclerotic plaque, leaving a smooth recanalized channel instead of remodeling of arterial wall by balloon angioplasty. To evaluate the effects of laser angioplasty on long-term vessel patency, further study including risk factors, percent residual stenosis, thermal damage, and subclassification of calcified lesion is needed in recanalized arteries treated only by laser angioplasty.

Coronary Laser Angioplasty

Based on experiences of laser angioplasty in peripheral vessels, several intraoperative studies of laser coronary angioplasty have been reported. In an initial report, argon lasing through a bare optical fiber at 5 W (60 to 1,231 J) recanalized three of five severely stenosed arteries.[42] One artery was perforated. On follow-up 10 to 25 days later, only one artery remained patent probably because of excessive thermal damage. In another study, coronary laser endarterectomy was performed using a handheld CO_2 laser with a hollow metal wave guide.[43] Recanalization was achieved in five of six coronary arteries, and all five were patent on 1-week follow-up. Recently clinically successful long-term laser coronary recanalization was reported.[44] Argon laser angioplasty with a hot-tip probe was done during coronary bypass surgery and recanalized a severe stenosis. The recanalized artery was patent at 5-month follow-up after laser angioplasty.

Percutaneous coronary laser angioplasty using a laser probe was performed by Sanborn et al. in patients with angina pectoris due to coronary arterial stenosis.[45] Argon lasing was done at 6 to 12 W. Initial attempt at laser coronary angioplasty showed that a 1.7-mm laser probe could recanalize four stenosed coronary arteries but failed in three instances in which vessel tortuosity and device profile prevented complete recanalization. The same technique was used by Cumberland et al. in four patients with high-grade stenosis and was technically successful in creating a channel.[46] However, two of those seemed to reocclude, with resulting myocardial infarction within 12 hours. In another study performed via percutaneous approaches,[47] laser thermal angioplasty was used to recanalize left anterior coronary artery stenosis; it recanalized three of six stenoses and resulted in one perforation. Failure was attributed to tortuous vessel, calcified lesion, and/or malalignment of the probe. Recently, Sanborn et al.[48] reported that percutaneous laser-assisted balloon angioplasty using a new flexible laser probe over a central guidewire increased the initial success rate (89% recanalization) in 19 patients. Complications were rare (no perforation, no embolization, and one abrupt reclosure).

Coronary laser balloon angioplasty (Spears laser balloon) has also been attempted in seven patients. Following percutaneous coronary balloon angioplasty, the laser balloon decreased the stenotic diameter. No change in diameter was noted at 1-month follow-up.[49] These recent data are encouraging; however, currently available devices are not very effective in calcified lesions, and small channels recanalized by the laser probe continue to require balloon angioplasty.

Improvement of laser devices is a prerequisite to increase the success rate, enlarge the vascular channel, and ablate calcified plaque and prevent complications. If thermal exposure of plaque by CW laser systems alters the pathophysiology of the atherosclerotic process, then restenosis may be potentially reduced with this approach.

LASER ABLATION IN CARDIAC ARRHYTHMIAS

Life-threatening ventricular arrhythmias, ventricular tachycardia, and certain intractable supraventricular arrhythmias are occasionally resistant to medical treatment. Surgical and electrical ablative procedures have been developed for the treatment of intractable arrhythmias. Laser ablation in cardiac arrhythmias has gained interest because it is a percutaneous approach. Argon and Nd:YAG lasers produced myocardial vaporization of variable depth including transmural lesions, depending on the amount of energy.[50–52] Preliminary studies using catheter-directed laser ablation systems suggested that laser ablation may have some advantages over electrical ablation, such as less adverse hemodynamic effects and more precise area of ablation.[52] Transection of the His bundle by catheter-directed argon laser energy has been demonstrated with development of complete atrioventricular block.[50, 52] This could be advantageous for patients with intractable supraventricular arrhythmias.[51, 53] Preliminary evidence in both experimental and clinical studies suggests that laser ablation can effectively abolish ventricular arrhythmias. Similar results have been obtained with electrical discharge or surgery. Further investigation is needed to define the advantages and risks of laser ablation of cardiac arrhythmias.

VALVULAR LASER ABLATION

The CW laser has been found to vaporize valvular tissue. Laser valvulotomy may be possible in congenital and rheumatic valvular stenosis.[54, 55] Isner et al.[56] demonstrated that calcified deposits may be ablated by CO_2 laser with little damage to surrounding valvular tissue. A special balloon catheter system for cardioscopy has been developed and used in a preliminary clinical trial.[57] In the future, it may be possible to perform safe percutaneous laser valvulotomy under cardioscopic guidance.

Laser Myectomy

In selected cases, myectomy for hypertrophic obstructive cardiomyopathy (HOCM) is an accepted form of treatment. Laser-guided energy can vaporize myocardium with considerable precision and may be used to perform myectomy. Intraoperative laser myectomy has been performed in patients with HOCM.[58] Percutaneous in vivo laser myectomy in clinical patients is feasible and may be further developed as a clinically accepted form of therapy.

LASER ENDARTERECTOMY

Open endarterectomy of atherosclerotic arteries is a standard surgical procedure. Laser endarterectomy using CW lasers has been performed and has provided surfaces at least as satisfactory as surgery.[59] Using this technique, the laser beam provides precise control over the plane of dissection, resulting in better defined edges. A potential advantage of laser endarterectomy might be heat sealing of the edges of the dissected surface, which might reduce the risk of thrombosis, but this remains to be determined.

GUIDANCE AND CONTROL SYSTEMS FOR LASER APPLICATION IN THE CARDIOVASCULAR AREA

As described before, CW laser energy can provide precise and efficacious ablation of cardiovascular tissue, but excessive damage to surrounding tissues may also result. Sophisticated guidance and control system may be necessary to achieve safe application of laser energy. Standard fluoroscopic and angiographic guidance imaging may not be reliable enough to avert vessel perforation. New methods for in vivo laser control are being investigated.

Recently, high-resolution, flexible, ultrathin angioscopes (0.5 to 1.4 mm in outer diameter [OD], Olympus Inc., Tokyo) were fabricated; these scopes are composed of 2,000 coherent optical bundles with illumination fibers. Angioscopy can provide cross-sectional topographic color views and evaluate cross-sectional area of the percent stenosis of the vessel lumen. It can detect atherosclerotic plaques or thrombus clearly. Angioscopy has been used for visualization of human coronary arteries,[60] evaluation and guidance of laser angioplasty,[10] visualization of thrombus formation and thrombolysis,[61, 62] evaluation of balloon angioplasty,[63] and characterization of the pathophysiology of ischemic heart disease.[64] Angioscopy requires a bloodless field, which is obtained by flushing the lumen with crystalloid solutions. This may be difficult using conventional percutaneous techniques. A special balloon-guiding catheter prevents antegrade flow and makes it easy to visualize the arterial lumen, cardiac valves, or cardiac chambers by flushing the target area with saline solution.[57] The problem of nonlinear magnification by angioscopy is being resolved by computerized quantitative methods.

Spectroscopic analysis or imaging of arterial wall tissues is being investigated during ablation of atherosclerotic plaques. Results from these studies suggest that the surface arterial fluorescence pattern returns to normal after laser ablation of atheromatous plaques.[65] A feedback mechanism also can be applied to stop lasing by recognition of the fluorescence pattern of normal arterial wall. However, for in vivo application this technique still has problems related to blood in the field of view and to having no control over the direction of laser beam. Leon et al.[66] attempted fluorescence-guided dye laser angioplasty in ten patients with peripheral arterial disease and achieved recanalization in 80%. The results are encouraging. Intravascular two-dimensional echocardiography may provide a cross-sectional image of arterial lumen as well as wall thickness to guide laser angioplasty,[67] but these systems remain to be developed. Finally, catheter systems with tip control may provide for more precise angioplasty vaporization.

FUTURE DIRECTIONS

Currently available laser devices have been found to provide safe and effective recanalization of totally occluded peripheral arteries in selected patients. However, conventional laser devices cannot be used easily for recanalization of small, tortuous, and/or calcific arterial segments. In addition, excessive thermal damage necessary for recanalization of calcified occlusions may result in arterial constriction, thrombosis, and/or arterial perforation. Finally, most recanalized channels created by laser angioplasty are too small for adequate blood flow to relieve symptoms, meaning that balloon angioplasty is frequently necessary. Possible solutions to these problems include: (1) more effective vaporization of heavily calcific lesions; (2) a more controllable catheter system; (3) limitation of thermal damage by monitoring probe and/or tissue temperature; (4) controlling the direction of the laser beam more precisely; (5) selective plaque ablation while simultaneously detecting tissue characteristics using spectroscopy; (6) vaporizing atherosclerotic plaques with an adequate wavelength that is selectively absorbed by the target tissue to spare normal vascular tissues; (7) enlarging the channel by improvement of the laser probe; and (8) developing photosensitive agents that localize plaque to reduce energy requirement.

As a CW laser angioplasty device, the hybrid probe has several properties that may overcome some of the problems with laser recanalization. It may be assumed theoretically that laser ablation of the atherosclerotic lesion could be done by the hybrid probe with less thermal energy than by a thermal laser probe alone. We achieved recanalization of occluded vessels at mean probe temperatures of 130°C, which is lower than those reported for the pure thermal laser probe. The hybrid probe has a guiding hole for a steerable guidewire, thus enhancing control of the probe. Large-sized probes and probes with a thermal monitoring and feedback system to prevent excessive thermal damage are being investigated. Thus the hybrid probe has potential for future improvement. To vaporize calcified tissue, pulsed laser energy is reported to be effective.[16] However, some investigators report that it cannot provide large-sized channels and perforations occur at high power in some devices.

CONCLUSIONS

The use of CW lasers in the cardiovascular area appears poised for rapid advancement in recanalization of occluded vessels, treatment of arrhythmias, myectomy, and valvulotomy. Experimental and clinical studies have demonstrated the potential advantage of laser ablation techniques over conventional intervention methods. New laser devices and guiding systems are also under development. The major problems for laser angioplasty at this point are defining an adequate wavelength for selective ablation of atheromatous plaque without damaging surrounding normal tissue and preventing complications including thrombosis, spasm, and perforation. Further studies and development of laser systems are required for ideal laser application in cardiovascular medicine and surgery.

REFERENCES

1. Abela GS, Normann S, Cohen D, et al: Effects of carbon dioxide, Nd:YAG and argon laser radiation on coronary atherosclerotic plaque. *Am J Cardiol* 1982; 50:1199–205.
2. Laurence PF, Dries DJ, Moatamed F, et al: Acute effects of argon laser on human atherosclerotic plaque. *J Vasc Surg* 1984; 1:852–859.

3. Abela GS, Normann S, Cohen DM, et al: Laser recanalization of occluded atherosclerotic arteries: An in-vivo and in-vitro study. *Circulation* 1985; 71:403–411.
4. Choy DSJ, Stertzer S, Rotterdam H, et al: Laser coronary angioplasty: Experience with nine cadaver hearts. *Am J Cardiol* 1982; 50:1206–1208.
5. Geschwind HJ, Boussignac G, Teisseire B, et al: Conditions for effective ND:YAG laser angioplasty. *Br Heart J* 1984; 52:484–489.
6. Barbieri E, Roxey T, Khoury A, et al: Evaluation of optical properties and laser effects on arterial tissue using a microlens tipped optical fiber. *Proc SPIE* 1986; 713:166–169.
7. Geschwind HJ, Blairr JD, Mongkolsmai D, et al: Development and experimental application of contact probe catheter for laser angioplasty. *J Am Coll Cardiol* 1987; 9:101–107.
8. Abela GS, Fenech A, Crea F, et al: "Hot-Tip": Another method of laser vascular recanalization. *Lasers Surg Med* 1985; 5:327–335.
9. Sanborn TA, Faxon DP, Haudenschild C, et al: Experimental angioplasty: Circumferential distribution of laser thermal energy with a laser probe. *J Am Coll Cardiol* 1985; 5:934–938.
10. Abela GS, Seeger JM, Barbieri E, et al: Laser angioplasty with angioscopic guidance in humans. *J Am Coll Cardiol* 1986; 8:184–192.
11. Isner JM, Clarke RH, Donaldson RF, et al: Identification of photoproducts liberated by in-vitro argon laser irradiation of atherosclerotic plaque, calcified cardiac valves and myocardium. *Am J Cardiol* 1985; 55:1192–1196.
12. Lee G, Ikeda RM, Stobbe D, et al: Effects of laser irradiation on human thrombus: Demonstration of a linear dissolution-dose relation between clot length and energy density. *Am J Cardiol* 1983; 52:876–877.
13. Choy DSJ, Stertzer S, Rotterdam HZ, et al: Transluminal laser catheter angioplasty. *Am J Cardiol* 1982; 50:1206–1208.
14. Lee G, Ikeda RM, Kozina J, et al: Laser dissolution of coronary atherosclerotic obstruction. *Am Heart J* 1981; 102:1074–1075.
15. Lee G, Ikeda RM, Herman I, et al: The qualitative effects of laser irradiation on human atherosclerotic disease. *Am Heart J* 1983; 105:885–889.
16. Grundfest WS, Litvack F, Forrester JS, et al: Laser ablation of atherosclerotic plaque without adjacent tissue injury. *J Am Coll Cardiol* 1985; 5:929–933.
17. Prevosti LG, Cook JA, Leon MB: Comparison of particulate debris size from excimer and argon laser ablation, abstracted. *Circulation* 1987; 76(suppl 4):410.
18. Abela GS, Crea F, Seeger JM, et al: The healing process in normal canine arteries and in atherosclerotic monkey arteries after transluminal laser irradiation. *Am J Cardiol* 1985; 56:983–988.
19. Lee G, Ikeda RM, Theis JH, et al: Acute and chronic complications of laser angioplasty: Vascular wall damage and formation of aneurysms in the atherosclerotic rabbit. *Am J Cardiol* 1984; 53:290–293.
20. Theis JH, Lee G, Chan MC, et al: Effects of simultaneous viewing and vaporization of plaques using steerable, laser-heated metal cap in the atherosclerotic monkey model. *Lasers Surg Med* 1987; 7:414–420.
21. Macruz R, Martins JRM, Tupinamba A, et al: Therapeutic possibilities of laser beams in atheromas. *Arq Bras Cardiol* 1980; 34:9–12.
22. Lee G, Ikeda RM, Dwyer RM, et al: Feasibility of intravascular laser irradiation for in-vivo visualization and therapy of cardiovascular diseases. *Am Heart J* 1982; 103:1076–1077.
23. Eldar M, Battler A, Neufeld HN, et al: Transluminal carbon dioxide laser catheter angioplasty for dissolution of atherosclerotic plaques. *J Am Coll Cardiol* 1984; 3:135–137.
24. Welch AJ, Bradly AB, Torres JH, et al: Laser probe ablation of normal and atherosclerotic human aorta in vitro: A first thermographic and histologic analysis. *Circulation* 1987; 76:1353–1363.
25. Crea F, Abela GS, Fenech A, et al: Transluminal laser irradiation of coronary arteries in live dogs: An angiographic and morphologic study of acute effects. *Am J Cardiol* 1986; 57:171–174.

26. Crea F, Fenech A, Smith W, et al: Laser recanalization of acutely thrombosed coronary arteries in live dogs: Early results. *J Am Coll Cardiol* 1985; 6:1052–1056.

27. Barbieri E, Abela GS, Khouri AL, et al: Temperature characteristics of laser thermal probes in the coronary circulation of dogs, abstracted. *Circulation* 1987; 76(suppl 4):409.

28. Sanborn TA, Haudenschild CC, Faxon DP, et al: Angiographic and histologic consequences of laser thermal angioplasty: Comparison with balloon angioplasty. *Circulation* 1987; 75:281–286.

29. Spears JR: Percutaneous transluminal coronary angioplasty restenosis: Potential prevention with laser balloon angioplasty. *Am J Cardiol* 1987; 60:61B–64B.

30. Litvack F, Grundfest WS, Forrester JS, et al: Effects of hematoporphyrin derivative and photodynamic therapy on atherosclerotic rabbits. *Am J Cardiol* 1985; 56:667–671.

31. Murphy-Chutorian D, Kosek J, Mok W, et al: Selective absorption of ultraviolet laser energy by atherosclerotic plaque treated with tetracycline. *Am J Cardiol* 1985; 55:1293–1297.

32. Abela GS, Barbieri E, Roxey T, et al: Laser enhanced plaque atherolysis with tetracycline, abstracted. *Circulation* 1986; 72(suppl 2):7.

33. Geschwind H, Bonsignac G, Teisseire B, et al: Percutaneous transluminal laser angioplasty in man, letter. *Lancet* 1984; 2:844.

34. Ginsburg R, Wexler I, Mitchell RS, et al: Percutaneous transluminal laser angioplasty for treatment of peripheral vascular disease: Clinical experience with sixteen patients. *Radiology* 1985; 156:619–624.

35. Fourrier JL, Brunetaud JM, Prat A, et al: Human percutaneous laser angioplasty with sapphire tip, abstracted. *Circulation* 1987; 76(suppl 4):231.

36. Nordstrom LA, Casteneda-Zuniga WR, Lindeke CC, et al: Direct argon laser exposure for recanalization of peripheral arteries: Early results. *Radiology* 1988; 168:359–364.

37. Sanborn TA, Cumberland DC, Greenfield AJ, et al: Percutaneous laser thermal angioplasty: Initial results and 1 year follow-up in 129 femoropopliteal lesions. *Radiology* 1988; 168:121–125.

38. Myler RK, Cumberland DA, Clark DA, et al: High and low power thermal laser angioplasty for total occlusions and restenosis in man, abstracted. *Circulation* 1987; 76(suppl 4):230.

39. Kreppel VM, van Andel GJ, van Erp WFM, et al: Percutaneous transluminal angioplasty of the femoropopliteal artery: Initial and long term results. *Radiology* 1985; 156:325–328.

40. Hewes RC, White RI Jr, Murray RR, et al: Long term results of superficial femoral artery angioplasty. *AJR* 1986; 146:1025–1029.

41. Murray RR, Hewes RC, White RI Jr, et al: Long-segment femoropopliteal stenosis: Is angioplasty a boon or a bust? *Radiology* 1987; 162:473–476.

42. Choy DSJ, Stertzer SH, Myler RK, et al: Human coronary laser recanalization. *Clin Cardiol* 1984; 7:377–381.

43. Livesay JJ, Leachman DR, Hogan PJ, et al: Preliminary report on laser coronary endoatherectomy in patients, abstracted. *Circulation* 1985; 72(suppl 3):302.

44. Lee G, Garcia JM, Chan MC, et al: Clinically successful long-term laser coronary recanalization. *Am Heart J* 1986; 112:1323–1325.

45. Sanborn TA, Faxon DP, Kellett MA, et al: Percutaneous coronary laser thermal angioplasty. *J Am Coll Cardiol* 1986; 8:1437–1440.

46. Cumberland DC, Oakly GDG, Smith GH, et al: Percutaneous laser assisted coronary angioplasty. *Lancet* 1986; 2:214.

47. Crea F, Davies G, McKenna WJ, et al: Laser recanalization of coronary arteries by metal-capped optical fibers: Early clinical experience in patients with stable angina pectoris. *Br Heart J* 1988; 59:168–174.

48. Sanborn TA, Bonan R, Cumberland DC, et al: Percutaneous coronary laser-assisted balloon angioplasty with flexible, central lumen laser probe catheters, abstracted. *Circulation* 1988; 78(suppl 2):295.

49. Spears JR, Reyes VP, James LM, et al: Laser balloon angioplasty: Initial clinical percutaneous coronary results, abstracted. *Circulation* 1988; 78(suppl 2):269.

50. Abela GS, Griffin JG, Hill JA, et al: Transvascular argon laser induced atrioventricular ablation in dogs, abstracted. *Circulation* 1983; 68(suppl 2):145.

51. Vincent GM, Hunter J, Dixon JA, et al: Nd:YAG laser ablation of simulated ventricular tachycardia in a canine model. *Lasers Surg Med* 1985; 5:168.

52. Lee BL, Bottdiner JS, Fletcher RD, et al: Transcatheter ablation: Comparison between laser photoablation and electrode shock ablation in the dog. *Circulation* 1985; 71:579–586.

53. Saksena S, Hussain SM, Gelchinsky I: Successful mapping-guided argon laser ablation of ventricular tachycardia in man, abstracted. *Circulation* 1986; 74(suppl 2):186.

54. Gessman LJ, Reno CW, Chang KS, et al: Feasibility of laser catheter valvulotomy for aortic and mitral stenosis. *Am J Cardiol* 1984; 54:1375–1377.

55. Reimenschneider TA, Lee G, Ikeda RM, et al: Laser irradiation of congenital heart disease: Potential for palliation and correction of intracardiac and intravascular defects. *Am Heart J* 1983; 106:1389–1393.

56. Isner JM, Michlewitz H, Clarke RH, et al: Laser assisted debridement of aortic calcium. *Am Heart J* 1985; 109:448–452.

57. Uchida Y, Tomaru T, Nakamura F, et al: Fiberoptic angioscopy of cardiac chambers, valves and great vessels using a guiding catheter in dogs. *Am Heart J* 1988; 115:1297–1302.

58. Isner JM, Clarke RH: Laser myoplasty for hypertrophic cardiomyopathy: In vitro experience in human postmortem hearts and in vivo experience in a canine model (transarterial) and human patients (intraoperative). *Am J Cardiol* 1984; 53:1620–1625.

59. Eugene J, McColgan SJ, Hammer-Wilson M, et al: Laser endoarterectomy. *Lasers Surg Med* 1985; 5:265–274.

60. Uchida Y, Tomaru T, Nakamura F, et al: Percutaneous coronary angioscopy in patients with ischemic heart disease. *Am Heart J* 1987; 114:1216–1222.

61. Tomaru T, Uchida Y, Masuo M, et al: Experimental canine arterial thrombus formation and thrombolysis: A fiberoptic study. *Am Heart J* 1987; 114:1216–1222.

62. Tomaru T, Uchida Y, Nakamura F, et al: Enhancement of arterial thrombolysis with native tissue plasminogen activator by pretreatment with heparin or batroxobin: An angioscopic study. *Am Heart J,* 1989; 117:275–280.

63. Uchida Y, Masuo M, Tomaru T, et al: Fiberoptic observation of thrombosis and thrombolysis in isolated human coronary arteries. *Am Heart J* 1986; 112:691–696.

64. Sherman CT, Grundfest WS, Lee ME, et al: Angioscopy in patients with unstable angina pectoris. *N Engl J Med* 1986; 315:913–919.

65. Leon MB, Lu DY, Prevosti LG, et al: Human arterial surface fluorescence: Atherosclerotic plaque identification and effects of laser atheroma ablation. *J Am Coll Cardiol* 1988; 12:94–102.

66. Leon MB, Almayer Y, Bartorelli AC, et al: Fluorescence-guided laser angioplasty in patients with femoropopliteal occlusions, abstracted. *Circulation* 1988; 78(suppl 2):294.

67. Yock PG, Linker DT, Thapliyal HV, et al: Real-time, two dimensional catheter ultrasound: A new technique for high resolution intravascular imaging, abstracted. *J Am Coll Cardiol* 1988; 11:130A.

68. Abela GS, Seeger JM, Pry RS, et al: Percutaneous laser recanalization of totally occluded human peripheral arteries: Technical approach. *Dynamic Cardiovasc Imaging* 1988; 1:302–308.

Chapter 9

Excimer Laser Angioplasty: Recent Development and Clinical Trials*

Warren S. Grundfest, M.D.

Frank Litvack, M.D.

Louis Adler, M.D.

Ann Hickey, M.D.

Jacob Segalowitz, M.D.

Lisa Hestrin, M.P.H.

James S. Forrester, M.D.

In previous chapters the theoretical basis of nonthermal ablation of tissue was discussed. Work from our laboratory at Cedars-Sinai[1] and the work of others[2, 3] have demonstrated that 308-nm excimer laser irradiation delivered via fiberoptics is capable of nonthermal tissue removal. This process may occur via photochemical mechanisms since ultraviolet photons possess sufficient energy to break organic bonds.[4] Whatever the mechanism, both in vivo and in vitro studies have demonstrated the ability of this wavelength to ablate tissue with minimal generation of heat. In vivo studies in canine aorta irradiated with 308-nm light revealed minimal thrombus formation after excimer irradiation at 72 hours.[5] In long-term studies healing at 30 days exhibited minimal changes over controls.[6] Additionally, through the choice of appropriate parameters, it is possible to ablate calcified material including bone and teeth without destroying the fiberoptic delivery system.[7]

*Supported in part by Clinical Investigator Award 5K08 HL01391 and 5K0 HL01522 (Drs. Grundfest and Litvack) and First Award R29 HL38948 (Dr. Hickey). Also supported in part by SCOR P50 HL17651 from the National Institutes of Health; Grand Sweepstakes, Medallions Imperial Grand Sweepstakes; and Merry Mary Charitable Organizations of Cedars-Sinai Medical Center, Los Angeles.

Because of its ability to debulk even calcified atheroma precisely, the excimer laser may provide a significant alternative energy source for laser angioplasty.

The goal of this chapter is to describe the recent changes in excimer laser technology that permit clinical application of this laser source and to present the acute results of the initial clinical trials using first-generation prototype 308-nm laser angioplasty systems.

METHODS

Our patient population consisted of 30 patients with 31 lesions. One patient had both legs treated. Nineteen men and 11 women were included in the study, with an age range of 41 to 85 years. All patients had symptomatic peripheral vascular disease. Rest pain or gangrene was present in 4 patients (13%). Twenty-nine patients (67%) had two block claudication, and six patients experienced claudication at more than two blocks. This last group of six patients had significant impairment of quality of life and were referred to vascular surgeons for bypass procedures.

Ten patients were active cigarette smokers at the time of excimer laser angioplasty. Nineteen patients had preprocedural color-flow Doppler (Acuson, Inc., Mountain View, Calif) for evaluation of their lower extremities. All patients had baseline ankle-brachial indices (ABI) prior to angioplasty. The mean ABI was 0.62 ± 0.10 (range, 0.41 to 0.75). All patients had diagnostic angiography to document extent and severity of disease. Nine patients had stenotic lesions, and 22 had femoropopliteal occlusions. Lesion characteristics are described in Table 9–1. The mean occlusion length was 10.9 ± 9.5 cm.

The energy source used for this study was a 308-nm, 140-nanosecond (nsec), 20-Hz pulsed xenon chloride laser. This prototype device was built and designed by the Laser Physics and Materials Science Division of NASA-Jet Propulsion Laboratories.[8] After transfer to Cedars-Sinai, the device was modified for medical application. Further changes in the laser system were performed at Advanced Interventional Systems, Inc., in Irvine, Calif. The laser operates off a single-phase current 208-V line and is self-cooled. This thyratron-driven, magnetically switched laser emits a high-quality beam with a very low divergence angle. The laser output is optically relayed to a specially designed fiberoptic coupler that delivers the energy into a fiberoptic wave guide. This coupler has the ability to accommodate all the fiberoptic catheters used in this study.

The laser discussed above is an interim prototype system. A new laser operating at 308 nm at 250 nsec at 250 mJ/pulse is capable of delivering 50 Hz. This new device is entirely self-contained and has all the elements of a clinical laser unit (Fig 9–1). The problems of dealing with the xenon/hydrogen chloride gas mix have been adequately and elegantly solved through the development of a ''gas cabinet.'' This adjunct device permits very easy maintenance of the gas system in the laser.

TABLE 9–1.
Characteristics of 31 Lesions Treated With Excimer Laser Angioplasty

Stenoses	N = 9
Diameter	= 93.5% ± 4.7% (range, 85%–99%)
Occlusions	N = 22
0– 5 cm	7
6–10 cm	8
11–15 cm	4
>15 cm	3
Mean length	= 10.9 cm ± 9.5 cm (range, 3%–40%)

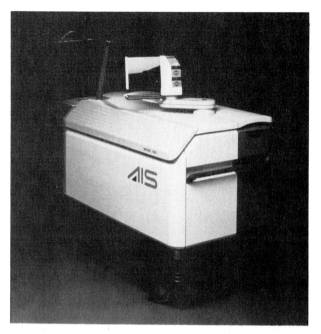

FIG 9–1.
Xenon chloride excimer laser.

CATHETER DELIVERY SYSTEMS

Extensive work in catheter and fiberoptic design has been done by our colleagues, Drs. Goldenberg and Laudenslager. In their chapters in this book, they describe the elements necessary to achieve clinical laser systems. Through their efforts, two distinct fiberoptic catheter delivery systems were developed. These prototype systems were used in this study. They are only the first developmental phase in the evolution of these devices. The first system is used exclusively for stenotic lesions. This is a 150-cm, 5 F polyethylene catheter with a centrally placed lumen for a 0.018-in. guidewire. Concentrically positioned around the guidewire lumen are seven 200-μm fibers (Fig 9–2). This catheter is front firing, and laser energy is emitted from the fiber tips and around the guidewire. For total vascular occlusions, a single laser fiber was used to create a channel through which a conventional balloon angioplasty catheter could be advanced. The 4-m-long fiberoptic has a 400-μm core and is coated with a flexible polyethylene material. The tip is modified so as to create a front-firing contact area of 1.2-mm diameter. The first 20 occlusions that were attempted incorporated this system positioned within an 8 F, multipurpose percutaneous transluminal coronary angioplasty (PTCA) guide catheter (Shiley, Inc., Irvine, Calif) as the delivery catheter. In the last two cases, a specially constructed 7 F modified PTA catheter was used (Fig 9–3). This catheter has a 2-cm-long balloon (4- to 6-mm indicated diameter) that is inflated during laser ablation for coaxial positioning of the laser fiber. This large lumen catheter permits insertion of the 1.2-mm tip fiberoptic device yet has sufficient lumen diameter to allow distal contrast injection. All laser catheter systems were calibrated to emit from 35 to 50 mJ/sq m for the procedures. Energy output was measured prior to and at the completion of each procedure.

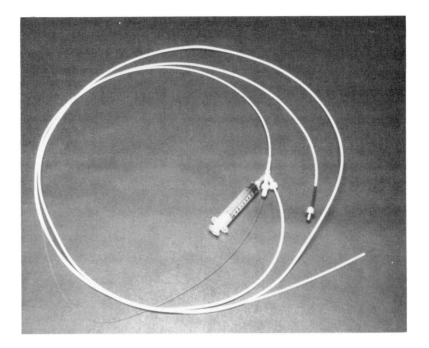

FIG 9–2.
Multifiber excimer laser angioplasty catheter.

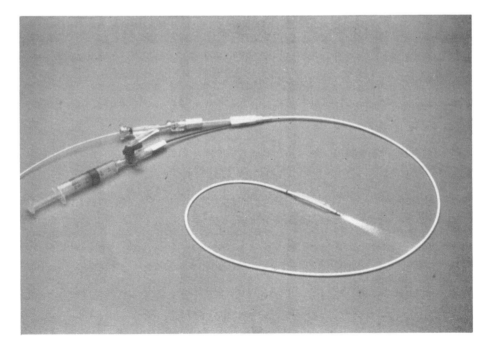

FIG 9–3.
Modified 7 F PTA catheter that permits passage of a laser fiber through the central lumen. This system ablates a 1.2-mm channel.

PROCEDURE

Thirty-one procedures were performed in 30 patients[9]; 28 were performed via percutaneous puncture of the ipsilateral femoral artery, and 3, via the contralateral femoral artery. Prior to puncture all patients were pretreated with aspirin, 325 mg/day. All procedures were performed in the Cardiac Catheterization Laboratory to take advantage of the best imaging system available in the institution. Consents were obtained from all individuals in this study using guidelines and a form approved by our Institutional Review Board, and the procedures are part of an FDA protocol to evaluate the device. Patients were given preoperative hydration and, where appropriate, hypertension was controlled using calcium channel blockers. All procedures were performed with the patients under local anesthesia with the aid of intravenous sedation with hydromorphone (Dilaudid). In all patients a baseline angiogram was performed to outline the lesion limits and determine lesion length. After determination that the lesion anatomy was appropriate for attempted excimer laser angioplasty, an 8 F introducer sheath was placed in the superficial femoral artery using standard technique and 2,500 to 7,500 units of heparin was given intravenously.

For dealing with stenoses a 0.018-in. directable guidewire (ACS, Mountain View, Calif) was advanced across the lesion under fluoroscopic control. The multifiber laser system was then passed to the proximal portion of the lesion. After confirmation of appropriate position by dye injection, laser angioplasty was begun under fluoroscopic control. The laser was activated only when the catheter is advanced. Activation of the system via a footpedal control allows precise delivery of the laser energy. The presence of blood tends to damp the effect of the laser unless the fiberoptic is in direct contact with the tissue to be ablated. This system is designed to ablate on contact. Since it is passed over a guidewire and the procedure is performed under fluoroscopic control, the catheter remains relatively coaxial with the vessel lumen. Upon recanalization of the lumen, the catheter was passed from one to five times back and forth across the lesion in an attempt to enlarge the channel. The progress of the procedure was monitored by using intermittent contrast injections through either the catheter or the sheath. The laser portion of the procedure was terminated when luminal improvement was no longer achieved by passage of the laser fiber. If the residual stenosis was greater than 50%, then balloon angioplasty was performed via standard techniques to finish the recanalization.

Treatment of total occlusions requires a different technique. Either the multipurpose guide catheter or the coaxial balloon system is advanced over a wire to the origin of the occlusion. The wire is withdrawn and replaced with a laser fiber. Under fluoroscopic control lasing is initiated, and the fiber is advanced out at the end of the catheter. In the initial segment of recanalization, repeated dye injections are made to ensure coaxial alignment of the system. Use of the balloon laser angioplasty catheter has greatly simplified this portion of the procedure and ensures the coaxial positioning of the laser fiber. When the lesion has been traversed, confirmatory angiograms are obtained and a 0.038-in. guidewire is exchanged for the laser fiber. Balloon angioplasty is then performed in the standard fashion. In noncalcified lesions laser recanalization of 40% to 70% of the original lumen is often achieved. This corresponds to a channel of 2.5 to 3.5 mm in a 5-mm vessel. Even in calcified lesions the laser fiber generates a 1.5- to 2-mm channel. Unless subintimal tracking has occurred, passage of the dilatation balloon is a relatively straightforward procedure. Final angiography is always performed to document the results. All intra-arterial sheaths were removed within 24 hours. In patients with long lesions (greater than 10 cm) and with intraluminal filling defects on x-ray films, heparinization is continued for 24 hours. In five patients it was elected to treated with oral warfarin (Coumadin) for 3 months because of significant residual luminal lucency.

Acute success is defined as a residual angiographic stenosis no greater than 50% and an ankle-brachial index increase of at least 0.5, combined with resolution of symptoms.

Restenosis is defined as recurrence of symptoms, a change in the ankle-brachial index to less than the 0.15 improvement, or a 50% loss of luminal diameter originally achieved as detected by angiography or color-flow Doppler.

Patients were followed up at 24 to 48 hours, 1 month, 2 months, 4 months, 6 months, and 1 year. At each interval, patients were seen by a team physician for evaluation of symptoms, pulses, and appearance of the leg. Ankle-brachial indices and color-flow Dopplers were obtained at the same time.

RESULTS

The procedure was successful in 7 of 9 stenotic lesions (78%). In one case, the superficial femoral artery of a 59-year-old woman was opened using 1,320 pulses at 35 mJ/sq m with the 5 F "over-the-wire" device. The lesion was taken from 85% to 10% stenosis. Of the two unsuccessful cases, one could not be completed because of thrombosis at the site of femoral artery puncture unrelated to the action of the laser, and the other case was complicated by an inability to puncture the ipsilateral femoral artery. The

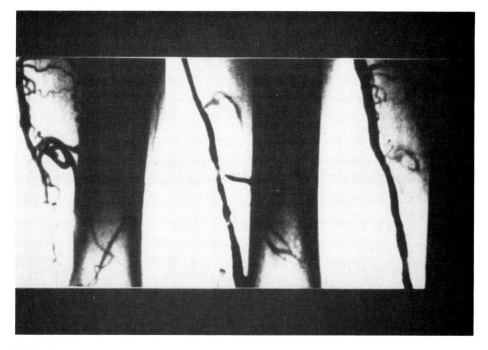

FIG 9–4.
A 57-year-old man who presented with one block claudication and a Doppler A/B ratio of 0.44. Angiography revealed a complex lesion in the midsuperficial femoral artery *(left)*. The middle figure demonstrates the results of excimer laser angioplasty using a single fiber system. The central portion of this lesion was heavily calcified. The figure on the right shows the appearance of the lesion following balloon angioplasty. The A/B ratio at one day and also at one year following the procedure was 0.88.

procedure was performed from the contralateral femoral artery and difficulty was encountered advancing the laser catheter through a femoral artery stenosis because of a tendency for the laser catheter to buckle at the aortic bifurcation. For the stenotic lesions, a mean of 1,911 ± 1,370 pulses (range, 335 to 4,676) of laser energy were used.

Initial success was achieved in 17 of 22 total occlusions (77%) (see Table 9–1). For these cases, a mean of 1,071 ± 561 (range 195 to 2,396) laser pulses were used. Failure to recanalize occurred in five cases, each time related to inability to maintain the fiber in a coaxial position with resultant subintimal tracking of the fiber without adverse clinical effect. In one of the unsuccessful attempts, a contralateral approach was attempted as a limb salvage in a 40-cm occlusion beginning at the common femoral artery and ending in the popliteal artery. Although 25 cm of femoropopliteal artery was successfully traversed, the final 15 cm could not be recanalized. Table 9–2 demonstrates results for total occlusions classified by lesion length. In occlusions less than 15 cm, success was 84% compared to an overall success of 77% including all lengths. Of note, the last two cases were successfully performed with the coaxializing balloon system. This system is particularly effective in heavily calcified lesions as it maintains the coaxial position of the fiber. In one patient, a 4-cm densely calcified occlusion required 800 pulses to achieve the last 1 cm of recanalization. Despite this prolonged lasing the fiber was held in a coaxial position, and the artery was successfully opened. Surprisingly, this calcified area dilated easily with subsequent balloon angioplasty. An additional case obtained with excimer laser angioplasty is shown (Fig 9–4).

Prior to the excimer laser procedures the mean ABI was 0.62 ± 0.10 (range, 0.41 to 0.75). After recanalization the ABI rose to a mean value of 0.86 ± 0.15 (range, 0.62 to 1.07; $P = 0.05$).

COMPLICATIONS

Four groin hematomas occurred following the procedure, perhaps in part due to aggressive heparinization and antiplatelet therapy. One diabetic patient developed transient renal failure that resolved spontaneously without the need for hemodialysis. Only one patient suffered an embolus. This embolus occurred at the time of passage of a 6-mm balloon catheter through a freshly recanalized segment of artery. An 8 F multipurpose PTCA guide catheter was advanced into the infrageniculate popliteal artery, and under fluoroscopic control a suction embolectomy successfully removed the atheroma. One patient developed an acute thrombosis of the proximal superficial femoral artery at the site of sheath insertion. This patient required femoropopliteal bypass grafting. One patient not receiving aspirin therapy developed an acute thrombosis 12 hours after recanalization of a 15-cm occlusion. Over the next 24 hours, infusion of 1.5 million units of intra-arterial urokinase successfully lysed the thrombus, and the patient is currently asymptomatic at 14 months.

FOLLOW-UP RESULTS

Of all the patients in whom angiographic success was achieved, all but one became asymptomatic. Despite successful recanalization of a long occlusion in the superficial femoral artery of an 85-year-old woman, persistent advanced gangrene of the foot and

TABLE 9–2.
Acute Success Classified by Lesion Length

Lesion Length, cm	No. (%)	
Occlusions		
0– 5	6/7	(86)
0–10	7/8	(88)
11–15	3/4	(75)
⟩15	1/3	(33)
Total	17/22	(77)

ankle eventually necessitated below-the-knee amputation. At a follow-up of 9.1 months ± 3 months, seven patients (28%) had developed restenosis. Table 9–3 describes the characteristics of these restenotic lesions. Of the four restenotic lesions in the total occlusion group, none was totally occlusive when discovered at follow-up. All of these lesions were successfully dilated with conventional balloon angioplasty techniques and remained patent. Of the original stenotic lesions that ultimately restenosed, two required bypass surgery and one was managed medically.

DISCUSSION

This chapter describes our initial experience with 308-nm excimer laser angioplasty. Due to the small numbers and the prototype nature of the catheter systems, conclusions from this study must be drawn carefully. Our initial success rate of 83% in all occlusions less than 15 cm is in part due to the ability of this system to ablate calcified material. We believe that we have achieved at least a partial solution to the problem of coaxial positioning of the fiberoptic element through the use of the coaxializing balloon. Our preliminary experience with this system is exciting and suggests that success rates of 90% to 95% should be possible in occlusive femoropopliteal lesions from 0 to 15 cm in length. In no patient was recanalization unsuccessful because of the inability to advance the laser fiber catheter through a hard or calcific occlusion.

Complications discussed above were largely procedural in nature and not related to the process of excimer laser angioplasty. The risk of embolization (3% in our study) is likely to be a significant hazard when recanalizing long occlusions. Although the incidence of this complication appears low, the potential for disastrous sequelae (amputation) is present. Inability to remove an embolus from a single vessel that is the only blood supply to the leg might well result in amputation. Therefore, we are excluding patients with single vessel infrageniculate run-off. Interestingly, subintimal tracking of the fiberoptic system occurred in five patients without clinical sequelae. Potential solutions for this problem, including both coaxializing balloon catheters and steerable catheters, are under development.

Careful follow-up of these patients tends to alert the physician to restenosis before symptoms appear. Aggressive intervention at this time usually leads to a successful balloon angioplasty of the recurrent lesion. Thus, of the 17 successfully treated total occlusions, all are currently patent.

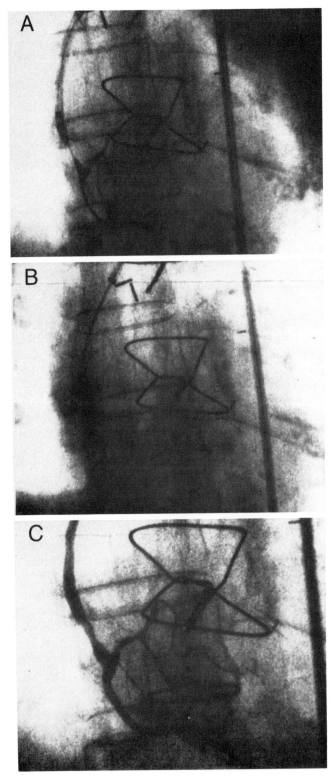

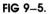

FIG 9–5.
Angiographic appearance of the subtotal occlusion of the saphenous vein graft at the previously dilated site (**A**). Excimer laser angioplasty reduced the stenosis to approximately 30% (**B**), and the patient has remained asymptomatic for 2 months following balloon angioplasty of the residual lesion (**C**).

CORONARY EXCIMER LASER ANGIOPLASTY

Recently, we have commenced a clinical trial using 308-nm percutaneous coronary excimer laser angioplasty.[10] To date, we have been successful in 12 of 16 attempted excimer laser coronary angioplasties. The device used is a 5 F polyethylene catheter consisting of the 12- to 200-μm fiber system concentrically arranged around the guidewire lumen. The use of the multiple fiber system allows a large area of plaque ablation without sacrifice of catheter flexibility. This catheter is front firing and contact dependent. Preclinical work using a porcine model has demonstrated that the over-the-wire system can safely track through tortuous coronary segments without inducing vascular perforation.[11] Figure 9–5 demonstrates the coronary angiograms from the first patient successfully treated with percutaneous coronary excimer laser angioplasty. This 85-year-old woman had two previous bypass surgeries and three balloon angioplasty procedures in the saphenous vein graft to her right coronary artery. She had restenosed after the first two balloon angioplasties within 3 months and on the current admission presented with sudden cardiac death. Angiography revealed a subtotal occlusion of the saphenous vein graft at the previously dilated site (see Fig 9–5). Excimer laser angioplasty was performed with the 12- to 200-μm fiber system at 40 mJ/sq m. After a total of 550 pulses, a residual stenosis of approximately 30% was obtained (see Fig 9–5,B). Follow-up balloon angioplasty was performed, and the patient has remained asymptomatic to this time (2 months) (see Fig 9–5,C). Further device modification is required to provide catheters with larger areas of ablation such that plaque debulking can be performed with the excimer laser without the requirement for adjunctive balloon angioplasty.

The combination of the new excimer laser previously described and the development of more sophisticated multifiber systems (Plate 12) that allow access to distal coronary and peripheral vessels with concomitant incorporation of spectroscopic guidance mechanisms should permit further advances in the development of clinically viable excimer laser angioplasty systems.

TABLE 9–3.
Description of Seven Patients Who Developed Restenosis

Lesion	Restenosis
Original stenoses	
1 below knee 99% (Proximal PTA-related SFA restenosis)	50% (laser only)
1 SFA* (3 mm) 90%	10% (laser and balloon)
1 SFA* (6 mm) 90%	10% (laser only)
Total	3/7
Original occlusions	
0– 5 cm	1/6
6–10 cm	1/7 (tip detachment)
11–15 cm	1/3
>15 cm	1/1
Total	4/17
*SFA = superficial femoral artery.	

REFERENCES

1. Grundfest WS, Litvack F, Morgenstern L, et al: Effect of excimer laser irradiation on human atherosclerotic aorta: Amelioration of laser-induced thermal damage. *IEEE-CLEEO Technical Digest* 1984; 248–249.
2. Singleton DL, Paraskevopoulos G, Jolly GS, et al: Excimer lasers in cardiovascular surgery: Ablation products and photoacoustic spectrum of arterial wall. *App Phys Lett* 1986; 48:878–880.
3. Srinivasan R: Ablation of polymers and biological tissue by ultraviolet lasers. *Science* 1986; 234:559–565.
4. Srinivasan R, Braren B, Dreyfus RW, et al: Mechanism of the ultraviolet laser ablation of polymethylate at 193 and 248 nm: Laser-induced fluorescence analysis, chemical analysis, and doping studies. *J Opt Soc Am (B)* 1986; 3:785–791.
5. Grundfest WS, Litvack F, Doyle L, et al: Comparison of in vitro and in vivo thermal effects of argon and excimer lasers for laser angioplasty, abstracted. *Circulation* 1986; 74(suppl 2):204.
6. Litvack F, Doyle L, Grundfest W, et al: In vivo excimer laser ablation: Acute and chronic effects on canine aorta, abstracted. *Circulation* 1986; 74(suppl 2):204.
7. Heme H, et al: Action of 308 mm pulsed light on dental enamel. *Calif Dental J,* in press.
8. Pacala TJ, McDermid IS, Laudenslager JB: Ultranarrow linewidth, magnetically switched, long pulse, xenon chloride laser. *Appl Phys Lett* 1984; 44:658–660.
9. Litvack F, Grundfest WS, Adler L, et al: Percutaneous excimer laser angioplasty of the lower extremities: Results of an initial clinical trial. *Radiology,* in press.
10. Litvack F, Grundfest WS, Segalowitz J, et al: Interventional cardiovascular therapy by laser and thermal angioplasty. *Circulation,* in press.
11. Grundfest WS, Litvack F, Goldenberg T, et al: Optical fibers in medicine III: Fiber imaging: New developments in angioscopy. *Proc SPIE* 88, Jan 10–17, 1988.

Chapter 10

Alternative Laser and Thermal Angioplasty Devices

Rodney A. White, M.D.

Warren S. Grundfest, M.D.

Initial clinical successes of laser angioplasty systems have encouraged the rapid development of additional prototype devices. This chapter briefly reviews alternative thermal and laser angioplasty devices that may not have been covered in preceding chapters and describes the current status of each system.

NONLASER THERMAL HOT-TIP ANGIOPLASTY

Following selection of the target, control of thermal injury and precise control of the ablative process are essential for successful angioplasty. Although there are a variety of solutions for laser angioplasty, including pulsed lasers and multiple fibers, the simplest solution thus far is the so-called hot-tip. The hot-tip, as first described by Sanborn, is a metal cap on the end of an optical fiber as opposed to a bare fiber. The metal cap rounded the edges of the fiber and reduced the rate of perforation. In a rabbit atherosclerotic model, Sanborn et al. were able to show that, as opposed to free argon laser energy emitted from a bare fiber, which makes a localized point injury with overlying thrombus, the hot-tip generated a circumferential injury.[1] The circumferential distribution of the heat allowed more precise delivery of the energy and therefore a lower perforation range. Newer hot-tip devices have improved efficacy because of olive-shaped tip configurations. In the initial series of 124 patients, Sanborn et al. achieved an overall 80% success rate, which is quite remarkable for the first clinical evaluation of a new device.[2]

However, using a $90,000 laser to generate the energy required to produce a hot-tip is a very expensive method to generate heat. Thus, several investigators have begun to evaluate other, more cost-effective power sources, with radiofrequency, electrical, and chemical systems being promising alternatives. Radiofrequency devices are potentially appealing because of lower cost, small portable size, and operation by conventional electric power. Theoretically the units could be air cooled and be solid-state design requiring minimal maintenance. Advanced Interventional Systems (Irvine, Calif.) has developed a radiofrequency generator that operates at 50 MHz and delivers up to 60 W via a coaxial cable into a metal-tipped catheter. Conversion of the radiofrequency energy to heat takes place entirely within the catheter tip. This device was tested at Cedars-Sinai Medical Center in an animal model that simulates human atherosclerotic disease typical of the superficial femoral artery. The model is prepared by embolizing autogenous fat wrapped in Gelfoam through a catheter introduced percutaneously into the vessel. The femoro-popliteal or iliac occlusions are matured over 3 to 6 months, resulting in firm, fibrotic lesions similar to those seen in noncalcified occlusions of the femoropopliteal arteries.[3] Lesions that contain calcifications can be produced by adding calcium sulfate to the embolized material. Following preparation of the lesions, thermal angioplasty was performed on the occlusions. Thirty-five animals were prepared in this fashion, creating 76 lesions in the femoropopliteal distribution.

The initial radiofrequency catheters were developed with a brass tip. Brass was chosen due to its low cost and easy machinability; however, the device frequently stuck to the vessel wall, resulting in perforation (four out of nine arteries). A silver-tipped device also had a significant perforation rate (3 out of 12 arteries). Measurements of the thermal rise time showed that these metals conducted heat slowly. Gold ultimately proved to be the best tip material because of improved conductivity. Using a 2.3-mm gold device, there were no perforations in 15 arterial recanalizations.

The tip size was determined by concomitant research that demonstrated that a 1:2 catheter tip-to-artery diameter ratio is optimal when the artery is 2 mm. As the vessel diameter increases to 3 mm, a ratio of 3:2 has been found to be appropriate. In vessels less than 6 mm and greater than 2 mm in diameter, the investigators found that the 3:2 ratio of vessel diameter-to-probe size is a reliable guide. In larger arteries the medial layer is thicker and the risk of perforation is less. In small vessels, the ability of the relatively thin arterial wall media to insulate the external elastic lamina from thermal damage is limited. Vaporization of the media invariably leads to perforation.

The first radiofrequency thermal angioplasty systems were activated by footpedal controls and achieved temperatures of 550°C at 60 W with a variety of catheter sizes. In subsequent experiments it was found that smaller, battery-powered units provided adequate energy (Plate 13). Battery-powered devices are inherently safer, since there is no direct contact between an electrical outlet and the patient. With 40 W of energy, the gold-tipped devices easily achieve 400°C. The current generation of catheters have a high temperature plastic coating that is in contact with the gold tip (Plate 14). The plastic insulation limits the axial temperature of the shaft to 90°C. In contrast, the metal connectors required to attach the laser-based hot tips to the fiberoptics can attain temperatures similar to the tip itself. This may result in excessive heating of the adjacent arterial wall.

Using an AGA infrared thermal camera and Omega rapid-response thermistors, the investigators at Cedars-Sinai examined the thermal profiles of both the argon laser-based and radiofrequency hot tips. Tissue in the proximity of comparably sized argon laser–energized hot-tips reaches approximately 136°C when the tips are passed through muscle. Similarly, radiofrequency hot-tips produce identical temperatures of 136°C (variance 107°C to 268°C) depending upon the test circumstances.[4] Temperature of the radiofrequency (RF) device rises rapidly (in air) and reaches a maximum temperature within 2 seconds. The radiofrequency catheter is designed to reach a predetermined maximum temperature and then shut off until the temperature falls below this level. A family of catheters set at various maximum temperatures is envisioned. At present, 350°C has been chosen as the maximum temperature.

On the basis of preliminary work, the Cedars-Sinai group began a collaborative clinical effort with Prof. Rothe at the Agerthal Clinic in West Germany. Initially five patients with total femoropopliteal occlusions of 4 to 17 cm in length were chosen for therapy. In four of these patients (80%), a successful recanalization of the occlusion was achieved.[5] In one case (the 4-cm occlusion), severe calcification prevented passage of the device. This occlusion was impervious to traditional wire and balloon methods as well.

Figure 10–1 demonstrates treatment of a 9-cm femoropopliteal occlusion in a 46-year-old patient with an ankle-brachial index of 0.47. Using standard angiographic techniques, an 8 F sheath was placed in the common femoral artery, and the patient was given 3,000 units of heparin. Under fluoroscopic guidance, the hot-tipped catheter was advanced to the point of occlusion. The device was energized and under gentle pressure was passed through the lesion in 13 seconds. Following the procedure the ankle-brachial index was 0.98. At 1-year follow-up the patient is asymptomatic with an ankle-brachial index of 0.97.

Subsequent FDA approval for clinical trials in the United States and additional patients (added through the efforts of Dr. Frederick Mohr of the University of Bonn, West Germany, and investigators in Canada and Australia) have led to more than 60 patients having been treated with this new device, with the initial success rate of approximately 75%. It should be noted that this device is not effective against calcified lesions. Case selection plays a major role in the successful outcome of the procedures. The rate of successful recanalizations is obviously dependent on lesion length and location. In our experience occlusions are recanalized quickly as long as they are noncalcified and in relatively large vessels (larger than 4 mm in diameter). To date, all radiofrequency recanalizations have been followed by balloon angioplasty.

In conclusion, the radiofrequency hot-tip device recanalizes occluded arterial lesions similar to laser devices and is a simple alternative to laser hot-tip systems.[6] Investigation of an electric thermal probe has recently been abandoned because of difficulties in controlling the maximum temperature.[7] An additional alternative is a hot-tip catheter system energized using chemical energy.[8] This prototype system has a metal probe that contains a particle of palladium that catalyzes an exothermic reaction between oxygen and hydrogen, generating high temperatures that are precisely controlled by adjusting gas flow.

ALTERNATIVE FREE-LASER ANGIOPLASTY SYSTEMS

Many investigators and manufacturers have attempted to improve the guidance of free-laser systems to improve the precision of ablation and help prevent perforations. One modification uses a pulsed Nd:YAG laser energy through a fiber positioned parallel to, but at a fixed distance from, the central guidewire. The catheter rotates the laser in a circle so that it affects a larger area. This laser catheter has been used in 14 patients with superficial femoral, popliteal, and tibial arterial stenosis and in 5 superficial femoral occlusions by Heintzen et al. of the University of Dusseldorf, West Germany.[9] Despite a reduction in the mean stenosis diameter from 91% to 30%, subsequent balloon dilatation was needed.

An excimer laser catheter (designed by Vaser, Inc., Indianapolis) functions in a fashion similar to the German device and features an occlusive balloon that aligns the fiber on an axis parallel to the vessel lumen. The catheter is rotated around a central axis while blood is irrigated from the field. Katzen et al. have reported on 22 patients with peripheral vascular lesions who were treated with a 351-nm excimer laser angioplasty

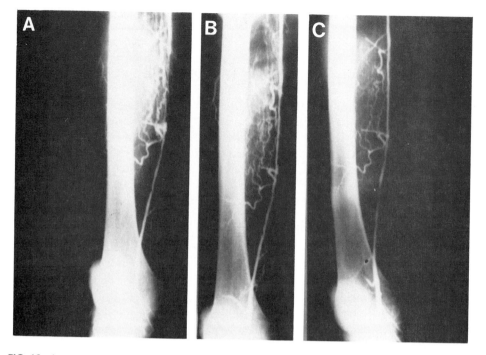

FIG 10–1.
A 46-year-old man who presented with a history of 1-block claudication. Angiography revealed a 9-cm midsuperficial femoral artery occlusion (**A**). A 2.3-mm gold-tipped RF hot-tip was used at 20 W and recanalized the lesion in 13 seconds (**B**). Results following balloon angioplasty are demonstrated (**C**). Following the procedure Doppler A/B ratio was 0.98.

device and a 6 F catheter suitable for both stenotic and occlusive lesions.[10] Laser ablation of plaque was combined with continuous suction to withdraw particulate debris. Successful plaque ablation sufficient to avoid adjunctive balloon angioplasty was achieved in 10 out of 12 patients and successful recanalization of occlusions was achieved in 9 out of 10 patients. A percutaneous atherectomy performed after one of the excimer procedures revealed no evidence of thermal injury.

A dilatation balloon with an argon laser fiber running through its core (LASTAC, GV Medical, Minneapolis) has been investigated by Dr. Leonard A. Nordstrom of Methodist Hospital, Minneapolis.[11] The balloon aligns the laser fiber coaxially in the vessel and stops blood flow to avoid blood absorption of the beam; it then enters the lased opening to dilate the artery. The laser fiber has been used against 20 occlusions and 14 stenoses in the superficial femoral artery (SFA) and iliac artery; one perforation occurred, with no sequelae. Ballooning followed in 32 patients, and 23 arteries remained patent during follow-ups lasting up to 9 months.

Target-specific laser angioplasty may become possible by analysis of the emitted fluorescent pattern from various tissues to differentiate normal from atherosclerotic tissue.[12] A dual laser catheter system controlled by a computer uses a signal from a lower-power 325-nm–induced fluorescence in the vessel wall. If the computer recognizes the unique spectroscopic pattern of atheroma, rather than of healthy tissue, it permits a second, higher-power laser to fire. This so-called smart laser (MCM Laboratories, Mountain View, Calif), used on chronic, total peripheral occlusions in approximately 35 patients, created a tiny channel that was enlarged with a balloon.[13]

The ablative laser for this system is a pulsed dye laser operating at 480 nm. Leon et al.[13] and Geschwind et al.[14] reported on the first 36 lesions in 35 patients treated with the MCM system. In the patient population studied, seven occlusions (20%) were treated with conventional guidewire-based balloon angioplasty technique. In the remaining 29 lesions in 29 patients, laser recanalization of total occlusions was attempted following inability to advance a guidewire. The average lesion length was 7.1 cm (range, 0.1 to 50 cm). The laser was delivered through a 200-μ fiber and successfully traversed 90% of these lesions. However, the channel was so small that successful balloon angioplasty was possible only in 21 of 29 patients. The majority of failures have been in heavily calcified lesions. Of 27 patients with successful primary laser recanalization, there were 6 perforations (21%) and 6 dissections (21%), while none of these complications were associated with clinical problems. The smart laser's fluorescent feedback depends upon being able to discriminate between healthy tissue and atheroma. Preliminary investigations have demonstrated the feasibility of in vivo fluorescence spectroscopic analysis of plaque. The perforation rate of 20% would imply that although this first system is promising, significant improvements in discriminatory ability and guidance systems are required. Inadequate guidance has also been proposed to be the cause of premature termination of the laser energy by the computer control when the catheter migrates away from the vascular lumen.

The use of laser-induced fluorescence as a guidance system may be limited to non-thermal ablative lasers. Specifically, ablation by argon, yttrium-aluminum-garnet (YAG), and carbon dioxide (CO_2) lasers changes the chemical nature of the arterial wall, thus altering the tissue's spectral characteristics.[15] The combination of thermal ablation and laser-induced fluorescence may therefore not be possible.

LASER HEATING DURING BALLOON DILATATION

Laser heating through the wall of a balloon during balloon dilatation is being evaluated as a method to weld or seal tears of the wall following dilatation.[16] Experimentally, aortic dissections have been irradiated with low-power neodymium:yttrium-aluminum-garnet (Nd:YAG) energy to seal the layers by the combination of laser heating and balloon pressure. A laser balloon angioplasty system developed by Dr. J. Richard Spears of Harper Hospital and Wayne State University, Detroit, features conventional balloon angioplasty followed by laser irradiation to a depth of 2 to 3 mm of the artery during a final balloon expansion. In this device, Nd:YAG laser energy is passed through an ultrathin central fiber and is transmitted through the balloon (Spears Laser Balloon, USCI, Billerica, Mass), entering the lesion as heat. Animal[17, 18] and cadaver[19] studies indicate that laser balloon angioplasty (LBA) decreases vessel elasticity at the treatment site, heat-molding and firming the arterial segment at about the size and shape of the balloon at final dilatation. Spears and Sinclair et al. have demonstrated that temperatures between 85° and 140°C consistently welded aortic separations effectively.[20, 21] It may also destroy smooth muscle cells that proliferate in response to injury, thereby discouraging restenosis.[22]

Initial trials of LBA have been started in the coronary arteries. To date 15 patients have received the LBA treatment. Complications have included severe arrhythmias, cardiac arrest, and infarctions. Also of note was the intense pain felt by the patient during irradiation. This has led to the use of general anesthesia during the procedure. In the first 15 patients, a restenosis rate of 33% was reported, although follow-up is not completed. At present, the role of this technique remains undefined.

SAPPHIRE-TIPPED DEVICES

Sapphire-tipped contact probes combine features of bare-fiber lasing with several of the advantages of thermal angioplasty and may be useful in creating wider channels. The sapphire tip permits generation of high temperatures at the tip/tissue interface. Sapphire is highly resistant to thermal damage and does not melt at the ablative temperatures achieved during laser angioplasty. Cooling by a saline infusion is required to prevent excessive thermal injury to adjacent arterial wall structures. The laser energy may be focused or diverged, depending on the shape of the sapphire lens. A large divergent angle of the beam allows rapid decrease in power density at a distance from the fiber, thus confining the ablative effects to a region quite close to the contact tip.[23] Initial clinical success has been reported in a small number of patients.[24-27] In initial studies, restenosis rates of 20% to 40% have been reported.

REFERENCES

1. Sanborn TA, Faxon DP, Haudenschild CC, et al: Experimental angioplasty: Circumferential distribution of laser thermal injury with a laser probe. *J Am Coll Cardiol* 1985; 5:934–938.
2. Sanborn TA, Cumberland DC, Greenfield AJ, et al: Percutaneous laser thermal angioplasty: Initial results and 1-year follow-up in 129 femoropopliteal lesions. *Radiology* 1988; 168:121–125.
3. Doyle L, Litvack F, Grundfest WS, et al: An in vivo model for testing laser angioplasty systems. *Circulation* 1986; 74(suppl 2):361.
4. Litvack F, et al: Percutaneous "hot tip" angioplasty in man by a radiofrequency catheter system, abstracted. *J Am Coll Cardiol* 1988; 11:103A.
5. Grundfest WS, Litvack F, Hickey A, et al: Radiofrequency thermal angioplasty for the treatment of peripheral vascular occlusive disease: Preliminary results of a clinical trial. *J Am Coll Cardiol,* in press.
6. Litvack F, Grundfest WS, Segalowitz J, et al: Interventional cardiovascular therapy by laser and thermal angioplasty. *Circulation,* in press.
7. Lu DY, et al: Electric thermal angioplasty: Catheter design features, in vitro tissue ablation studies and in vivo experimental findings. *Am J Cardiol* 1987; 9:187A.
8. Lu DY, et al: A prototype catalytic thermal tip catheter: Design parameter and in vitro tissue studies, abstract. *J Am Coll Cardiol* 1987; 9:187A.
9. Heintzen MP, et al: Percutaneous peripheral laser angioplasty by a novel bare fiber catheter: Initial clinical results, abstract. *Circulation* 1987; 76:IV–231.
10. Katzen, et al: Initial experience with an excimer laser in peripheral lesions. *Circulation* 1988; 78(suppl 2):417.
11. Nordstrom LA, Castaneda-Zuniga WR, Lindeke CC, et al: Laser angioplasty: Controlled delivery of argon laser energy. *Radiology* 1988; 167:463–465.
12. Sartori MP, Bossaller C, Weilbacher D, et al: Detection of atherosclerotic plaques and characterization of arterial wall structure by laser induced fluorescence, abstracted. *Circulation* 1986; 74(suppl 2):7.
13. Leon MB, et al: Human arterial surface fluorescence: Atherosclerotic plaque identification and effects of laser atheroma ablation. *J Am Coll Cardiol* 1988; 12:94.
14. Geschwind HJ, et al: Percutaneous pulsed laser angioplasty with atheroma detection in humans, abstract. *J Am Coll Cardiol* 1988; 11:107A.
15. Chaudhry H, et al: Alteration of artery wall fluorescence due to excessive laser irradiation. *J Am Coll Cardiol* 1988; 11:49A.
16. Hiehle JF, Bourgelais DBC, Shapshay S, et al: Nd-YAG laser fusion of human atheromatous plaque-arterial wall separations in vitro. *Am J Cardiol* 1985; 56:953–957.

17. Jenkins RD, et al: Laser balloon angioplasty vs. balloon angioplasty in normal rabbit iliac arteries, abstract. *Circulation* 1987; 76:IV–47.
18. Sinclair IN, et al: Effect of laser balloon angioplasty on normal dog coronary arteries in vivo, abstract. *J Am Coll Cardiol* 1988; 11:108A.
19. Jenkins RD, et al: Laser balloon angioplasty: Effect of exposure duration on shear strength of welded layers of postmortem human aorta, abstract. *Circulation* 1987; 76:IV–46.
20. Spears JR: Percutaneous laser treatment of atherosclerosis: An overview of emerging techniques. *Cardiovasc Intervent Radiol* 1985; 9:303–312.
21. Sinclair IN, Anand R, Spears JR: Laser balloon angioplasty: Thermal profile for in vitro welding of neointimal arterial separations, abstract. *J Am Coll Cardiol* 1987; 9:105A.
22. Spears JR: Percutaneous transluminal coronary angioplasty restenosis: Potential prevention with laser balloon angioplasty. *Am J Cardiol* 1987; 60:61B.
23. Verdaadonk RM, Cross FW, Borst C: Physical properties of sapphire fibertips for laser angioplasty. *Lasers Med Sci* 1987; 2:183–188.
24. Fourner JL, Brunetaud JM, Prat A, et al: Percutaneous laser angioplasty with sapphire tip. *Lancet* 1987; 1:105.
25. Cross FW, Bowker TJ: Percutaneous laser angioplasty with sapphire tips. *Lancet* 1987; 1:350.
26. Fourrier JL, et al: Human percutaneous laser angioplasty with sapphire tips: Results and follow up, abstract. *Circulation* 1987; 76:IV–231.
27. Geschwind HJ, et al: Efficiency and safety of optically modified fiber tips for laser angioplasty. *J Am Coll Cardiol* 1987; 10:655.

Chapter 11

Laser-Assisted Vascular Anastomoses*

Rodney A. White, M.D.

George E. Kopchok, B. S.

Geoffrey H. White, M.D.

Roy M. Fujitani, M.D.

Jerry W. Vlasak, M.D.

Louann W. Murray, Ph.D.

Shi-Kaung Peng, M.D., Ph.D.

Vascular surgery has developed rapidly as a specialized field over the past 30 years. Many of the advances have relied on development of blood-compatible, synthetic polymers for use as suture and prosthetic materials. Current areas of development in the repair of vascular lesions with a smaller internal diameter require miniaturization of sutures, needles, prosthetic materials, and instruments to yield continued satisfactory results. Development of an expedient nonsuture technique for repairing arterial lesions and making anastomoses would be cost-effective and time-effective, would reduce the technical difficulty of procedures, and would improve the quality of patient care. Ideally, new technology would extend to smaller vessels, would reduce the trauma of surgery, and would enhance the healing to alleviate many long-term complications, such as mechanical mismatch and myointimal hyperplasia.

Preliminary experimental and clinical testing have shown that laser tissue fusion has possible specific advantages over conventional suture methods, such as healing without foreign-body reaction, better compliance, and limited intimal hyperplasia at anastomoses. The technique is currently limited by: (1) a lack of understanding of the biologic mechanism of laser tissue fusion; (2) inadequate knowledge of the independent laser parameters

*The experimental work described in this chapter was supported in part by PHS grant HL-32622 from the National Institutes of Health.

(i.e., wavelength, energy fluence, etc.) required to make fusions with maximal strengths in the shortest time interval; (3) inadequate fusions approximately 20% to 25% of the time, requiring sutures to maintain hemostasis; (4) a limited length (0.5 to 1.0 cm) over which fusions can be made reliably between aligning sutures; and (5) false aneurysms that have been noted to occur on a long-term basis with some types of laser fusions, in particular, those formed with the carbon dioxide (CO_2) laser.

This chapter reviews the current status of laser vascular tissue fusion and identifies the areas that require investigation before this technology can be adapted to clinical practice.

TECHNIQUE

Vascular tissue fusion or welding by lasers is performed by directing low-power, continuous wave laser energy at the opposed edges of the repair. The energy is applied by moving the beam back and forth along the fusion line or in certain cases by delivering the energy by "spot" application. Vessel sealing is apparent to the trained eye in the majority of instances, as is nonunion caused by inadequate energy delivery, tissue coagulation or vaporization from excessive exposure. Laser repairs can be fashioned in time intervals comparable to or slightly longer than those required for suture repairs.

LASER FUSION OF MICROVESSELS

The CO_2, neodymium:yttrium-aluminum-garnet (Nd:YAG) (1,060 and 1,320-nm), and argon laser welds in microvessels have adequate tensile strength compared to sutured wounds.[1-3] Frazier et al. performed microvascular anastomoses of femoral arteries in growing miniswine and reported that CO_2 laser anastomoses grew normally in diameter while sutured controls had restricted growth.[4] McCarthy et al. reported patency comparable to sutured repairs and 22% aneurysms at 1 year in rabbit carotid artery anastomoses made with the CO_2 laser at 60 to 70 mW power.[5] Other investigators have noted that the aneurysms observed for CO_2 repairs have not been apparent in fusions made using different laser parameters and tissue alignment techniques.[1-3, 6]

LASER FUSION OF MEDIUM-SIZED VESSELS

Experiments performed in our laboratory demonstrated that CO_2, Nd:YAG (1.06 um), and argon lasers can all be used to seal longitudinal openings in 6- to 8-mm internal diameter canine femoral and jugular veins.[7, 8] Using 1-W power over 25 seconds for CO_2, 1 W over 40 seconds for Nd:YAG (1.06 μm), and 0.5 W over 240 seconds for argon laser, 2-cm long venotomies were fused. All repairs were patent at 1 to 4 weeks without evidence of aneurysms or luminal narrowing. Laser repair of venotomies were compared to suture controls and found to have similar healing by biochemical analysis and tensile strength determinations. Histologic examination of the sutured wounds had granulomatous reaction around the sutures with areas of excessive collagen accumulation. In contrast, the laser-welded wounds had minimal inflammatory response and near normal collagen content, with minimal residual disorientation and breaks in the elastic fiber continuity (Fig 11–1).

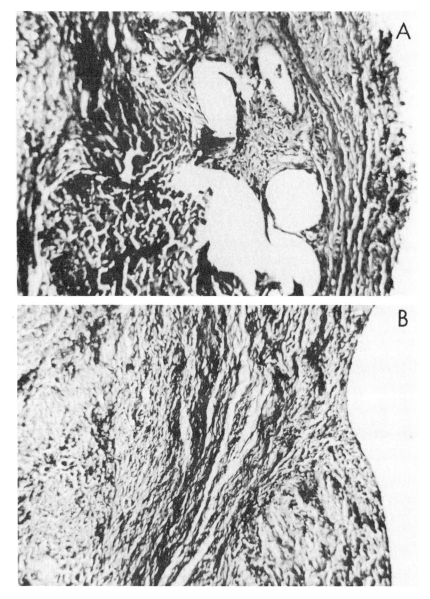

FIG 11–1.
Histologic appearance of sutured and Nd:YAG laser-welded venotomies at 5 weeks. Sutured wounds
(A) had granulomatous reaction around the sutures, areas of excessive collagen accumulation, and
a broad gap in elastin continuity, whereas laser welds **(B)** had near-normal vein architecture (Verhoeff–van Gieson's stain; × 100). (From White RA, Abergel RP, Lyons R, et al: Laser welding–An
alternative method of venous repair. *J Surg Res* 1986; 41:260–263. Used by permission.)

Laser welding of medium-sized arteries (>3 mm) that are pulsatile and have intraluminal pressures of 100 to 150 mm Hg presents several unique problems. In initial
canine studies we have observed that the CO_2 laser did not produce seals that could
withstand larger diameter arterial pressure. The Nd:YAG (1.06 μm) laser welds in large
arteries were initially successful, but the majority failed within 20 to 40 minutes. In

contrast, the argon laser uniformly sealed 2-cm long arteriotomies that healed rapidly within 4 to 6 weeks.[9]

An additional study compared the histology, tensile strength, and collagen synthesis of welded and sutured arteriotomies performed with the argon laser.[10] Bilateral canine femoral or carotid arteries (2 cm in length) were evaluated at 1,2,3, and 4 weeks post-operatively, with one vessel (control) closed with interrupted 6–0 polypropylene sutures and the contralateral vessel (experimental) welded with an argon laser (0.5 W, 240-second exposure per 1-cm length of repair). Laser anastomoses required an average of 1 suture per repair, while 13 sutures per repair were used for sutured arteriotomies. At removal, all experimental closures were patent without hematomas, aneurysms, or luminal dilatation. Histologic examination revealed that laser-welded arteriotomies have less inflammatory reaction, more normal collagen and elastin reorientation, and similar endothelial continuity when compared to that of the control, sutured wounds (Fig 11–2; Plate 15). The tensile strength of the 1- and 2-week laser specimens was less than sutured wounds and became approximately equal to sutured repairs at 3 and 4 weeks. There were no significant differences in the rate of collagen synthesis.

Based on our preliminary success using the argon laser to seal arteriotomies in medium-sized vessels, we have directed our investigations to performing vein-to-artery anastomoses.[11] The first series of experiments evaluated 2-cm long, bilateral canine femoral arteriotomies anastomosed to a venotomy in the adjacent femoral vein, thus producing arteriovenous fistulas, with one anastomosis (control) being closed with running 6–0 polypropylene sutures and the contralateral repair (experimental) welded with the argon laser. Laser welds were fashioned using 0.5-W power, 0.066-sq cm spot size, 0.3-mm fiberoptic spot, 7.6 W/sq cm power density, 1,830 J/sq cm energy fluence, and 240-second exposure time per 1 cm length of anastomosis, and 5-second pulses with 0.2-second intervals. The edges of the laser-welded arteriovenous fistulas were approximated by single 6–0 polypropylene sutures at the apexes of the incisions and by a suture at the midportion of the back and front wall of the repairs (Fig 11–3). The traction sutures were used to oppose the edges of the vessels during laser fusion. The wounds were continuously irrigated during the fusions with saline at room temperature to prevent thermal damage. In these experiments, laser welding of 10 fistulas was accomplished by sealing segments, each 1 cm long, i.e., four segments per anastomosis. Seven of the 40 laser-fused segments required one or two additional interrupted sutures to close small holes that did not fuse adequately.

Experimental and control arteriovenous fistulas were removed from 1 to 8 weeks and were evaluated by histologic examination and for tensile strength. Histologic examination of the arteriovenous repairs removed from 1 to 4 weeks were similar to those described previously for argon-laser–welded veins and arteries. At eight weeks, three sets of anastomoses demonstrated intimal hyperplasia in the sutured repairs and minimal or no abnormal finding at the luminal surface in the laser welded specimens. This finding implicates the sutures in the development of intimal lesions and suggests that laser artery-vein anastomoses may have delayed or minimized intimal hyperplastic response (Fig 11–4). The tensile strength of both sutured and laser-welded specimens was essentially equivalent from 2 to 8 weeks. The appearance of a canine femoral laser-welded arteriovenous (AV) fistula at 16 weeks is shown in Figure 11–5.

More recent work has examined vein-to-artery anastomoses in canine, reversed-vein, femoral artery bypasses.[12] One anastomosis of the vein bypasses was performed using running 6–0 polypropylene sutures, and the other anastomosis was formed using the same methodology and laser parameters described for fashioning laser-welded AV fistulas.

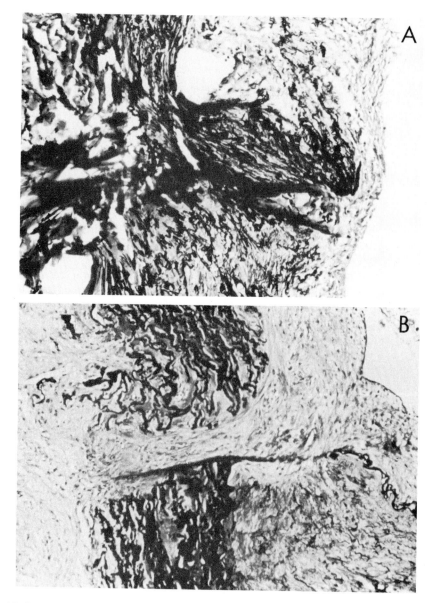

FIG 11–2.
Histologic appearance of sutured **(A)** and argon laser-welded **(B)** arteriotomies at 4 weeks. Sutured wound shows granulomatous reaction around sutures and disorientation of elastin fibers, whereas laser-welded wound has minimal foreign body response and reorienting fibers (Verhoeff–van Gieson's stain, ×100). (From White RA, Kopchok G, Abergel RP, et al: Comparison of laser-welded and sutured arteriotomies. *Arch Surg* 1986; 121:1133–1135. Used by permission.)

Laser seals have required only occasional reinforcing sutures, and patency and healing of the bypass grafts have been successful and followed up to 12 weeks. Figure 11–6 displays a laser-welded vein-artery anastomosis immediately following fusion. Figure 11–7 compares the healing of sutured and laser-fused vein-artery anastomoses at 12 weeks. This study supports the feasibility of using laser fusion to form vein-artery anastomoses if the laser technology can be shown to provide long-term improvement in healing.

An appealing addition to the laser vascular fusion technique would be elimination of the nonresorbable aligning sutures that have been used to oppose the tissue edges in the experiments that have been described. Although we would like to remove the long-term presence of the foreign-body, sutures have been found to be the most convenient method to attain alignment of the edges of the vessels during fusions and to assure the initial strength of the fusions until healing occurs. An alternative method to fulfill these needs was investigated in a study that evaluated the feasibility of forming vascular anastomoses using combined argon laser fusion and absorbable, monofilament suture (PDS, Ethicon).[13] Femoral arteriovenous fistulas 2 cm in length were created bilaterally in each of ten dogs and were studied histologically at 2, 4, 8, 16, and 24 weeks (2 animals for each interval). In each animal, one anastomosis (control) was formed with continuous 6–0 polypropylene suture and the contralateral anastomosis (experimental) was performed with an argon laser (0.5 W, 5-minute exposure, energy fluence 2,600 J/sq cm, utilizing stay sutures of 5–0 PDS at 0.5-cm intervals. At removal, all anastomoses were patent without hematomas, aneurysms, or luminal narrowing. Histologic examination at 2 and 4 weeks demonstrated persistence of suture material surrounded by a local inflammatory reaction in laser-fused specimens and a diffuse reaction to the permanent sutures in the sutured controls. At 8 and 16 weeks, there was no gross physical evidence of residual PDS suture material in experimental repairs, although on histologic examination some fragments remained, surrounded by a resolving inflammatory response. Suture control

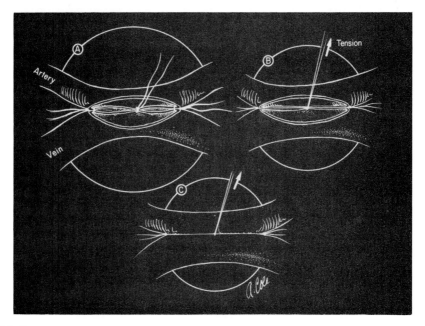

FIG 11–3.
Technique of laser welding of vein-artery anastomoses. **A**, sutures are placed at the apexes of the incisions and at the middle of the posterior wall; **B**, tension on the suture at the middle of the posterior wall opposes the edges of the repair for welding; **C**, a suture is placed in the middle of the anterior wall and opposes the edges for welding. (From White RA: Technical frontiers for the vascular surgeon: Laser vascular anastomotic welding and angioscopy-assisted intraluminal instrumentation. *J Vasc Surg* 1987; 5:673–680. Used by permission.)

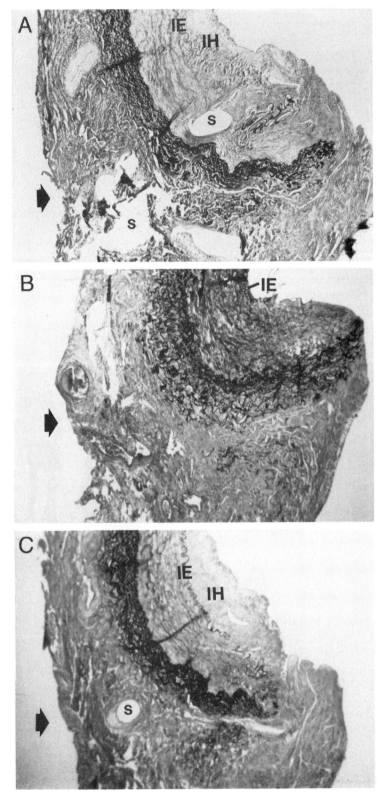

FIG 11–4.
Arteriovenous fistulas at 8 weeks: suture (**A**), argon-laser–sealed (**B**), and argon-laser–sealed at the site of a traction suture (**C**). In each illustration the artery is on the top and the vein is on the bottom. Note that sutured areas in both the suture control (**A**) and lasered specimen at the site of a traction suture (**C**) were associated with a marked intimal response. Line of artery vein fusions are marked (*arrows*); *IE* = internal elastic laminae; *IH* = intimal hyperplasia; *S* = suture holes. (Verhoeff–van Gieson's stain; ×40). (From White RA, Kopchok GE, Donayre C, et al: Argon laser-welded arteriovenous anastomoses. *J Vasc Surg* 1987; 6:447–453. Used by permission.)

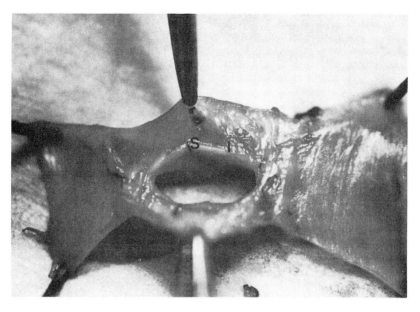

FIG 11–5.
Gross appearance of an argon-laser-welded, canine arteriovenous fistula at 16 weeks; *S* indicates traction sutures; *l*, 1-cm lengths of laser fusion.

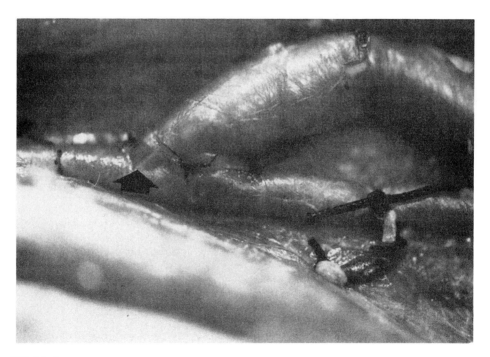

FIG 11–6.
Laser-welded vein-artery anastomosis immediately following fusion. Laser-fused segment is indicated *(arrow).* (From White RA, Kopchok GE, Donayre CE, et al: Mechanism of tissue fusion in argon laser–welded vein-artery anastomoses. *Lasers Surg Med* 1988; 8:83–89. Used by permission.)

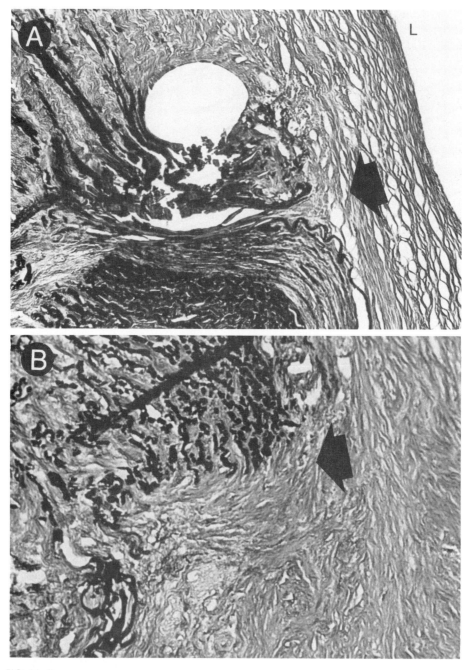

FIG 11–7.
Histology of artery-vein anastomoses at 12 weeks; sutured **(A)**, argon laser-welded **(B)**. *L* = luminal surface. The sites of vein-artery fusion are indicated *(arrows)*. Verhoeff–van Gieson's stain; × 40. (From White RA, Kopchok GE, Donayre CE, et al: Mechanism of tissue fusion in argon laser-welded vein-artery anastomoses. *Lasers Surg Med* 1988; 8:83–89. Used by permission.)

specimens at the same intervals exhibited an ongoing, foreign body response at the suture line. At 24 weeks the laser-fused specimens had no evidence of suture material at the anastomotic line and healing consisted of a bond between artery and vein wall tissues (Fig 11–8).

It is apparent from this preliminary study that we may be able to form laser fusions using biodegradable aligning sutures and eliminate the foreign body reaction that persists surrounding permanent sutures. This method may help improve the healing and long-term patency at the anastomotic site by eliminating the tissue response to permanent suture materials.

EXPERIMENTS ADDRESSING THE MECHANISM AND METHODS OF MAXIMIZING THE STRENGTH OF LASER FUSIONS

Although the majority of large vessel argon laser fusions have been successful, approximately 20% fail when exposed to systemic arterial pressures. For this reason, a series of experiments have been performed to determine the parameters that enhance the maximum strength and healing of fusions. Specimens have been examined immediately following fusions and at various intervals following fabrication by histologic examination, electron microscopy, tensile strength testing, and by measuring the formation of [³H]-hydroxyproline as an index of collagen synthesis. Ultrastructural and histologic exami-

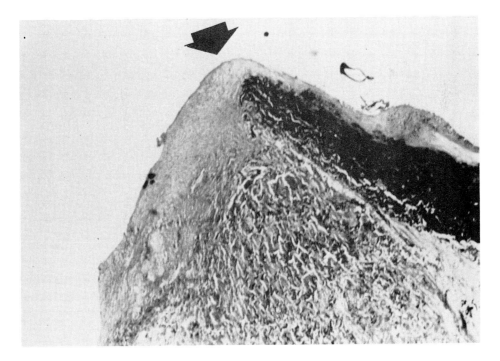

FIG 11–8.
Histology of arteriovenous anastomosis formed by a combination of argon laser-fusion and biodegradable sutures at 24 weeks. Note the absence of suture material and bonding of vein to artery wall tissues. The *arrow* indicates the site of vein-artery fusion (Verhoeff–van Gieson's stain; × 40).

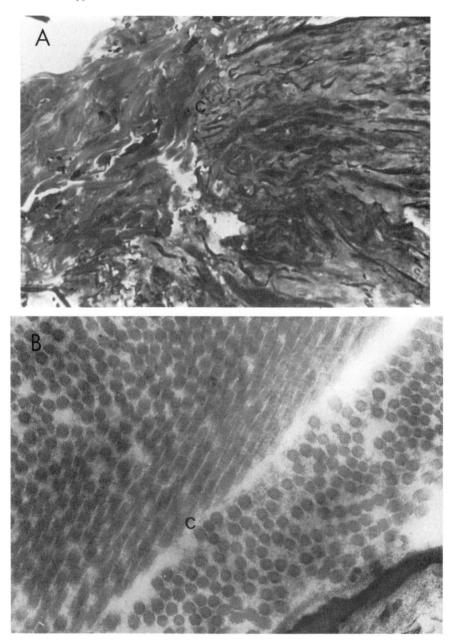

FIG 11–9.
A, histologic examination showing collagen-collagen *(C)* apposition in the media of the vessels (toluidine blue, × 100). **B,** electron micrograph of a collagen-collagen bonding *(C)* (× 27,000). (From White RA, Kopchok G, Peng S: Laser vascular welding—How does it work? *Ann Vasc Surg* 1987; 1:461–464. Used by permission.)

nation of successful laser welds immediately after they were formed showed apparent bonding of collagen to collagen and elastin to collagen[14] (Figs 11–9 and 11–10). For this reason, the precision of tissue apposition at the time of fusion is a critical parameter that affects the rate of healing and tensile strength of tissue fusions. A gap between the vessel edges or blood at the interface compromises weld strength.

An additional study was designed to determine optimal argon laser parameters for maximal strength of repairs as measured by bursting pressures.[15] Longitudinal incisions measuring either 2.5 or 5 mm in length were performed in canine femoral, carotid, and jugular veins and arteries (4 to 7 mm diameter); after placement of apical sutures for apposition, they were fused with the argon laser at 0.3, 0.5, 0.7, or 0.9 W of power. The laser beam was delivered via a 300 μm quartz fiber and at 1 cm from the vessel surface resulted in a spot size of 0.066 sq cm. Total exposure time for each repair (50 to 80 sec/0.5 cm) was adjusted to yield identical energy fluences of 1,100 J/sq cm. A continuous drip of room-temperature normal saline (1 drop/sec) was applied to the tissue during fusion for cooling. Isolated segments containing the repairs were then burst in vivo by infusion of anticoagulated blood while intraluminal pressure was continuously monitored. Mean bursting pressures for venous and arterial repairs were significantly higher in the 2.5-mm as compared to the 5-mm segments. Venous and arterial repairs of equal length performed at each power resulted in equivalent bursting strengths. However, 5-mm venous segments fused with 0.9 W withstood lower pressures than all other venous repairs and 5-mm arterial segments were in turn significantly weaker at 0.3 W. We concluded from this work that argon laser fusion is equally suitable for repair of medium-sized veins and arteries and that immediate strength decreases with increasing length of repair. To maximize strength of longer repairs, venotomies should be welded at power settings between 0.3 and 0.7 W, while arteriotomies should be fused between 0.5 and 0.9 W. These power discrepancies may be explained by different wall composition and thickness in veins and arteries. More study is required to determine optimal laser wavelength, exposure time, and energy fluence and to develop techniques for fusing incisions of increasing length.

There are conflicting opinions regarding the mechanism of fusion of vascular tissue

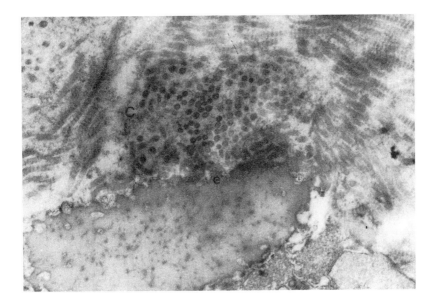

FIG 11–10.
Electron micrograph demonstrating collagen-collagen *(C)* and collagen-elastin *(e)* bonding in fusion between media of vein and adventitia of artery (× 8,000). (From White RA, Kopchok G, Peng S: Laser vascular welding—How does it work? *Ann Vasc Surg* 1987; 1:461–464. Used by permission.)

by lasers and concomitantly about the cause of failures due to weak seals or formation of anastomotic aneurysms. In order to address the etiology of these failures, we have performed additional experiments to examine the thermal and thrombogenic aspects of argon laser fused and sutured repairs. The first group of experiments examined the independent effect of tissue temperature on fusions produced by argon laser welding of femoral and carotid arteriovenous fistulas.[16, 17] Detailed analysis of the thermal images recorded using a digital thermographic camera revealed that the maximal and mean temperatures of the tissues increased with greater laser power. We have found that the rise in tissue temperature can be limited by saline irrigation, as cooling to 37°C occurs with each drop of saline irrigation. Of the welds performed using powers of 0.50, 0.75, and 1.00 W and saline irrigation, the 0.50- and 0.75-W fusions were all successful with temperatures of 44.2° ± 1.6°C and 55.0° ± 3.6°C, with maximal temperatures of 47.9° and 59.9°C, respectively (Plate 16). At 1 W, the tissue was desiccated and the welds disrupted when exposed to blood flow with temperatures measured at 63.7 ± 10.0°C and maximum of 88.0°C. Of the welds attempted without saline irrigation at 0.25 and 0.50 W, the tissue fusion achieved at 0.2 W disrupted when exposed to blood flow, and no fusion was achieved at 0.50 W because of drying and retraction of the vessel edges after 5 pulses of 5 seconds' duration, and separation of the edges at 10 pulses with temperatures measured at greater than 125°C (Plate 17). From these experiments we concluded that argon laser vascular tissue welding occurs optimally at temperatures between 44° and 60°C, that saline irrigation limits the maximum temperature and prevents drying and retraction of tissue edges, and that welding at powers greater than 0.75 W may have deleterious effects. These studies address the problem of weld failure, but more work is needed to define the effect of temperature on the mechanism of fusion.

An additional study measured the thermal properties and thrombogenicity of argon-laser–assisted and sutured vascular repairs in canine veins and arteries.[18] The results suggest that temperatures less than 60°C did not have a detrimental effect on hemodynamic integrity or thrombogenicity. Arterial argon laser anastomoses with the energy applied from the adventitial surface had significantly less platelet deposition when compared with sutured repairs in the canine model. However, no significant difference in thrombogenicity was demonstrated between venous repairs.

In a pilot study, we have also compared the thermal properties of various types of laser fusions in an attempt to relate any differences to the observed patterns of healing.[19] The thermal properties and maximum temperatures attained during CO_2-and argon-laser–welded repair of arteries were compared in a canine model. With CO_2 laser welding, temperature increased quickly to 60.7° ± 9.8°C (maximum 84.0°C), which was maintained as the laser energy moved slowly (0.1 cm/second) along the vessel edges. This temperature will denature type I collagen, but not type VI collagen. In contrast, the argon laser welding temperatures rose to only 45.1° ± 2.7°C (maximum, 48.8°C) and returned to a baseline temperature with each drop of saline. Type I collagen in solution will denature at 40°C, but in a fiber form, it will return to its native configuration after a brief exposure to these temperatures. The thermal difference with these two laser wavelengths may bring about different welding mechanisms and provide an explanation for the increased incidence of thrombus and aneurysm formation that has been reported in CO_2 laser fusions.

We have begun further studies to evaluate the role of extracellular matrix components in laser tissue fusions.[20] The extracellular matrix components from untreated and laser welded guinea pig skin and blood vessels were extracted with guanidine hydrochloride and separated by SDS PAGE. The laser treated samples showed definite electrophoretic alterations in the profiles. The skin was treated with an argon laser at 1 W, for 5 seconds, without saline drip cooling, while the blood vessels were treated at 0.5 W, with saline drip cooling. In both skin and blood vessel, the concentration of a high molecular weight, pepsin-sensitive protein decreased in laser treated samples. This protein migrated on SDS PAGE just below the 200k dalton beta chains of type I collagen and may represent fibronectin or the high molecular weight form of type VI collagen. The protein may have been cross-linked and therefore shifted to a higher molecular weight region of the gel, or degraded, and shifted to a lower molecular weight region of the gel. In the laser treated, but not control, skin samples, there was a large amount of very high molecular weight protein that was in the stacking gel. This indicates that a high degree of crosslinking (or coagulation of protein) has occurred. However, in the blood vessel samples, this high molecular weight aggregate did not appear. Instead, a large amount of material was seen at the dye front of the gel, indicating that significant degradation had occurred. These results suggest that protein cross-linking and degradation can be induced with laser treatment. We do not know if the differences observed are due to tissue differences or to differences in the laser treatment.

SUMMARY OF THE CURRENT UNDERSTANDING OF THE MECHANISM OF LASER VASCULAR TISSUE FUSION

The mechanism of vessel sealing by lasers is presently not understood. Most studies propose that "collagen" is involved, but a systematic survey of predominant tissue components of the vessel including collagen types I, III, IV, and VI as well as elastin and other extracellular matrix molecules has not been performed. Serure et al. proposed that tissue adhesion in CO_2 laser welds of microvascular anastomoses resulted from collagen denaturation in the media and adventitia of the vessel, as well as fibrin polymerization.[2] Badeau et al. reported that CO_2-laser–assisted microvascular anastomoses were sealed at temperatures within the range of 80 to 120°C.[21] Epstein and Cooley demonstrated that seals in CO_2 laser welded microvessels consist of nonviable cells and collagen that reorganize over the first 2 to 4 weeks of healing.[22] They experienced a significant incidence of aneurysm formation (approximately 10%) in the early postoperative period and proposed that this was caused by breaks in elastin fibers due to laser damage. The 10% to 20% incidence of aneurysms in CO_2-laser–welded microvessels has been confirmed by other investigators.[23] Quigley et al. have shown that the welded areas in CO_2 laser microanastomoses retain a 200- to 300-μm separation of the internal elastic lamina for up to 1 year and that this gap is filled with spindle-shaped cells and hyperplasia of intimal tissue on the luminal surface.[24] The break in the elastic lamina of the CO_2 laser repairs may be due to tissue necrosis produced by the 80° to 120°C temperatures generated during the fusion. Recently, Ashworth et al. have reported successful end-to-end laser assisted vascular anastomoses of canine carotid arteries using a milliwatt CO_2 laser (150 to 175 mW, 2,400 to 3,500 J/sq cm energy fluence) with no aneurysms noted up to 4 weeks.[25] These investigators attributed the absence of aneurysms in the larger vessels sealed with the milliwatt CO_2 laser compared to the high incidence of aneurysms reported in microvessels to lesser degrees of thermal damage of the vessel wall seen in the large artery repairs.

Based on preliminary studies in our laboratory, our current hypothesis to explain the success of argon laser welding of medium-sized vein-artery anastomoses is that argon laser fusion occurs by reestablishing covalent bonds in the extracellular matrix proteins, particularly collagen. Histologic and electron microscopic examinations of successful fusions have demonstrated alignment and apparent bonding of collagen fiber.[12, 14] We have also observed that argon laser welds are improved by maintaining the temperature at the anastomosis between 43 and 48°C with a constant irrigation of saline solution. At temperatures greater than 60°C, collagen is damaged and welding is unsuccessful.[17] Tissue desiccation occurred at approximately 125°C without saline irrigation.[16] These observations suggest that molecular bonding occurs if tissue apposition is precise and the temperature is controlled to prevent denaturation of the proteins and disruption of the tissue. Interestingly, laser fusion is successful at temperatures below the denaturation temperature of type VI collagen (63°C). Further, preliminary attempts to fuse tendons that have little or no type VI collagen is generally unsuccessful. This suggests that type VI collagen plays a role in the fusion process. The collagen bonding theory is also supported by Schober et al. who observed a homogenizing change in periodically banded collagen with interdigitation of altered individual fibers that appeared to be the structural basis of the welding effect in microvessels fused with the 1,319-nm Nd:YAG laser.[26] Type VI collagen coats the outside of the periodically banded Type I fibers and may be involved in the interdigitation of those fibers.

PRELIMINARY HUMAN CLINICAL EVALUATION OF LASER TISSUE FUSION

A carefully controlled human protocol approved by the institutional review board (IRB) at our hospital has evaluated the adaptability of the initial experimental data regarding argon laser vascular tissue fusions to human vessels. Forearm Brescia-Cimino arteriovenous fistulas were chosen as a low-risk site for the initial clinical evaluation of argon-laser–assisted anastomosis of human vessels.[27] Ten patients (6 men, 4 women; 37.2 ± 12 years), with renal failure caused by diabetes (2); systemic lupus erythematosus (SLE) (2); nephritis (1); and unknown (5) had side-to-side radial artery (2.5- to 4.0-mm diameter) to cephalic vein (3.0 to 6.0 mm) fistulas welded by laser. Incisions of 1.2- to 1.5-mm length were made in adjacent segments of artery and vein and were positioned for application of laser energy by 4-quadrant simple, interrupted sutures so that each fistula was divided into four segments of 5- to 6.5-mm length. Each segment was sealed satisfactorily in 75 to 100 seconds using 0.5 W, 1,130 to 1,520 J/sq cm energy fluence argon laser energy. Seven (17.5%) of 40 welds required an additional 7–0 biodegradable suture to close small gaps that did not fuse adequately. The fistulas were observed at regular intervals postoperatively by physical examination, duplex scanning, and selected magnetic resonance imaging (MRI). Eight of the 10 patients were started on dialysis at 1 to 6 weeks. Serial follow-up examinations of the patients at 12 to 20 months (15.4 ± 2.8) postoperatively have demonstrated uniformly patent, compliant anastomoses and no evidence of hematomas, false aneurysms, or luminal narrowing. Figure 11–11 demonstrates the appearance of one of the fistulas on duplex scan at 1 year. Two patent fistulas were revised at 4 and 5 months because of inadequate development or thrombosis of the cephalic vein proximal to the fistula. Figure 11–12 demonstrates the gross appearance of a fistula excised at 5 months postoperatively. Histology from the fistulas at revision demonstrated healing of the entire circumference of the anastomosis similar to that noted in our extensive preclinical canine AV studies (Fig 11–13). We conclude from these preliminary results that argon laser vascular tissue fusion is possible in humans with reliable primary sealing of vascular anastomoses and that healing occurs without aneurysms on careful serial follow-ups of up to 20 months.

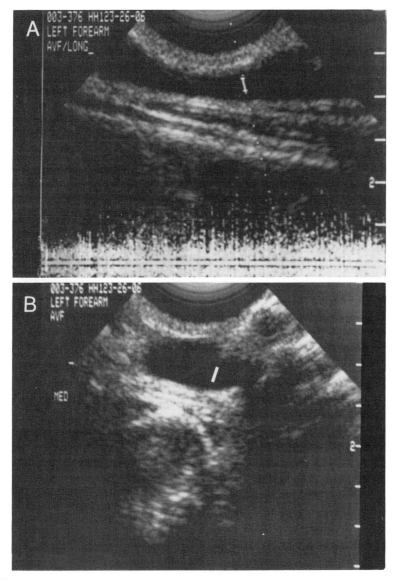

FIG 11–11.
Duplex scan in longitudinal (A) and cross-sectional (B) projections of a laser-fused fistula at 1-year postoperatively. The *white line* marks the line of anastomosis. (From White RA, White GH, Fujitani RM, et al: Initial human evaluation of argon laser-assisted vascular anastomoses. *J Vasc Surg,* in press. Used by permission.)

Four additional patients have had Cimino AV fistulas formed using combined argon laser fusion and absorbable, 5–0 monafilament sutures (PDS, Ethicon). The methodology for establishing fistulas was identical to that used to form similar fistulas in our canine model that was described previously in this chapter. Serial follow-up of these patients from 4 to 10 months by physical examination and duplex scanning demonstrated uniformly patent anastomoses and no evidence of hematomas, false aneurysms, of luminal narrowing. One patient expired 10 months after the procedure and at autopsy the fistula was excised and examined histologically. Gross examination revealed a widely patent anas-

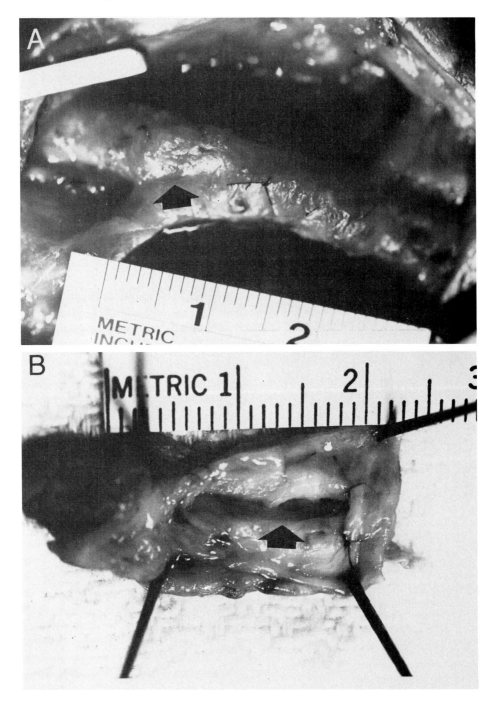

FIG 11–12.
External **(A)** and intraluminal **(B)** appearance of an excised arteriovenous fistula 5 months postoperatively. Areas of laser fusion are identified *(arrows)*. (From White RA, White GH, Fujitani RM, et al: Initial human evaluation of argon laser-assisted vascular anastomoses. *J Vasc Surg*, in press. Used by permission.)

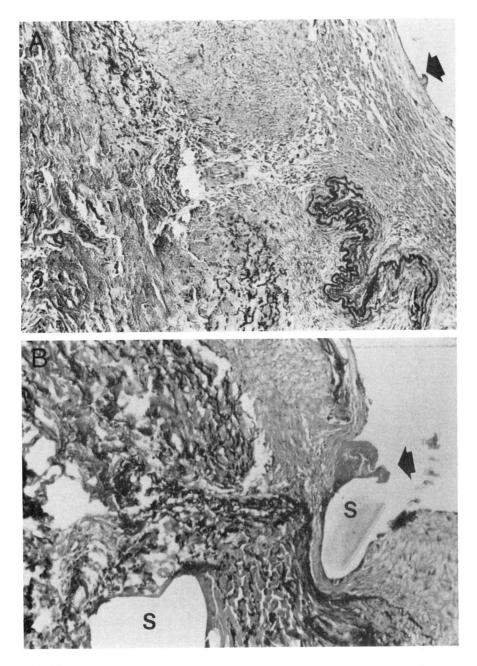

FIG 11–13.
Laser-fused arteriovenous fistula excised 5 months postoperatively. Laser fused segments **(A)** showed regular orientation of the vascular wall architecture and normal repair with no inflammation and **(B)** sutured segments showed foreign body reaction and tortuosity and disorientation of the elastin, collagen, and wall constituents. Site of anastomosis at the luminal surface is marked *(arrows)*; s = sutures. (Verhoeff–van Gieson's stain; × 40) (From White RA, White GH, Fujitani RM, et al: Initial human evaluation of argon laser-assisted vascular anastomoses. *J Vasc Surg*, in press. Used by permission.)

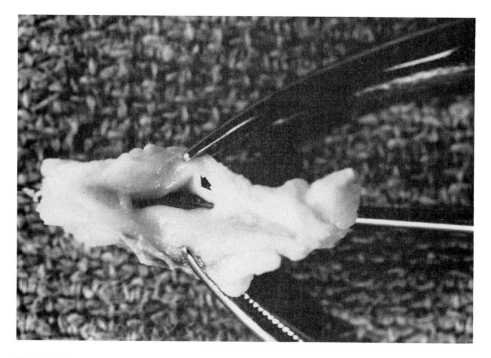

FIG 11–14.
Intraluminal appearance at 10 months after operation, of a human argon laser–welded arterio-venous fistula that initially had the edges of the anastomosis opposed by biodegradable traction sutures at 0.5 mm intervals. The line of fusion is marked (arrow).

tomosis as depicted in Figure 11–14. Histologic examination showed no evidence of remaining suture material and approximation of the healed tissues at the line of fusion (Fig 11–15). This preliminary work demonstrates the feasibility for combining laser tissue fusion and biodegradable sutures as a possible method to eliminate healing abnormalities at the anastomotic line caused by an ongoing foreign body reaction to the suture material.

CONCLUSIONS

At present, it is known that approximation of tissue in a bloodless interface and low energy (approximately 0.5 to 1 W) are required for vascular welding of medium-sized arteries by laser. Possible advantages of laser fusion over suture techniques may include (1) healing without foreign body reaction related to sutures; (2) preserved mechanical properties at anastomoses; (3) decreased incidence of intimal hyperplasia; and (4) unrestricted enlargement of growing vessels. Possible areas for clinical use of laser fusion of vascular tissue are in pediatric surgery, in sealing intimal flaps in endarterectomies, and in forming artery-vein anastomoses. Additional work is needed to determine the mechanism and the optimal laser parameters and wavelengths required for vascular tissue fusion by laser; in particular, work is needed to identify the characteristics needed to seal large diameter arteries uniformly and to fashion welds that withstand systemic arterial pressures.

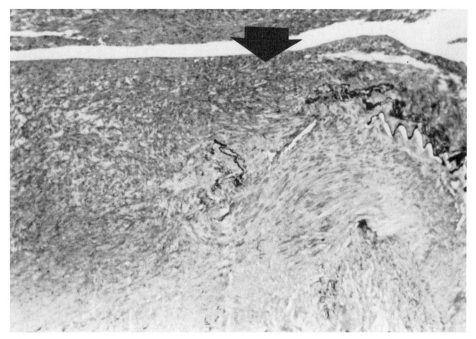

FIG 11–15.
Histologic appearance of line of tissue fusion from the human fistula displayed in Figure 11–14. The *arrow* marks the site of vein-to-artery anastomosis at the luminal surface.

REFERENCES

1. Dew DK, Serbent R, Hart WS, et al: Laser assisted microvascular anastomoses using argon and CO_2 lasers. *Lasers Surg Med* 1983; 3:135.
2. Serure A, Withers EH, Thomsen S, et al: Comparison of carbon dioxide laser assisted microvascular anastomosis and conventional sutured anastomosis. *Surg Forum* 1984; 34:634–636.
3. Jain KK: Sutureless microvascular extra-intracranial anastomoses with Nd:YAG laser. *Lasers Surg Med* 1984; 3:311–312.
4. Frazier OH, Painvin GA, Morris JM, et al: Laser assisted microvascular anastomoses: Angiographic and anatomopathologic studies on growing microvascular anastomoses: Preliminary report. *Surgery* 1985; 97:585–590.
5. McCarthy WJ, Lo Cicero J, Hartz RS, et al: Patency of laser-assisted anastomoses in small vessels: One year follow-up. *Surgery* 1987; 102:319–326.
6. White RA: Technical frontiers for the vascular surgeon: Laser anastomotic welding and angioscopy assisted intraluminal instrumentation. *J Vasc Surg* 1987; 5:673–680.
7. White RA, Abergel RP, Klein SR, et al: Laser welding of venotomies. *Arch Surg* 1986; 121:905–907.
8. White RA, Abergel RP, Lyons R, et al: Laser welding: An alternative method of venous repair. *J Surg Res* 1986; 41:260–263.
9. White RA, Abergel RP, Lyons R, et al: Biological effects of laser welding on vascular healing. *Lasers Surg Med* 1986; 6:137–141.
10. White RA, Kopchok G, Abergel RP, et al: Comparison of laser welded and sutured arteriotomies. *Arch Surg* 1986; 121:1133–1135.
11. White RA, Kopchok G, Donayre C, et al: Argon laser welded arteriovenous anastomoses. *J Vasc Surg* 1987; 6:447–454.

12. White RA, Kopchok GE, Donayre CE, et al: Mechanism of tissue fusion in argon laser welded vein-artery anastomoses. *Lasers Surg Med* 1988; 8:83–89.
13. White RA, Kopchok GE, Vlasak J, et al: Experimental evaluation of combined argon laser-fused, biodegradable suture vascular anastomoses. *J Vasc Surg,* submitted for publication.
14. White RA, Kopchok G, Peng SK, et al: Laser vascular welding: How does it work? *Ann Vasc Surg* 1987; 1:461–464.
15. Vlasak J, White RA, Kopchok GE, et al: Argon laser vascular fusion-venous and arterial bursting pressures. *Lasers Surg Med,* submitted for publication.
16. Kopchok G, Grundfest WS, White RA, et al: Argon laser vascular welding: The thermal component. *Proc Soc Photo-optical Instr Engineers* 1986; 712:260–263.
17. Kopchok G, White RA, Grundfest WS, et al: Thermal studies of in vivo vascular tissue fusion by argon laser. *J Invest Surg* 1988; 1:5–12.
18. Fujitani RM, White RA, Kopchok GE, et al: Comparison of indium [111] oxine labelled platelet aggregation between sutured and argon laser-assisted vascular anastomoses. *J Vasc Surg* 1988; 8:274–280.
19. Kopchok G, White RA, Fujitani R, et al: Laser vascular welding: A comparison of thermal properties of argon and CO_2 energy. *Proc Soc Photo-optical Instr Engineers* 1988; 907:72–74.
20. Su L, Murray L, Kopchok G, et al: Laser induced biochemical changes in the extracellular matrix of welded tissues. *Proc Soc Photo-optical Instr Engineers,* in press.
21. Badeau AF, Lee CE, Morris JR, et al: Temperate response during microvascular anastomosis using milliwatt CO_2 laser. *Lasers Surg Med* 1986; 6:179.
22. Epstein M, Cooley CB: Electron microscopic study of laser dosimetry for microvascular tissue welding. *Lasers Surg Med* 1986; 6:202.
23. McCarthy WJ, Hartz RS, Yao JST, et al: Vascular anastomoses with laser energy. *J Vasc Surg* 1986; 3:32–41.
24. Quigley MR, Bailes JE, Kwaan HC, et al: Microvascular laser-assisted anastomosis: Results at one year. *Lasers Surg Med* 1986; 2:179.
25. Ashworth EM, Dalsing M, Olson J, et al: Laser assisted vascular anastomoses of larger arteries. *Arch Surg* 1987; 122:673–677.
26. Schober R, Ulrich F, Sander T: Laser induced alteration of collagen substructure allows microsurgical tissue welding. *Science* 1986; 232:1421–1422.
27. White RA, White GH, Fujitani RM, et al: Initial human evaluation of argon laser-assisted vascular anastomoses. *J Vasc Surg,* in press.

Chapter 12

Laser Endarterectomy*

John Eugene, M.D.

Yvon Baribeau, M.D.

Michael W. Berns, Ph.D.

Endarterectomy is one of the fundamental techniques of reconstructive cardiovascular surgery. It is usually performed to remove an obstructing or ulcerating atheroma from an artery.[1-3] The diseased intima and underlying internal elastic lamina are dissected away from the wall of the artery to leave a luminal surface lined by the innermost fibers of the media. Since the introduction of endarterectomy 40 years ago, it has become evident that removing the intima of a diseased artery enables one to restore normal blood flow and achieve long-term patency of the artery.[4] This chapter describes work performed at the University of California, Irvine, evaluating the treatment of atherosclerotic cardiovascular disease using laser endarterectomy.

TECHNIQUE OF LASER ENDARTERECTOMY

To perform a laser endarterectomy, the artery is dissected free from surrounding tissues and exposed in the standard surgical fashion. Following systemic anticoagulation with heparin, proximal and distal vascular control of the artery is obtained and a longitudinal arteriotomy is made to visualize the atheroma. A line of laser craters is created at the proximal and the distal ends of an atheroma using individual laser exposures. The lines of laser craters are connected by constant laser radiation to form the sites for future proximal and distal end points. This maneuver loosens the atheroma from the artery just beneath the internal elastic lamina and exposes the cleavage plane. The plaque is dissected free from the artery by using constant laser light to dissect within the cleavage plane while the plaque is being gently retracted. Once the plaque is removed, any particles of atheromatous debris remaining on the endarterectomy surface can be vaporized by individual exposures or welded into place along the endarterectomy surface. The end points

*The experimental works cited in this chapter were supported by NIH grants RRO-1192 and HL-31318.

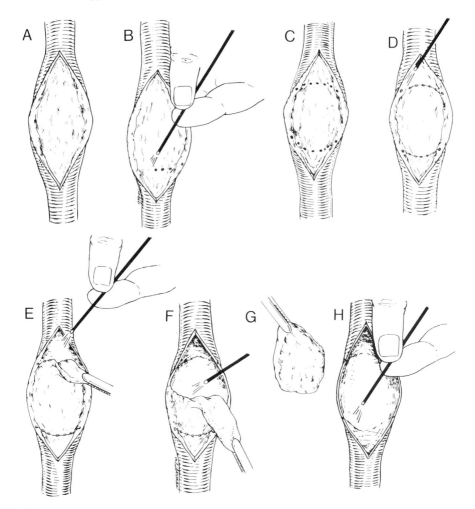

FIG 12–1.
A, artist's drawing of an arteriosclerotic artery opened longitudinally to expose an atheroma. **B,** lines of laser craters are being created at one end of the atheroma by individual laser exposures. **C,** individual laser exposures have been applied to create lines of laser craters at both ends of the atheroma. **D,** the lines of laser craters are connected by continuous laser radiation to loosen the atheroma and create the sites for the proximal and distal end points. **E,** the atheroma is being elevated away from the artery by continuous applications of laser light. **F,** continuous laser exposures are used to develop the cleavage plane within the media and dissect the atheroma from the artery. **G,** the dissection is completed and the atheroma is removed from the artery. **H,** the proximal and distal end points are welded by continuous laser radiation. (From Eugene J, McColgan SJ, Hammer-Wilson M, et al: Laser endarterectomy. *Lasers Surg Med* 1985; 5:265–274. Used by permission.)

are welded for a smooth and secure transition from endarterectomy surface to intima. This technique is illustrated in Figure 12–1 and Plates 18 and 19.

The laser endarterectomy technique was developed using the rabbit arteriosclerosis model and the argon ion laser (488 and 514.5 nm).[5, 6] Arteriosclerosis was created in adult New Zealand white rabbits by inflicting balloon catheter trauma to the thoracoabdominal aorta with the rabbits under general anesthesia (intramuscular acepromazine, 0.5 mg/kg; xylazine, 3.0 mg/kg; ketamine, 50 mg/kg) and maintaining them on a 2% cholesterol diet for 18 weeks. Early in our experience, we performed angiography on the rabbits to evaluate the severity of arteriosclerosis, and we learned that significant arteriosclerotic lesions were produced in 86% of surviving rabbits. Grossly, the diseased aortas are thickened and discolored (white with yellow streaks) and the disease is uniform throughout the traumatized aorta. Microscopically, each atheroma has a fibrous cap that overlies areas of fatty infiltration (foam cells), inflammation, and focal calcifications with fracture of the internal elastic lamina and extension into the superficial fibers of the media.

LASER ENDARTERECTOMY VS. CONVENTIONAL ENDARTERECTOMY

Although we had demonstrated that laser radiation could be used to perform an endarterectomy, there was no proof that it was any different from standard endarterectomy. A series of experiments was performed to compare endarterectomy by laser and endarterectomy by knife.[7] Under general anesthesia (intramuscular acepromazine, 0.5 mg/kg; xylazine, 3.0 mg/kg; ketamine, 50 mg/kg), a thoracoabdominal exploration was performed in 16 arteriosclerotic rabbits. The aorta was isolated and heparin (3.0 mg/kg intravenously) was administered. Proximal and distal vascular control was obtained and the aortas were opened longitudinally. In eight rabbits, open laser endarterectomy was performed with an argon ion laser (Coherent INNOVA 20) with mixed wavelengths 488 and 514.5 nm. Laser light was directed through a 400-μm quartz fiberoptic at a power of 1.0 W to perform open laser endarterectomy. In the remaining eight rabbits, standard surgical endarterectomy was performed using an endarterectomy knife and vascular instruments.

On completion of the endarterectomies, the aortas were removed, preserved, serially sectioned at 6-μm intervals, and stained with hematoxylin and eosin for histologic examination. The specimens were assigned a point score determined by the gross and microscopic surface characteristics (1, arterial perforation; 2, the wrong cleavage plane; 3, rough surface; 4, smooth surface) and by the type of transition at the endarterectomy end points (1, arterial perforation; 2, intimal flap; 3, rough transition; 4, smooth transition).

By gross appearance, satisfactory endarterectomy surfaces were obtained with both techniques. The end points following laser endarterectomy appeared to be more even and more well defined than the end points following conventional endarterectomy. By microscopic appearance, both techniques showed that the endarterectomy surfaces were in the proper cleavage plane and were relatively smooth and free of debris (Figs 12–2 and 12–3). The end points, however, were quite different. The conventional endarterectomy end points exhibited a rough transition from media to intima (Fig 12–4), and in two cases intimal flaps were seen (Fig 12–5). The laser endarterectomy end points were welded in place. Most of the laser end points exhibited a smooth transition from media to intima, and there were no distal intimal flaps (Fig 12–6). When the surfaces were graded, both conventional and laser endarterectomy specimens achieved identical scores of 3.6. When the end points were graded, the conventional endarterectomy specimens achieved a score of 2.8 and the laser endarterectomy score was 3.6 ($P<.05$). These experiments demonstrated that laser endarterectomy offers the distinct advantage of welding the end points for a secure transition from endarterectomy surface to arterial lumen.

Subsequently the surface thrombogenicity of laser endarterectomy and conventional endarterectomy were compared in the rabbit arteriosclerosis model.[8] Twelve arteriosclerotic rabbits underwent thoracoabdominal exploration while under general anesthesia. The aortas were dissected free; proximal and distal vascular control was obtained, and

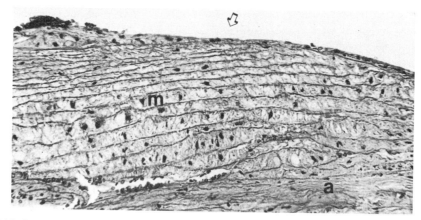

FIG 12–2.
Longitudinal section of an arteriosclerotic rabbit aorta following conventional endarterectomy showing that the atheroma and internal elastic lamina have been removed. The endarterectomy surface *(open arrow)* is smooth and the elastic fibers of the media *(m)* retain their normal configuration; a = adventitia (hematoxylin-eosin, ×40).

longitudinal arteriotomies were performed to expose atheromatous plaques. Several conventional surgical endarterectomies and laser endarterectomies were performed in each arteriosclerotic rabbit, leaving a segment of atheroma intact between each endarterectomy. The conventional endarterectomies were performed using an endarterectomy knife and standard vascular instruments. The laser endarterectomies were performed using an argon ion laser (Coherent INNOVA 20) at 488 and 514.5 nm. The laser beam was delivered through a 400-μm quartz fiberoptic to perform the laser endarterectomies. Blood (0.05 ml) from normal rabbits was placed on the laser and conventional endarterectomy surfaces, and the clotting times were determined. Surface thrombogenicity was calculated as the ratio of the clotting time of the endarterectomy surfaces to the clotting time of normal intima. Both types of endarterectomy achieved identical surface thrombogenicity scores of 0.46 ± 0.08. Ragimov and associates have reported similar results for laser treated

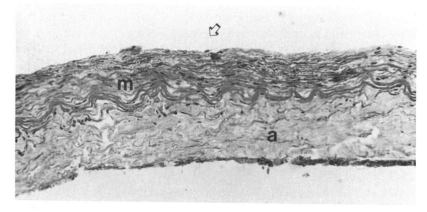

FIG 12–3.
Longitudinal section of an arteriosclerotic rabbit aorta following argon ion laser endarterectomy showing smooth endarterectomy surface *(open arrow)*. The atheroma and the internal elastic lamina have been removed, leaving the elastic fibers of the media *(m)* undisturbed; a = adventitia (hematoxylin-eosin, ×40).

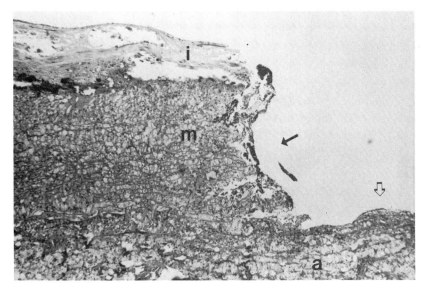

FIG 12–4.
Longitudinal section of a distal end point following conventional endarterectomy in an arteriosclerotic rabbit aorta showing an abrupt transition from endarterectomy surface *(open arrow)* to atheroma *(closed arrow)*; *i* = intima; *m* = media; *a* = adventitia (hematoxylin-eosin, ×10).

surfaces.[9] It appears that both the laser endarterectomy and conventional endarterectomy surfaces are thrombogenic. The cause of the thrombogenicity is not related to the way in which the atheroma is removed but rather to the loss of normal endothelium.

EXPERIMENTAL ENDARTERECTOMY COMPARING LASERS

The technique of laser endarterectomy was developed with the argon ion laser because

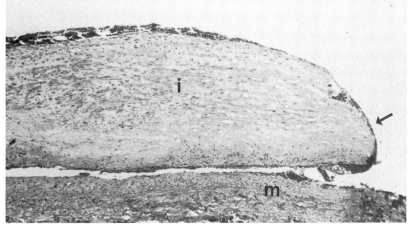

FIG 12–5.
Longitudinal section of a distal end point following conventional endarterectomy in an arteriosclerotic rabbit aorta showing separation of the layers of the arterial wall at the transition from media *(m)* to intima *(i) (arrow)*. This represents a distal intimal flap (hematoxylin-eosin, ×10).

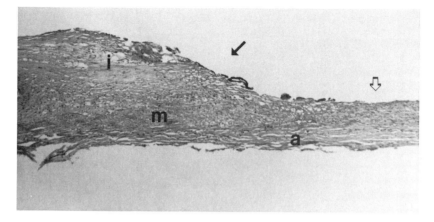

FIG 12–6.
Longitudinal section of a distal end point following argon ion laser endarterectomy in an arteriosclerotic rabbit aorta showing a smooth transition from endarterectomy surface *(open arrow)* to intima *(closed arrow)*. The layers of the end point are welded together to prevent an intimal flap; *i* = intima; *m* = media; *a* = adventitia (hematoxylin-eosin, × 10).

its beam is within the visible spectrum (488 and 514.5 nm), permitting the surgeon to direct the beam accurately to the target tissue and observe if there is any scatter or transmission of laser light. Other lasers that have been evaluated for the treatment of arteriosclerosis include the neodymium:yttrium-aluminum-garnet (Nd:YAG) laser (1.06 μm) and the carbon dioxide laser (10.6 μm).[10–12] These lasers are usually operated as continuous wave lasers, and they have different standard applications in surgery. Additional studies were performed to compare the laser-atheroma interaction of all three lasers by their ability to perform laser endarterectomy in arteriosclerotic rabbit aortas.[13–15]

The argon ion laser (Coherent INNOVA 20) beam was delivered through a 400-μm quartz fiberoptic at a power of 1.0 W. The Nd:YAG laser (Molectron Medical Model 8000-3) beam was delivered through a 600-μm quartz fiberoptic with an integral aiming light at a power of 10 to 20 W. Carbon dioxide laser (Directed Energy Model Systems LS 20-H) radiation was delivered directly from the laser head to the aorta at a power of 10 W for 10 msec (0.01 J). Laser endarterectomy was performed in arteriosclerotic rabbits with each of the lasers, and the aortas were resected for histologic studies following the procedures.

Grossly, the argon ion laser endarterectomies appeared satisfactory. The surfaces were smooth, without residual atheroma, and the end points were welded in place. Grossly, the Nd:YAG laser endarterectomies appeared unsatisfactory. The surfaces were desiccated and the end points were burned. Significant thermal injury was seen in the adventitia of the aortas and in surrounding structures, such as the inferior vena cava, indicating transmission of Nd:YAG radiation through the arteriosclerotic aortas. The carbon dioxide laser endarterectomies appeared generally satisfactory by gross inspection; however, closer inspection under a dissecting microscope revealed that fragments of intima and internal elastic lamina were left on the surfaces, and there were minute perforations at the end points.

Microscopically, the argon ion laser endarterectomy surfaces showed the cleavage plane to be just beneath the internal elastic lamina in all of the experiments. The surfaces all appeared relatively smooth. The end points were welded securely for an even transition from media to intima. The Nd:YAG laser endarterectomy surfaces showed thermal changes

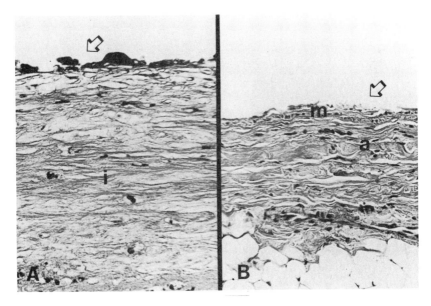

FIG 12–7.
Longitudinal sections of arteriosclerotic rabbit aortas following Nd:YAG laser endarterectomy. **A,** cleavage plane superficial to the media with charring of the surface; *i* = intima. **B,** cleavage plane deep within the media *(m)* almost to the adventitia *(a)*; (hematoxylin-eosin, ×40).

manifested as charring and discoloration. The depth of the cleavage plane was irregular and was seen to be superficial to the media or too deep within the media (Fig 12–7). Perforation occurred at the distal end points in 75% of the experiments (Fig 12–8). Despite the fact that the gross appearance of the carbon dioxide laser endarterectomy surfaces and the end points were satisfactory, microscopically the surfaces were uneven

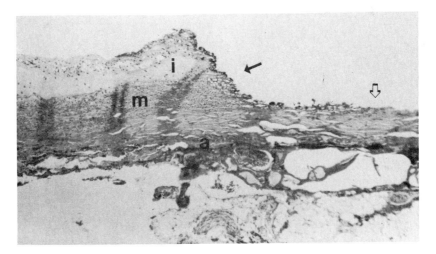

FIG 12–8.
Longitudinal section of a distal end point following Nd:YAG laser endarterectomy in an arteriosclerotic rabbit aorta showing an abrupt transition from endarterectomy surface *(open arrow)* to arterial surface *(closed arrow)*. There is a full-thickness injury (perforation) to the arterial wall at the transition of the end point; *i* = intima; *m* = media; *a* = adventitia (hematoxylin-eosin, ×10).

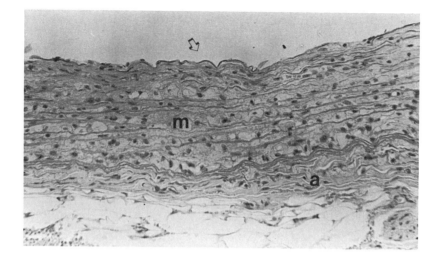

FIG 12–9.
Longitudinal section of an arteriosclerotic rabbit aorta following carbon dioxide laser endarterectomy shows an uneven surface with fragments of the internal elastic lamina left in place *(arrow).* This endarterectomy surface is in the wrong cleavage plane; *m* = media; *a* = adventitia (hematoxylin-eosin, × 40).

and were often in the wrong cleavage plane (Fig 12–9). Perforations occurred at the distal end points in 80% of the carbon dioxide endarterectomies (Fig 12–10).

Argon ion laser endarterectomy achieved a surface score of 3.6 and an end point score of 3.5. The Nd:YAG laser endarterectomy achieved a surface score of 2.6 and an end point score of 1.5. Carbon dioxide laser endarterectomy achieved a surface score of 2.3 and an end point score of 1.3. Argon ion laser endarterectomy required an average

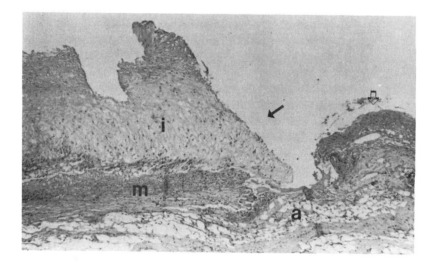

FIG 12–10.
Longitudinal section of a distal end point following carbon dioxide laser endarterectomy in an arteriosclerotic rabbit aorta. The transition from endarterectomy surface *(open arrow)* to arterial surface *(closed arrow)* is uneven and irregular. There is a full-thickness injury (perforation) at the transition of the end point; *i* = intima; *m* = media; *a* = adventitia (hematoxylin-eosin, × 40).

energy density of 100 ± 12 J/sq cm. The Nd:YAG laser endarterectomy required an average energy density of 1147 ± 120 J/sq cm, and carbon dioxide laser endarterectomy required a mean energy density of 38 ± 5 J/sq cm. These data showed that argon ion and carbon dioxide laser radiation were well absorbed by atheromas, but Nd:YAG laser radiation was not well absorbed and was transmitted and scattered to surrounding tissues. The excellent interaction between atheromas and carbon dioxide laser energy did not result in a satisfactory endarterectomy because the beam could not be accurately delivered without fiberoptics. The poor laser-atheroma interaction observed with the Nd:YAG laser led to unsatisfactory endarterectomy, even though fiberoptic delivery was available. Satisfactory endarterectomy was performed only with the argon ion laser because the energy was well absorbed by arteriosclerotic rabbit aortas and the beam was accurately directed through a fiberoptic.

The excellent results seen with argon ion laser radiation for endarterectomy of experimental atheromas may have been due to the wavelength of the argon ion laser (488 and 514.5 nm). A similar wavelength laser was studied. The second harmonic of the Nd:YAG laser, the KTP laser (Laserscope, Inc.) delivers a wave length of 532 nm in pulsed or continuous wave mode. Laser endarterectomies were performed in arteriosclerotic rabbits at an average power output of 1 W.[16] Power was delivered through a 300-μm quartz fiberoptic in either the pulsed or continuous mode to perform laser endarterectomy. Using the continuous wave mode, smooth endarterectomy surfaces and secure welded end points were obtained in all experiments. Using a pulsed mode, perforations occurred at the end points and the end points could not be welded in place.

Laser endarterectomy has also been performed in the arteriosclerotic rabbit model with the excimer laser (xenon chloride, 308 nm). Laser radiation was delivered through a 600-μm quartz fiberoptic at an energy density of 50 mJ/pulse, 120 nsec pulses, and 15 pulses/second.[16, 17] Smooth endarterectomy surfaces were seen in 75% of experiments. The end points were not welded in place, however, and intimal flaps as well as perforations were seen in 30% of experiments. The pulsed mode does not appear suitable for laser endarterectomy because of the inability to weld the end points reliably with pulsed laser radiation. The best results for laser endarterectomy of experimental atheromas have been obtained with the argon ion laser.

CONTACT LASER ENDARTERECTOMY

The laser endarterectomy operation has been described using free beam laser radiation. This eliminates tactile feedback. Contact laser surgery has been described in other fields of surgery using laser knives made of artificial sapphire crystals (Al_2O_3). Experiments were performed in arteriosclerotic rabbits using sapphire crystal laser knives (SLT, Inc.) to perform laser endarterectomy. Conical-shaped knives with rounded tips of 0.2, 0.4, 0.6, and 0.8 mm were used.[18] They were powered by argon ion (488 and 514.5 nm) or Nd:YAG (1.06 μm) lasers, with the beam delivered through 400-μm fiberoptics. Power of 1.0 W to 4.0 W was used to perform the endarterectomies. The endarterectomy surfaces showed uneven plaque removal and gross irregularities in 50% of the experiments. The end points were not welded in place and frequent perforations were seen. The atheromatous plaques tended to adhere to the sapphire crystals and this sticking tended to disrupt the endarterectomy. Laser endarterectomy is best performed as a free beam laser surgery operation.

PHOTOSENSITIZATION OF ATHEROMAS

Neoplasms are known to accumulate hematoporphyrin derivative (HPD), and this accumulation of HPD can be detected by fluorescence of the tumor under ultraviolet light. When neoplasms are photosensitized with HPD, exposure to specific wavelengths of laser light causes a cytotoxic reaction that destroys the tumor. Theoretically, if atheromas can be photosensitized in a similar fashion, selective ablation of atheromas could be accomplished with laser light using energy levels so low that injury to adjacent tissue would be eliminated and the threat of arterial preformation would be greatly reduced.

Fluorescence of arteriosclerotic arteries that have been treated with HPD has been described in rabbits, a Patas monkey, and human cadaver aortas.[19-22] An additional study was performed to determine the site of localization of porphyrins in arteriosclerotic arteries.[23] Photofrin II was used instead of HPD because it is a standard commercial preparation used for photodynamic therapy of cancer. Four groups of rabbits were studied: normal rabbits; normal rabbits given 5 mg/kg of Photofrin II intravenously; arteriosclerotic rabbits; and arteriosclerotic rabbits given 5 mg/kg of Photofrin II intravenously. Within 48 hours the rabbits underwent surgical exploration, and multiple full-thickness biopsies of their aortas were obtained. These biopsies were immediately frozen and sectioned at 4-μm intervals. Adjacent alternate sections were either stained with hematoxylin and eosin or prepared for fluorescence microscopy to quantitate porphyrin fluorescence. Paired sections were matched so that the sites of fluorescence could be localized to a specific histologic region of the arteries. A marked increase in fluorescence was seen in the intima of the arteriosclerotic arteries, proving that porphyrins localized within atheromas (Plate 20).

With the knowledge that porphyrins localized in atheromas, laser endarterectomy was used to determine if the atheromas were photosensitized by porphyrin accumulation. Laser endarterectomy was performed in arteriosclerotic rabbits given 5 mg/kg of intravenous Photofrin II 48 hours preoperatively, and arteriosclerotic rabbits without Photofrin II pretreatment. An argon ion laser was used because the wave lengths (488 and 514.5 nm) are in the range of one of the best absorption peaks of porphyrins. Laser endarterectomy in arteriosclerotic rabbits required an average energy density 103 ± 3 J/sq cm, and laser endarterectomy in arteriosclerotic rabbits given photofrin II required an average energy density of 33 ± 3 J/sq cm ($P < .01$). Since the technique of laser endarterectomy requires atheromas to be dissected from the artery, the significant changes in energy density show that porphyrin localization in atheromas does indeed sensitize atheromas to selective laser ablation.

CLINICAL INVESTIGATIONS OF LASER ENDARTERECTOMY

Investigational laser endarterectomy operations are currently being performed in the peripheral circulation[24] and in the carotid circulation.[25] These trials are conducted under FDA approval and University of California, Irvine Human Subjects Committee approval. An argon ion laser (Trimedyne Optilase, Model 900) has been used for the clinical trials.

The clinical technique of argon ion laser endarterectomy is similar to the laboratory technique. Laser radiation is delivered through a 300-μm quartz fiberoptic at an average power of 1.0 W. The fiber is positioned so that the spot size of the beam is approximately 0.5-mm diameter. The fiber is never allowed to touch the target tissue. The direction of the beam is changed during the operation in order to perform the different parts of the operation. For vaporization, the beam is directed at right angles to the target. For dissection, the beam is directed tangentially, and for welding, the beam is kept moving over the arterial surface while a saline drip is applied. The endarterectomy dissection is usually begun with an endarterectomy knife to expose the cleavage plane. The atheroma is grasped with instruments and laser light is directed at the cleavage plane to dissect the plaque from the artery. The dissection continues for the length of the arteriotomy in order to remove the plaque and, as the end point is approached, the angle of incidence of the laser beam is changed so that the plaque can be transected at a low angle to leave a smooth transition. The end point is then welded in place under a constant saline drip. The arterial surface is inspected for any residual atheromatous debris. Remaining debris can be vaporized with individual laser exposures or welded in place to the endarterectomy surface. Laser endarterectomy has been performed in the aorto-iliac system, the common femoral artery, the profunda femoris artery, the superficial femoral artery, the popliteal artery, and the posterior tibial artery. The endarterectomies have ranged in length from 10 to 60 cm. The atheromas have ranged in consistency from fibrous plaques to densely calcified plaques. In all cases, an average power of 1.0 W was used. This is the same power output that was used to perform the laser endarterectomy operation in arteriosclerotic rabbits.

The carotid artery laser endarterectomy is performed in the same fashion as the peripheral vascular laser endarterectomy. The plaque is initially elevated with a dissector and then it is dissected from the artery with continuous wave argon ion laser radiation at power at 1.0 W. At the end point, the direction of the laser beam is changed to transect the plaque at an acute angle, and the distal end point is welded in place with 1.0-W argon ion laser power under a saline infusion. The constant saline infusion maintains the low temperature necessary for arterial welding without protein denaturation. The initial clinical results are satisfactory and long-term results are pending (Plate 21).

FUTURE DIRECTIONS FOR LASER ENDARTERECTOMY

Large-scale clinical trials of laser endarterectomy will be necessary to refine the operation and evaluate the clinical efficacy of the operation. Long-term studies comparing laser endarterectomy to other forms of arterial reconstruction will be necessary.

As new lasers are developed and new information is learned about the atheromatous response to lasers, it may be advantageous to perform laser endarterectomy with a different laser or with a combination of lasers. It may become advisable to use a pulsed laser for dissection and then a continuous wave laser to weld the end points. The operation could be improved if laser radiation could be used to weld the arteriotomy closed following the endarterectomy instead of suturing the arteriotomy closed. This is being evaluated in the laboratory, but it has not yet been attempted in the clinical setting.

Finally, laser endarterectomy can be advanced to the coronary artery system. Laser endarterectomy offers a safe way to apply laser radiation to the treatment of arteriosclerotic cardiovascular disease. The procedure is performed under vascular control and direct observation in order to minimize complications. Laser endarterectomy is a modern refinement of one of the fundamental operations of reconstructive cardiovascular surgery and may find a place in the future treatment of cardiovascular disease.

REFERENCES

1. Wiley EJ, Kerr E, Davies O: Experimental and clinical experiences with use of fascia lata applied as graft about major arteries after thromboendarterectomy and aneurysmorrhaphy. *Surg Gynecol Obstet* 1951; 93:257–272.
2. Wiley EJ: Thromboendarterectomy for atherosclerotic thrombosis of major arteries. *Surgery* 1952; 32:275–292.
3. Szilagy DE, Smith RF, Whitney DG: The durability of aortoiliac endarterectomy. *Arch Surg* 1964; 89:827–839.
4. Dos Santos JC: From embolectomy to endarterectomy or the fall of a myth. *J Cardiovasc Surg* 1976; 17:113–128.
5. Eugene J, McColgan SJ, Hammer-Wilson M, et al: Laser endarterectomy. *Lasers Surg Med* 1985; 5:265–274.
6. Eugene J, McColgan SJ, Hammer-Wilson M, et al: Laser applications to arteriosclerosis: Angioplasty, angioscopy and open endarterectomy. *Lasers Surg Med* 1985; 5:309–320.
7. Eugene J, McColgan SJ, Pollock ME, et al: Experimental arteriosclerosis treated by conventional and laser endarterectomy. *J Surg Res* 1985; 39:31–38.
8. Pollock ME, Eugene J, Hammer-Wilson M, et al: The thrombogenic potential of argon ion laser endartectomy. *J Surg Res* 1987; 42:153–158.
9. Ragimov SE, Andrey AB, Igor AV, et al: Comparison of different lasers in terms of thrombogenicity of the laser-treated vascular wall. *Lasers Surg Med* 1988; 8:77–82.
10. Geschwind HJ, Boussignac G, Teisseire B, et al: Conditions for effective Nd:YAG angioplasty. *Br Heart J* 1984; 52:484–498.
11. Livesay JJ, Leachman DR, Hogan PJ, et al: Preliminary report on laser coronary endarterectomy in patients, abstracted. *Circulation* 1985; 72(suppl 3):302.
12. Abela GS, Seeger JM, Barbieri E, et al: Laser angioplasty with angioscopic guidance in humans. *J Am Coll Cardiol* 1986; 8:184–192.
13. Eugene J, Pollock ME, McColgan SJ, et al: Fiber optic versus direct laser delivery for endarterectomy of experimental atheromas. *Proc Int Soc Opt Eng* 1985; 576:55–58.
14. Eugene J, McColgan SJ, Pollock ME, et al: Experimental arteriosclerosis treated by argon ion and neodymium-YAG laser endarterectomy. *Circulation* 1985; 72(suppl 2):200–206.
15. Eugene J, Pollock ME, McColgan SJ, et al: Comparison of continuous wave lasers for endarterectomy of experimental atheromas. *J Thorac Cardiovasc Surg* 1987; 93:494–501.
16. Baribeau Y, Eugene J, Firestein SL, et al: Comparison of pulsed lasers for endarterectomy of experimental atheromas. *Lasers Surg Med,* submitted for publication.
17. Baribeau Y, Eugene J, Firestein SL, et al: Excimer laser radiation for endarterectomy of experimental atheromas. *Lasers Surg Med,* submitted for publication.
18. Baribeau Y, Eugene J, Firestein SL, et al: Comparison of contact and free beam laser endarterectomy. *Lasers Surg Med,* submitted for publication.
19. Spears JR, Serur J, Shropstire D, et al: Fluorescence of experimental atheromatous plaques with hematoporphyrin derivative. *J Clin Invest* 1983; 71:395–399.
20. Cortis B, Harris DM, Principe J: Angioscopy of hematoporphyrin derivative in experimental atherosclerosis. *Proc Int Cong Appl Lasers Electro-Opt* 1984; 43:128–130.
21. Kessel D, Sykes E: Porphyrin accumulation by atheromatous plaques of the aorta. *Photochem Photobiol* 1984; 40:59–64.
22. Litvak F, Grundfest WS, Forrester JS, et al: Effects of hematoporphyrin derivative and photodynamic therapy on arteriosclerotic rabbits. *Am J Cardiol* 1985; 56:667–671.
23. Pollock ME, Eugene J, Hammer-Wilson M, et al: Photosensitization of experimental atheromas by porphyrins. *J Am Coll Cardiol* 1987; 9:639–646.
24. Eugene J, Carey JS, Cukingnam RA, et al: Fiber optic delivery of argon ion laser radiation for open endarterectomy. *Proc Int Soc Opt Eng* 1988; 906:310–312.
25. Eugene J, OH RA, Baribeau Y, et al: Argon ion laser radiation for carotid endarterectomy. *Lasers Surg Med,* submitted for publication.

PART III

Angioplasty Guidance Systems and Ancillary Devices

Chapter 13 _____

Angioscopy

Geoffrey H. White, M.D.

Angioscopy may be defined as the endoscopic inspection of the interior of blood vessels. Improvements in fiberoptic imaging and a strong interest in less invasive methods of treatment are bringing about rapid developments in this field. With new intravascular techniques such as balloon angioplasty, atherectomy, and laser ablation, there is now a strong desire to characterize the disease process visually and monitor the effects of these various interventions. Initial investigations showed that it was possible to aim lasers by the use of an angioscope and produce accurate ablative effects on atherosclerotic plaque. The inability to control the depth of laser penetration and the narrow recanalization channels were limiting factors.

Early attempts at vascular endoscopy were hampered by poor instrumentation; large, rigid tubes with inadequate methods of clearing blood from their field of view were of little clinical value. Development of narrow fiberoptics and flexible instrumentation allowed surgeons to visualize the lumen after endarterectomy or anastomosis.[1-3] Interest in the possibilities of viewing the interior of the heart and blood vessels has been further revived by the rapid growth of interventional cardiology and vascular radiology and an increased interest in therapy by less invasive, percutaneous techniques.[4]

Intraoperative applications of angioscopy are aided by the fact that the cardiovascular surgeon has direct control of blood flow within the vessel that is to be inspected in most situations. Retrograde or collateral blood flow can usually be overcome temporarily by infusion of a transparent solution or by use of various occlusion balloon techniques. To be of value in cardiology or interventional radiology, however, percutaneous instrumentation and techniques are necessary. Recent development of ultrathin optical bundles, less than half a millimeter in diameter, now allows good quality viewing through a delivery catheter system and it seems likely that percutaneous angioscopy will soon be developed to the stage where it may become a widespread diagnostic tool and an adjunct to many therapeutic procedures.

Angioscopy was first performed with rigid 5- to 8-mm diameter choledochoscopes or arthroscopes.[5-7] Now, flexible angioscopes are available in diameters ranging from 0.8 to 3.3 mm. They have fiberoptic light sources and coherent fiber bundle imaging systems that provide images via a handheld eyepiece that may preferably be connected to a video camera for recording and magnification onto a television monitor.[8, 9] Angioscopes 2 to 3 mm in diameter are best suited for most peripheral vascular procedures, whereas 0.80- to 1.7-mm diameters are required for coronary and tibial vessels.[10, 11]

Intraoperative angioscopy is performed through an opening in the artery after proximal clamping. An infusion of saline through the scope flushes blood away from the viewing lens. Collateral blood flow may be occluded by a balloon near the tip of the angioscope. Newer, ultrathin angioscopes sacrifice the added bulk of the irrigation and balloon channels; during coronary angioscopy chilled cardioplegia solution or heparinized saline is perfused via a separate cannula. Percutaneous angioscopy is technically more difficult and requires efficient mechanisms for removing blood from the field of view. For coronary application, complex balloon catheter systems are under investigation but those reported have required rapid infusion of large amounts of fluid, "monorail" guidewire introduction, slow motion photography or digital image analysis, and excessive time.[12, 13]

Several investigators have reported intraoperative applications and benefits of angioscopy during peripheral vascular anastomosis,[14, 15] embolectomy and thrombectomy procedures,[16] and preparation of the saphenous vein for in situ bypass.[17, 18] Recently, laser angioplasty,[19, 20] vascular brushing,[21] placement of intravascular stents,[22] and atherectomy instrumentation[23] have each been developed and evaluated with the aid of angioscopic monitoring.

It has been reported that in 15% to 30% of vascular operations angioscopy reveals clinically relevant information that is not apparent by external visualization, flow studies, or angiography.[9, 10] In our prospective study at Harbor-UCLA Medical Center, angioscopic findings differed from preoperative or intraoperative angiograms in 24% of cases, resulting in an alteration in the operation in 17%.[8] With an average procedure time of only 5 to 10 minutes, angioscopy provides an alternative to completion angiography during bypass operations and eliminates the need for radiation exposure, contrast media, and a technician. Thrombectomy under direct vision may be accomplished with a Fogarty catheter adjacent to the angioscope, providing a three-dimensional view to identify critical stenoses and demonstrate residual thrombus missed by angiography.[16] Potential complications include vessel perforation, intimal trauma, infection, and embolization. Introduction of the angioscope into vessels whose diameters are close to or smaller than that of the scope produces spasm and possible thrombosis. The clarity of video angioscopic images is usually excellent, but adequate clearing of blood flow by fluid infusion and techniques for manipulation of the angioscope must be learned. Future prospects include smaller angioscopes with improved optics and steerable components, percutaneous introduction catheters incorporating efficient occlusion balloon techniques, and the development of microinstruments that can be passed through a channel in the angioscope. A disposable optical catheter has recently been marketed.

ANGIOSCOPY EQUIPMENT

For angioscopy of the peripheral vascular system, we advocate a multichannel design of flexible, endoscopic catheter that, in particular, incorporates a relatively large fluid channel for irrigation of the vessel lumen to keep the field of view and lens free of blood. This fluid channel, or "working" channel, increases the diameter of the fine fiberoptic instruments to a size of approximately 2.5 mm and may also be used for passage of guidewires or laser fibers (Fig 13–1). Smaller endoscopes are also available, but these sacrifice the fluid lumen in return for a narrower catheter diameter.

Video coupling is used; an adapter connects the angioscope catheter to a video camera and enlarges the image (Fig 13–2). The final image, projected on a television monitor,

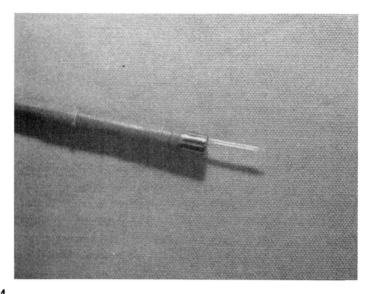

FIG 13–1.
A 2.8-mm diameter angioscope with a laser fiberoptic passed through a channel in the scope.

is magnified 40 to 100 times. A high-power light source of at least 300-W output is required to provide illumination of sufficient intensity through the ultrafine light fiber; most light sources available in the hospital for gastrointestinal and surgical endoscopy are usually of 100- to 150 W power.

Fluid irrigation solutions are infused under pressure through the working lumen to achieve flow rates of 30 to 75 ml/minute. A pressure bag of the Fenwal type is satisfactory; alternative commercial irrigation flush pump systems are being introduced, with footpedal rate control. We use heparinized saline solution (heparin, 5,000 units per liter of normal saline) and have found this to be very satisfactory. Papaverine may also be added.

The angioscope, video camera, and cables are all gas sterilizable and are set up on a sterile field next to the operating table. These instruments must be handled with great care because of the fragility of the optical fibers. Blood is cleared from the tubing and internal channels immediately after use to avoid deterioration of the optics. Ethylene oxide gas sterilization and airing procedures take 6 to 12 hours, so the angioscope may usually be used only once each day.

APPLICATIONS OF ANGIOSCOPY

Specific and theoretical applications of endoscopy have been described for coronary, peripheral vascular, carotid, visceral, and pulmonary arteries and for the venous system.[24] These applications can be defined as diagnostic or therapeutic.

Diagnostic use includes identification of luminal and surface pathologies such as thrombus, plaque, hemorrhage, ulceration, atherosclerotic occlusion, or embolus. It is feasible that new syndromes will be identified by further recognition of the roles of these various factors in the pathogenesis of cardiovascular diseases. Endoscopic biopsy of atheromatous lesions may come to play a role in determining prognosis and appropriate treatment including drug selection.[25] Angioscopy may also be used for validation of other imaging techniques such as ultrasound, duplex Doppler, and magnetic resonance imaging.

Therapeutic applications in clinical practice include the monitoring of many intravascular procedures that are performed at a remote site within the vessel. Laser angioplasty is a prime example of this capability. Direct information may be collected regarding the immediate and long-term effects of various instruments on the arterial lumen and intima, including a comparison of new techniques and immediate correction of detected faults or complications.

INTERPRETATION OF THE ANGIOSCOPIC IMAGE

As with any imaging technique, interpretation of the observed endoscopic findings and determination of which of these require intervention will be somewhat subjective and dependent on the experience of the angioscopist. The image projected on the video monitor is a relative field, with size changes being dependent on the distance of a lesion from

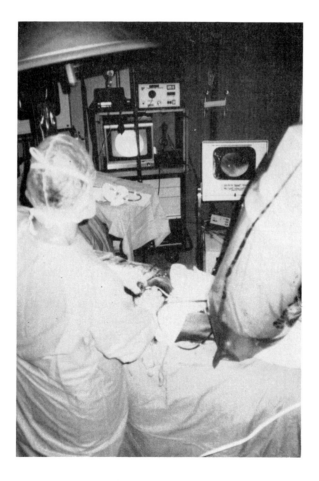

FIG 13–2.
Coupling of the angioscope to a high-resolution on-line video monitor enhances visualization of intraluminal images.

the objective lens. A minor abnormality that is examined from a distance of just a few millimeters may be distorted out of proportion.

Many investigators have reported a high incidence of retained fragments, debris, intimal fibrinous strands, and webs within peripheral arteries, especially following endarterectomy, thrombectomy, or angioplasty.[8–10, 14] The true clinical significance of these findings is often unclear. Perhaps no intervention is indicated, although such observations may often result in revision of the vascular procedure or further attempts at improving the result. Accurate interpretation of the observed abnormal angioscopic findings and correct management will rely on careful recording of a large experience, objectively correlated with early and late outcomes.[26] Angioscopy will likely be shown to have a prognostic role, with specific visual appearances correlating with an unsatisfactory result or early failure. Spectroscopic analysis of reflected light from atherosclerotic lesions may provide more complex data.[27]

ANGIOSCOPIC MONITORING OF LASER ANGIOPLASTY

Angioscopy may be used as a direct visual control for aiming laser fibers and immediately monitoring the results on the target tissue. Angioscopy is an effective method of inspection of the laser-treated vessel for evaluation of residual stenosis and the presence or absence of complications including plaque dissection, intimal flap, vessel perforation, thrombosis, or embolus (Plate 22). This capability for immediate, three-demensional assessment of vessel morphology allows rapid correction of defects while the access to the vessel is maintained, and it may lead to repeat procedure or alternative therapy by atherectomy or balloon angioplasty if the results of the laser procedure are judged to be inadequate.

The most valuable use for angioscopy would be as a replacement for fluoroscopy during intraoperative laser angioplasty performed by surgical exposure of the vessel. In this setting the radiologic monitoring is often limited by inadequate equipment; the possibility of contaminating sterile fields; x-ray exposure to the patient, surgeon, and operating room personnel; and the requirement for contrast media that may cause nephrotoxic or anaphylactic responses. As early as 1982, Lee and co-workers studied the feasibility of precise delivery of laser energy to atherosclerotic plaque by simultaneous angioscopic visualization and intravascular irradiation with bare-tip argon lasers.[28, 29] Abela and associates reported that vascular endoscopy could also be used in conjunction with metallic-tipped thermal laser probes of 2-mm diameter, to position the probe tip precisely and to observe the process of recanalization of occluded superficial femoral arteries.[30]

The role of angioscopic monitoring and aiming for control of laser intervention in the vascular system was further investigated in our research laboratory in 48 vessels in 33 canines, and the techniques were then applied to 20 humans undergoing intraoperative or percutaneous laser probe angioplasty.[31, 32] These studies, in summary, gave the following results: Experimental bare argon fiber laser application in 20 normal canine arteries in vivo demonstrated that small diameter fibers fed through the internal channel of a 2.5-mm diameter angioscope could be aimed by manipulations of the scope but resulted universally in perforation. Laser hot-tip probes positioned centrally within undiseased arteries produced intense spasm, thermal ulceration, thrombosis, and probe adherence to the wall with 5 or 8 W power. Continuous infusion of saline reduced these destructive thermal effects. In 28 canine and 1 human vein, angioscope-guided metallic-tipped laser probes were used to divide 82 valve cusps in preparation for in situ bypass, with satis-

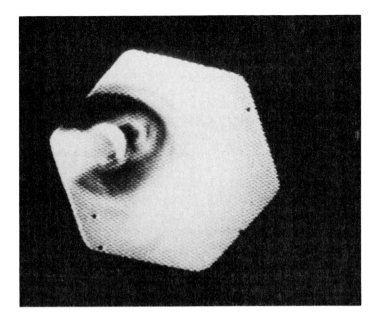

FIG 13–3.
Angioscopic monitoring of venous valve ablation in an in situ vein bypass using a metal-tipped laser probe.

factory aiming and monitoring achieved expeditiously by manipulations of the angioscope (Fig 13–3).[33,34]

Adapting these techniques to intraoperative laser angioplasty in atherosclerotic human arteries produced several difficulties.[35] In these selected patients with long or multisegmental arterial occlusions, proximal stenosis or tapering in the superficial femoral artery prevented the angioscope from reaching the site of occlusion before laser activation in 70% of cases. Perforation of the adductor canal segment occurred in 4 of 20 cases but was only observed angioscopically in 1 instance.[35] Percutaneous angioscopy was performed in selected patients, with access via the 8.5 F delivery sheath used for the laser probe. Postprocedural angioscopy was successful in 87% and revealed wall thermal damage, fragmentation, and mural thrombus. The findings were particularly prevalent in previously occluded segments of arteries. In all, four patients with these severe changes had early occlusion.

Preliminary conclusions from these experimental and clinical studies are: (1) Angioscopic aiming of lasers is feasible in normal veins and arteries. (2) In contrast, angioscopy has a restricted role for guidance of laser angioplasty in atherosclerotic, occluded arteries, and it does not prevent perforation. (3) Postprocedural inspection is valuable for immediate detection of inadequate recanalization or complications and may have prognostic value.

ANGIOSCOPIC MONITORING OF CORONARY LASER ANGIOPLASTY

Coronary angioscopy has been shown to be a useful technique in the intraoperative setting, where cardiac standstill associated with heart lung bypass and cardioplegia make safe cannulation of the small coronary arteries by ultrafine angioscopes a relatively uncomplicated procedure.[11] Monitoring the result of operative laser angioplasties by immediate inspection is therefore quite feasible.[27, 28]

However, the problems of successful angioscopy within the fine, tortuous vessels of the beating heart make angioscopic laser application in the coronary arteries little more than a difficult experimental program at present.

ANGIOSCOPY USED TO MONITOR ATHERECTOMY

Angioscopy may be employed in a similar fashion for monitoring atherectomy procedures, especially intraoperative atherectomy.[36] The diseased vessel is inspected before atherectomy to determine the severity, distribution, and character of the occluding or stenotic lesion. In selected cases, the drill or burr may be observed during its action or on repeated attempts. Of particular interest and value is the postprocedural inspection of the recanalized artery or graft to assess the lumen caliber and determine the presence of complications.

LIMITATIONS OF ANGIOSCOPY

Some of the possible disadvantages of angioscopy are listed in Table 13–1. In particular, these fine fiberscopes are delicate instruments that require meticulous care in handling, usage, and cleaning. Proper techniques will greatly reduce the need for costly repair and will prolong the life of the instruments.

Small and tortuous or branched vessels present special difficulties for cannulation and inspection. It is often not possible to monitor endovascular procedures directly since the angioscope will not fit comfortably into the lumen at the same time as the therapeutic device in use. In these cases, the inspection is limited to examination of the effects at the conclusion of treatment. Development of microinstruments that may be passed through the angioscope working channel has commenced.

The limitations of the use of angioscopy are mainly related to the time, cost, and design constraints of the present technology, and there is a potential for vessel trauma caused by the angioscope itself if great care is not exercised. There may be a tendency to overestimate the severity of the observed abnormalities, with resultant overtreatment of minor faults.

Angioscopy cannot be regarded as a total replacement for intraoperative arteriography since the angioscopes used generally do not pass safely into the smaller vessels and thus there is no information conveyed regarding the status of the runoff beyond the examined area. There is also no quantification of the flow through the anastomosis or vessels. In

TABLE 13–1.
Limitations of Angioscopy

Instrument fragility
Costs of equipment and accessories
Space requirements and set up time
Limited life span of the fiberoptic catheters
Necessity for gas sterilization
Vessel size and tortuosity
Potential for vessel trauma and complications
Image interpretation
Subjective measurement, affected by distance from lens
No quantification of flow
Requires experience for technical proficiency

cases in which these are an important consideration, intraoperative angiograms still play a valuable role and may be obtained by infusion of contrast via the fluid channel.

Training and experience are certainly necessary to achieve sufficient technical skill and interpretive ability and to aid in the selection of appropriate instrumentation. As experience grows and the technology becomes more refined, angioscopy will come to occupy a more important role in the management of cardiovascular disease.

REFERENCES

1. Crispin HA, Van Baarle AF: Intravascular observation and surgery using the flexible fiber-scope. *Lancet* 1973; 1:750–751.
2. Vollmar JF, Storz LW: Vascular endoscopy. *Surg Clin North Am* 1974; 54:111–122.
3. Towne JR, Bernhard VM: Vascular endoscopy: Useful tool or interesting toy. *Surgery* 1977; 82:415–419.
4. Spears JR, Marais HJ, Serur J, et al: In vivo coronary angioscopy. *J Am Coll Cardiol* 1983; 1:1311–1314.
5. Vollmar JF, Storz LW: Vascular endoscopy. *Surg Clin North Am* 1974; 54:111–122.
6. Towne JB, Bernhard VM: Vascular endoscopy: Useful tool or interesting toy. *Surgery* 1977; 82:415–419.
7. Goldstone SM, Shore JM, Heringman EC, et al: Arterial endoscopy (arterioscopy). *Arch Surg* 1966; 93:81–83.
8. White GH, White RA, Kopchok GE, et al: Intraoperative video angioscopy compared with arteriography during peripheral vascular operations. *J Vasc Surg* 1987; 6:488–495.
9. Mehigan JT, Olcott C: Video angioscopy as an alternative to intraoperative arteriography. *Am J Surg* 1986; 152:139–145.
10. Grundfest WS, Litvack F, Sherman T, et al: Delineation of peripheral and coronary detail by intraoperative angioscopy. *Ann Surg* 1985; 202:394–400.
11. Sherman CT, Litvack F, Grundfest W, et al: Coronary angioscopy in patients with unstable angina pectoris. *N Engl J Med* 1986; 315:313–319.
12. Tanabe T, Yokata A, Sugie A: Cardiovascular endoscopy: Development and clinical application. *Surgery* 1980; 87:375–379.
13. Forrester JS, Litvack F, Grundfest W, et al: A perspective of coronary disease seen through the arteries of living man. *Circulation* 1987; 75:505–513.
14. Seeger JM, Abela GS: Angioscopy as an adjunct to arterial reconstructive surgery: A preliminary report. *J Vasc Surg* 1986; 4:315–320.
15. Matsumoto T, Hashizuze M, Yang Y, et al: The use of angioscopy in vascular surgery. *Contemp Surg* 1986; 29:31–35.
16. White GH, White RA, Kopchok GE, et al: Angioscopic thromboembolectomy: Preliminary observations with a recent technique. *J Vasc Surg* 1988; 7:318–325.
17. Fleischer HL, Thompson BW, McCown TC, et al: Angioscopically monitored saphenous vein valvulotomy. *J Vasc Surg* 1986; 4:360–364.
18. White RA, Kopchok GE, White GH, et al: Valvulotomy in in-situ vein bypass by angioscopy-assisted laser probe. *J Surg Res* 1987; 42:440–445.
19. Abela G, Seeger JM, Barbieri E, et al: Laser angioplasty with angioscopic guidance in human. *J Am Coll Cardiol* 1986; 8:184–192.
20. Forrester JS, Litvack F, Grundfest WS: Laser angioplasty and cardiovascular disease. *Am J Cardiol* 1986; 57:990–992.
21. Crispin HA: Experience with the vascular brush. *J Cardiovasc Surg* 1987; 28:45–49.
22. Sigwart V, Puel J, Mirkovitch V, et al: Intravascular stents to prevent occlusion and restenosis after transluminal angioplasty. *N Engl J Med* 1987; 316:701–706.
23. Simpson JB, Zimmerman JJ, Mathews R, et al: Transluminal atherectomy: Initial clinical results in 27 patients, abstract. *Circulation* 1986; 74(suppl 2):203.

24. White GH, White RA (eds): *Angioscopy: Vascular and Coronary Applications.* Chicago, Year Book Medical Publishers Inc, 1988.

25. Looking inside arteries. *Lancet* 1987; 2:374–375.

26. Bernhard VM: Endoscopy and vascular surgery, editorial. *J Vasc Surg* 1986; 4:415.

27. Kittrell C, Willett RL, Santos-Pancheo C, et al: Diagnosis of fibrous arterial atherosclerosis using fluorescence. *Appl Optics* 1985; 24:2280–2281.

28. Lee G, Ikeda RM, Dwyer RM, et al: Feasibility of intravascular irradiation for in-vivo visualization and therapy of cardiocirculatory diseases. *Am Heart J* 1982; 103:1076–1077.

29. Lee G, Ikeda RM, Stobbe D, et al: Laser irradiation of human atherosclerotic obstructive disease: Simultaneous visualization and vaporization achieved by a dual fiberoptic catheter. *Am Heart J* 1983; 105:163–164.

30. Abela G, Seegar JM, Barbieri E, et al: Laser angioplasty with angioscopic guidance in humans. *J Am Coll Cardiol* 1986; 8:184–192.

31. White GH, Kopchok GE, White RA: Angioscopic monitoring for intraoperative laser angioplasty, abstract. Proceedings of the International Congress on Laser Applications in Vascular Surgery. Scottsdale, Ariz, 1988, V1–3.

32. White RA, White GH: Angioscopic monitoring of laser angioplasty, in White GH, White RA (eds): *Angioscopy: Vascular and Coronary Applications.* Chicago, Year Book Medical Publishers Inc, 1988.

33. White RA, Kopchok G, Donayre C, et al: Valvulotomy in in-situ vein bypass performed by angioscopy-assisted laser probe. *J Surg Res* 1987; 42:440–445.

34. White GH, Kopchok GE, Fujitani RM, et al: Valvulotomy within in-situ vein bypass grafts: A comparison of laser and instrument techniques (abstract). *J Cardiovasc Surg* 1987; 28:27.

35. White GH, Kopchok GE, White RA: Experimental and clinical applications of angioscopic guidance for laser angioplasty. *Am J Surg,* submitted for publication.

36. Ahn SS, Auth DP, Marcus DL, et al: Removal of focal atheromatous lesions by angioscopically guided high speed rotatory atherectomy: Preliminary experimental observations. *J Vasc Surg* 1988; 7:292–300.

Chapter 14

Spectroscopy

Michele Sartori, M.D.

FLUORESCENCE OF VASCULAR TISSUE

Laser spectroscopy has been used extensively to investigate the chemical structure and the energy transfer processes of organic and inorganic materials. This chapter only reviews data concerning its application and its potential relevance to cardiovascular disease and laser angioplasty.

Two factors contribute to perforation of the arterial wall during laser angioplasty: the sharp tip and stiffness of optical fibers, and the extension of the laser ablation process across the arterial wall.[10, 17] The transmural extension of the laser injury is the result of an incomplete control of the ablation process. In order for laser angioplasty to become a safe procedure, it appears that a monitoring device is needed, one that yields instantaneous feedback information concerning the targeting of the laser and the overall process of ablation. The device would distinguish between atherosclerotic and nonatherosclerotic tissue and provide an estimate of wall thickness. Although angioscopy of the intimal surface may be useful for detecting ruptured atherosclerotic plaques and thrombi,[15, 39] mere surface imaging may not give the structural information required to make laser ablation safe and predictable.[1]

Over the past few years, several research groups have been investigating the use of laser spectroscopy as a potential monitor for laser angioplasty.

BACKGROUND

The interaction of a low-power laser beam with tissue results in scattering of laser light. The scattered light may be divided into three types: In Rayleigh scattering the scattered light has the same wavelength as the incident laser light; in Raman scattering and fluorescent light the scattered light's wavelength has been changed by an amount corresponding to the energy characteristic of the tissue. The wavelength of the Raman scattered light can vary and its intensity is usually minimal, whereas the fluorescent light is characterized by a stronger intensity and by wavelengths (invariably) longer than the wavelength of the exciting beam. Thus, due to its easily detectable nature and the obvious

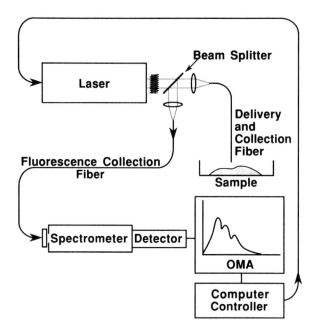

FIG 14–1.
Instrumental setup for fluorescence detection and spectroscopic control of ablation. (Modified from Pettit GH, Pini R, Sauerbrey R, et al: Excimer laser induced autofluorescence from arteriosclerotic human arteries. *IEEE J Quan Elec*, submitted for publication.)

advantages that this offers, laser-induced fluorescence has been used for many years as an important probe to characterize the molecular structure and energy reactions of biologic tissues.

The power density of the laser beam used to excite the fluorescence is several orders of magnitude below the power necessary to ablate the tissue. Thus, the process of "interrogating the tissue" is safe in that it does not alter the anatomic integrity of the tissue. Furthermore, both the exciting beam and the fluorescent light can be carried in the very same optical fiber used for ablating the tissue.

Therefore, in a system aimed at laser angioplasty, laser spectroscopy offers two potential advantages:

1. It is safe since it occurs well below the ablation energy threshold of the tissue.
2. It is efficient in that the same intravascular catheter used for plaque ablation can be used for fluorescence collection.

The main components of the instrumental setup for laser spectroscopy are illustrated in Figure 14–1. The laser, used as a source for the fluorescence excitation or ablation, is coupled into an optical fiber and delivered to the tissue sample. The fluorescence emitted from the tissue surface is collected by the same fiber and diverted, through a beam splitter, to a spectrometer in line with an Optical Multichannel Analyzer (OMA). The OMA analyzes the fluorescence radiation by counting the photons of light according to their energy, that is their wavelengths. The result is a plot of the fluorescence intensity over the spectrum of wavelengths investigated. The display of the fluorescence spectrum is nearly instantaneous to the excitation process and can take place fractions of a second before or after ablation. By comparing the collected spectrum to reference spectra stored in a computer, fluorescence characterization of the arterial tissue in real time is possible.

an important probe to characterize the molecular structure and energy reactions of biologic tissues.

AUTO-FLUORESCENCE OF HUMAN ARTERIES IN VITRO

Several investigators have conclusively demonstrated that the fluorescence spectra of postmortem human atherosclerotic arterial segments are significantly different from the spectra of normal arterial segments.* The vast majority of the spectra have been obtained with either a visible laser such as argon ion laser radiating blue light, or an ultraviolet (UV) laser such as helium-cadmium laser and excimer gas laser.

Figure 14–2,A illustrates a typical example of the fluorescence spectrum of a segment of normal coronary artery excited with an argon ion laser tuned at 458 nm. Shown on the abscissa is the wavelength in nanometers (nm); on the ordinate is the intensity of the fluorescence in arbitrary units (OMA counts). Notice the artifact due to the sharp small peak at the left corner of the spectrum corresponding to the wavelength of the exciting argon ion laser at 458 nm. Three broader peaks representing the fluorescence are seen at longer wavelengths of approximately 520, 550, and 600 nm. The fluorescence spectra collected from a lipid-rich atheroma and a calcified atheroma of the same coronary artery are also illustrated (see Fig 14–2,B and C). Compared to Figure 14–2,A, the spectra in Figures 14–2,B and C differ by exhibiting increased 550-nm peaks that fuse with the peaks at 520 nm. Apart from this spectral change common to both lipid-rich and calcified tissue, the calcified coronary sample is characterized by a pronounced increase in fluorescence intensity. The fluorescence of the calcified sample (see Fig 14–2,C) is four times more intense than the fluorescence originating from the normal tissue (see Fig 14–2,A) or the lipid-rich plaque (see Fig 14–2,B). The peak at 520 nm reaches 16,000 OMA counts in the calcified tissue compared to only 4,500 in the normal and 3,000 in the lipid-rich tissue. Virtually identical relationships between spectral profile and its intensity and tissue composition are demonstrable for aortic samples, which suggests that the fluorescence-tissue relation depicted has general validity for the characterization of arterial tissue.

Differences in the spectral profile of normal and atherosclerotic arteries are similarly detected by using a UV laser as excitation source. Figure 14–3 is the representation of the spectra of different tissue types excited with a UV laser tuned at 325 nm. The fluorescence peaks occurring at 520, 550, and 600 nm as a result of blue argon laser light are in this case substituted by peaks at shorter wavelengths with a maximum at 462 nm. The spectral profiles by the UV laser clearly differ for: normal specimen (Fig 14–3,A), lipid-rich atheroma (Fig 14–3,B), fibrous plaque (Fig 14–3,C), and plaque with subintimal hemorrhage (Fig 14–3,D). In Figure 14–4, the spectrum profile of a calcified atheroma is compared to normal tissue. The spectrum of the calcified sample exhibits a broader peak, the distinction is not striking. The difference can be enhanced if the normal trace is subtracted from the abnormal, as is shown in the lower section of the illustration. This type of subtraction analysis can be performed only if both spectra are normalized to the same intensity scale. Normalization entails that each intensity value of a spectrum

*References 11, 12, 19, 22, 26, 35–38.

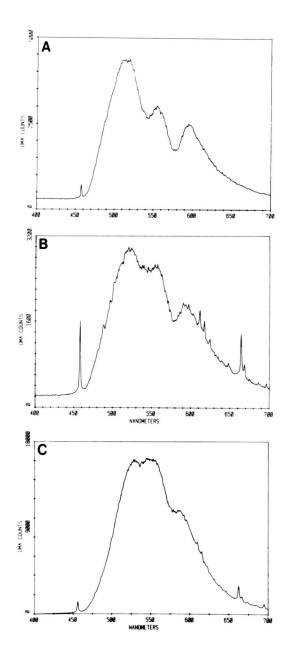

FIG 14–2.
Fluorescence spectra of human arteries excited with visible argon ion laser (458 nm). **A,** normal left anterior descending artery. **B,** lipid-rich plaque. **C,** calcified atheroma. The intensity of the fluorescence of the calcified plaque is remarkably higher than in normal and lipid-rich tissue; 16,000 vs. 4,500 and 3,000, respectively. (From Sartori M, Weilbaecher D, Henry P: Laser induced autofluorescence of human arteries. *Circ Res* 1988; 63:1053–1059. Used by permission.)

is divided by the intensity value at a normalizing wavelength and multiplied by a constant according to the formula

$$\frac{x}{y} \times 10^4$$

where x is the intensity in OMA counts on the spectrum profile at a given wavelength, y is the OMA counts at the normalizing wavelength, and 10^4 is the amplification constant. For the spectrum of Figure 14–4, 470 nm is chosen as normalizing wavelength since peaks of maximum intensity of both spectra (normal and calcified) occur near this wavelength, thus decreasing the chances that the intensity of the fluorescence at this wavelength is due to artifact. Thus, as one can resolve from the formula, the arbitrary value of 10^4 is assigned to the intensity at 470 nm.

Normalization removes differences in absolute magnitudes between spectra and leaves a pure comparison of curve shapes. Since the absolute intensity of the fluorescence spectra is affected by the distance of the optical fiber tip to the tissue (a parameter difficult to control in a tortuous blood vessel in vivo), only the comparison of spectral profile might, at least initially, be possible in vivo. On the other hand, mere comparison of profiles can severely limit identification of the highly fluorescent calcified atheroma. Furthermore,

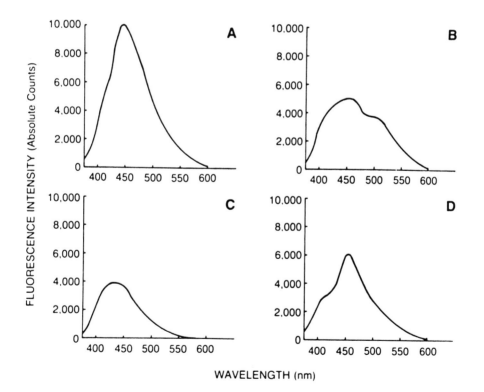

FIG 14–3.
Fluorescence spectra of human aorta excited with UV helium-cadmium laser (325 nm): normal (**A**); lipid-rich plaque (**B**); fibrous atheroma (**C**); and atheroma with subintimal hemorrhage (**D**). (From Leon MB, Lu DY, Prevosti LG, et al: Human arterial surface fluorescence: Atherosclerotic plaque identification and effects of laser atheroma ablation. *J Am Coll Cardiol* 1988; 12:94–102. Used by permission.)

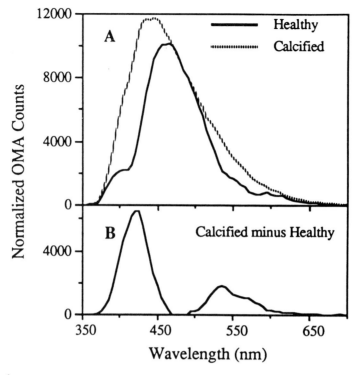

FIG 14–4.
Autofluorescence spectra of normal and calcified arterial tissue excited with UV excimer laser (XeF 3,512 nm). (From Pettit GH, Pini R, Sauerbrey R, et al: Excimer laser induced autofluorescence from arteriosclerotic human arteries. *IEEE J Quan Elec,* submitted for publication. Used by permission.)

the presence of a relatively thin fibrous cap or intimal hemorrhage overlying the calcium deposits is sufficient to change the spectral profile of calcified plaques. This problem is more apparent when using UV lasers, indicating that it probably depends on the progressively shallower tissue penetration of UV compared with visible light.

Quantitative parameters such as the area of subtraction shown previously (see Fig 14–4) have been derived from the spectra and show a consistent correlation between fluorescence signatures and histologic features of the tissue. Figure 14–5 represents the ratio (R) of the height of the peaks at 550 nm obtained with the argon laser to those at 520 nm for normal tissue (NL), lipid-rich (L), and calcified (C) atheromas. The R values for atherosclerotic samples are significantly higher than those for normal samples. Accordingly, it appears that R values in excess of 0.8 are characteristic of atherosclerotic plaques. The intensity values (PI) of the maximum fluorescence peak at 520 nm for the three tissue types are also illustrated (see Fig 14–5,B). Peak intensity values for calcified atheromas are significantly higher than normal and lipid-rich tissue. This indicates that calcified tissue, in addition to exhibiting an abnormal spectral profile, is characterized by high fluorescence intensity as compared to noncalcified tissue. Thus, by combining both parameters (R and PI), all tissue types can be correctly identified with the argon blue excitation light at 458 nm. Similarly, Leon and co-workers[22] have determined parameters derived from the spectra obtained with a UV laser: area within the spectra, spectral width at 25%, 50%, and 75% of the normalized maximal peak intensity; normalized intensities at ±40 and ±80 nm from the fluorescence maximum. These param-

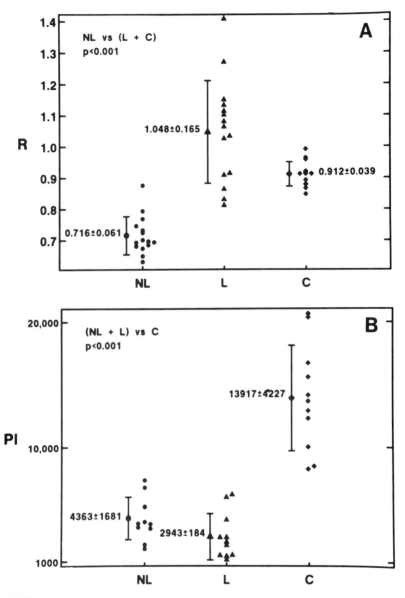

FIG 14–5.
A and B, values in arbitrary units of the parameters derived from the spectra of arteries radiated with 458-nm argon ion laser (see Fig 14–2). R = ratio of peak intensities 550/520 nm; PI = absolute intensity of the 520-nm peak; NL = normals; L = lipid rich; and C = calcified arterial samples. (From Sartori M, Weilbaecher D, Henry P: Laser induced autofluorescence of human arteries. *Circ Res* 1988; 63:1053–1059. Used by permission.)

eters consistently lead to the identification of noncalcified atherosclerotic tissue. On the other hand, calcified atheromas are not identified on the basis of these parameters. Their spectral profile appear not significantly different than lipid-rich atheromas (Fig 14–6) and, as mentioned above, it is dependent on the location of the calcium within the arterial wall.

In summary, from the available data on the autofluorescence of arteries in vitro, the following conclusions can be inferred:

1. Both argon ion blue laser at 458 nm and UV laser at 325 and 351 nm can correctly discriminate between normal and atherosclerotic tissue in vitro on the basis of parameters derived from the spectral profiles.
2. Lipid-rich plaques exhibit a lower peak intensity than normal arterial tissue, and they exhibit a secondary peak that significantly broadens their spectrum profile.
3. Fibrous plaques have the lowest fluorescence of all, usually exhibiting a poorly differentiated spectral profile.
4. Grossly calcified plaques exhibit a broader spectral profile and peak fluorescence intensity higher than any other tissue atheromas.
5. The presence of thrombotic, necrotic, or fibrotic tissue overlying a calcified atheroma makes the characterization of the tissue less reliable.

ORIGIN OF THE FLUORESCENCE

Identification of the fluorophores present in the arterial tissue has been predominantly studied under UV light.

The main source of arterial wall autofluorescence appears to be elastin contained in the media.[5, 7] The intensive blue fluorescence of elastin is most likely responsible for a great part of the maximum peak intensity of the arterial spectra occurring at 450 nm under UV light. Additional fluorophores are the flavins exhibiting green fluorescence, probably responsible for the longer secondary peak at 500 to 600 nm.

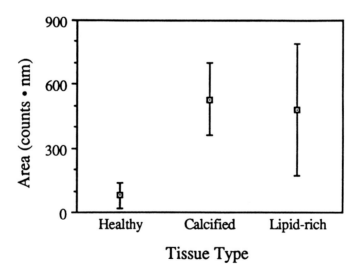

FIG 14–6.
Mean values of the areas of the normalized spectra obtained with UV laser (351 nm) for three histologic tissue types. (From Pettit GH, Pini R, Sauerbrey R, et al: Excimer laser induced autofluorescence from arteriosclerotic human arteries. *IEEE J Quan Elec,* submitted for publication. Used by permission.)

The diminution and change of fluorescence intensity observed in lipid-rich and fibrous noncalcified atheromas can be attributed to the destruction of elastin by the atherosclerotic material infiltrating the media,[5] growth of collagen,[20] increased amount of carotenoids,[5] and small layers of blood contained within the plaque.[16] The surface fluorescence is most likely the result of radiation from multiple fluorophores (elastin, flavins, etc.) in the media and absorption or "filtering" by overlying materials within the intima.

While the origin of fluorescence may not be of primary concern to the "laser angioplaster," its implications for the monitoring of the ablation process with laser spectroscopy are relevant. Removal of the atherosclerotic intima by microdissection and by laser ablation results in a return to the normal arterial spectra profile and intensity (Fig 14–7).[22, 31, 38] In normal tissue, increase in fluorescence intensity and a narrowing of the spectrum profile occur after shallow ablation of the intima, persisting unchanged until wall perforation occurs (Fig 14–9,A). In atherosclerotic tissue, progressive ablation results in proportional increase of the fluorescence intensity (Fig 14–8), but a change of the spectral profile is only reached at the intima-media interface (Fig 14–9,B). Other newer parameters of time-resolved fluorescence can further increase the potential of the monitoring of ablation by laser spectroscopy.[30]

AUTOFLUORESCENCE OF ARTERIES IN VIVO

The collection of fluorescence spectra in vivo has been performed only very recently. Using UV excitation at 325 nm during aorta coronary bypass surgery Leon and co-workers at the NIH found good correlation between the macroscopical and visual identification of atherosclerotic plaques and fluorescence signals.[3] Parameters derived from the fluorescence spectra similar to the ones from the in vitro experiments showed high sensitivity and specificity (91% and 100%, respectively) in recognizing atherosclerotic plaques. All sites not detected by the laser were from calcified lesions.

The group at the NIH and the Geschwind group in Europe recently reported the initial results of percutaneous laser angioplasty guided by real time spectroscopy.[13, 21]

Helium-cadmium laser (325 nm) and a pulse dye laser (480 nm) were used for excitation and ablation, respectively.

While mechanical perforation due to lack of steerability of the laser catheter still remained a problem, laser perforation appeared to be decreased comparing with previous reports.

EXOGENOUS FLUOROPHORES

Since the absorption of light by a fluorophore is markedly increased at its excitation wavelength, the use of exogenous fluorophores selectively absorbed by atherosclerotic plaques can provide a double advantage in a fluorescence-guided laser angioplasty system:

1. Enhanced detection of plaques.
2. Decreased ablation threshold of plaques.

Two series of compounds have been investigated for this purpose: hematoporphyrin derivative (HPD) and tetracycline.

The HPD is prepared by treating hematoporphyrin with acetic and sulfuric acids and

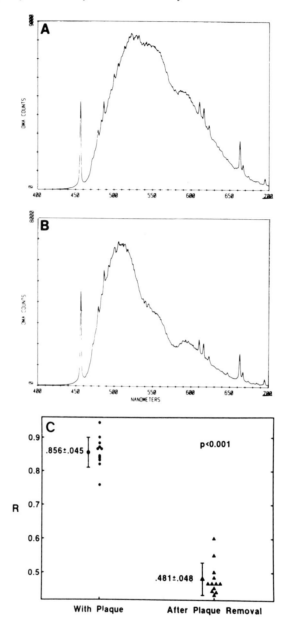

FIG 14–7.
Argon ion (458-nm laser-excited fluorescence spectroscopy before **(A)** and after **(B)** removal of the plaque by microdissection; values of R (550/520 nm) for ten sample sites before and after removal **(C)**. (From Sartori M, Weilbaecher D, Henry P: Laser induced autofluorescence of human arteries. *Circ Res* 1988; 63:1053–1059. Used by permission.)

then precipitating with sodium acetate. The HPD has three characteristics: (1) it selectively localizes in rapidly proliferating cells such as tumor cells; (2) it produces oxygen-free radicals when activated by the light; and (3) it fluoresces in red when irradiated with UV light.

The maximum absorption is between 350 and 450 nm, with emission of pink fluorescence at approximately 650 nm.

Spears et al.[41] have shown that atherosclerotic rabbits sacrificed 24 hours after injection of 2.5 to 10 mg of HPD, exhibit selective concentration of the fluorophore in the atheromatous lesions. Under UV light, the lipid-rich, fatty streaks of the rabbit aortas, characteristically fluoresce with red light. The fluorescence is more intense at the intimal surface and progressively diminishes toward the media.[25]

The fluorescence reaches a maximum at 2 days and persists for 1 to 2 weeks. The mechanism of the selective accumulation is not definitely established. The rapidity of concentration and the particular distribution within the arterial layers suggest that HPD passes across the endothelial cells in virtue of its structure. Accumulation by active uptake by rapidly proliferating smooth muscle cells contained in the plaque has been proposed, but it seems less likely since no HPD is present at 24 hours inside the gastrointestinal mucosa, which is composed of the fastest proliferating cells. Regardless of the mechanisms responsible for the accumulation in plaques, the experimental data indicate that:

1. The lipid-rich atheromas containing HPD have fluorescence spectra significantly different than that of the control.

2. In vivo low-energy radiation of atherosclerotic rabbit aortas at selected wavelengths (about 635 nm) causes inflammatory changes in the lipid-rich lesions and results in reduction of the intima.

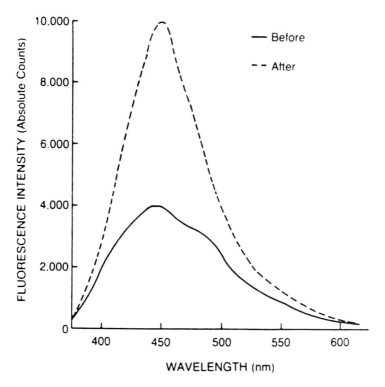

FIG 14–8.
Helium-cadmium (325-nm) laser excited fluorescence spectroscopy before and after atheroma ablation using a 480-nm pulsed dye laser. The spectrum after ablation closely resembles a normal tissue spectrum (see Fig 14–3,A for comparison). (From Leon MB, Lu DY, Prevosti LG, et al: Human arterial surface fluorescence: Atherosclerotic plaque identification and effects of laser atheroma ablation. *J Am Coll Cardiol* 1988; 12:94–102. Used by permission.)

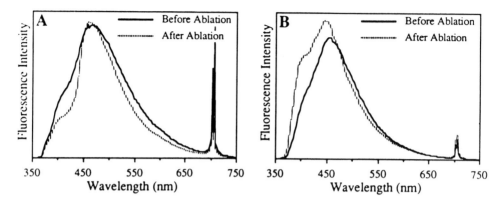

FIG 14–9.
Spectra profile obtained before and after radiation with excimer at 351 nm. **A**, normal tissue. **B**, calcified atheroma. (From Pettit GH, Pini R, Sauerbrey R, et al: Excimer laser induced autofluorescence from atherosclerotic human arteries. *IEEE J Quan Elec*, submitted for publication. Used by permission.)

It is unclear at this time whether such photodynamic therapy can be effectively and safely performed, but it is clear that detection of lipid atheromas is enhanced. Skin phototoxicity and poor penetration in calcified or fibrotic plaques may, however, represent a limitation to their clinical use.

Tetracycline has been known to accumulate in atherosclerotic plaques since 1966.[23] It localizes in the proximity of phospholipids, suggesting that its lipophilic structure is probably at the origin of its selective concentration in plaques. These initial observations have been recently confirmed by Murphy-Chutorian et al. at Stanford.[26] Atherosclerotic plaques of human aortic segments soaked in isotonic saline solution containing 16 μg/cc of tetracyclines for 2 hours exhibit a characteristic yellow fluorescence when exposed to UV light that is not present in control normal segments. Tissue uptake study with H^3-radiolabeled tetracycline shows the uptake to be maximum after 10 minutes of incubation and to persist unchanged for 2 hours. According to the Stanford group, similar results were obtained with samples of carotid artery of two patients given 1 gm of IV tetracycline prior to surgical endarterectomy. Ablation with UV laser at the peak of maximum absorption of tetracycline (355 nm) resulted in a depth of tissue penetration of the atherosclerotic sites double that of the normal tetracycline-treated and untreated sites (2.2 $\pm$ 0.24 vs. 1.2 $\pm$ 0.29 and 1.0 $\pm$ 0.8 mm).

Figure 14–10 represents the spectra of normal and calcified tissue upon UV excitation before and after incubation with tetracycline. It is evident how the fluorophore has remarkably increased the difference of the two spectra that would be naturally overlapping.

Spectroscopy of Plasma Emission

As stated elsewhere in this book, when a high-power excimer laser beam interacts with tissue, a process of "photoablation" takes place. Ablation in air is accompanied by an audible snap and brief formation of a bright plume extending away from the sample surface.

Figure 14–11 shows a spectrum taken during emission of the plasma from a calcified atheroma. Analogous lines are not seen at any normal tissue site during ablation. Only vaguely similar number lines are found in the plume using a different laser source.[34]

Many of the spectral lines in the plume fluorescence can be attributed to electronic transitions in excited-state calcium, magnesium, or phosphorus. Since the sharp lines only appear during plasma formation in the calcified tissue, plume spectroscopy may have source utility as an in vitro method of determining with high special resolution the pathologic calcium deposition in tissue. Currently, such analysis requires electron mi-

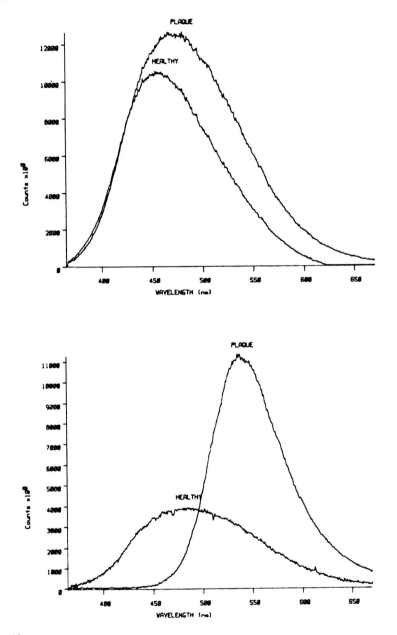

FIG 14–10.
Fluorescence of normal and disease tissue sites from an aortic valve leaflet before *(top)* and after *(bottom)* staining with chlorotetracycline. Notice that the peak of maximum intensity of the atherosclerotic site has shifted to a longer wavelength, 550 nm. (From Clarke RH, Isner JM, Gauthier T, et al: Spectroscopic characterization of cardiovascular tissue. *Lasers Surg Med* 1988; 8:45–59. Used by permission.)

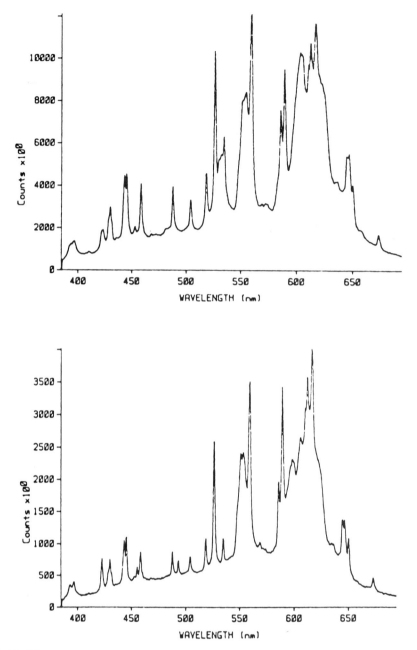

FIG 14–11.
Spectroscopy of plasma emission obtained by ablating hydroxyapatite crystals *(top)* and a calcified atheroma *(bottom)*. (From Clarke RH, Isner JM, Gauthier T, et al: Spectroscopic characterization of cardiovascular tissue. *Lasers Surg Med* 1988; 8:45–59. Used by permission.)

croprobe or atomic absorption analysis. Unfortunately, this effect cannot be reproduced with samples submerged in saline. This could confine the potential use of this technique only to conditions in which laser ablation is performed in air.

In conclusion, laser spectroscopy seems to offer a great potential for laser angioplasty. Better characterization of the tissue structure and plaque recognition through a single fiber is possible. Parameters for fluorescence monitoring of the ablative process are continuously developed. Enhancement of detection and selective removal of atherosclerotic tissue by tagging technique is promising.

Whether the maps shown in Plates 23 and 24 will remain a dream or whether they will become part of our diagnostic and therapeutic modalities, the years to come will disclose.

REFERENCES

1. Abela GS, Seeger JM, Barbieri E, et al: Laser angioplasty with angioscopic guidance in humans. *J Am Coll Cardiol* 1986; 8:184–192.
2. Banga I, Bihari-Varga M: Investigations of free and elastin-bound fluorescent substances present in the atherosclerotic lipid and calcium plaques. *Connect Tissue Res* 1974; 2:237–241.
3. Bartorelli AL, Almagor Y, Prevosti LG, et al: In vivo coronary plaque recognition by laser-induced fluorescence spectroscopy. *Circulation* 1988; 78:II–294.
4. Benson RC, Meyer RA, Zaruba ME, et al: Cellular autofluorescence: Is it due to flavins? *J Histochem Cytochem* 1978; 27:44–48.
5. Blankenhorn DH, Braunstein H: Carotenoids in man: III. The microscopic pattern of fluorescence in atheromas and its relation to their growth. *J Clin Invest* 1958; 37:160–165.
6. Blomfield J, Farrar JF: Fluorescence spectra of arterial elastin. *Biochem Biophys Res Commun* 1967; 28:346–351.
7. Bloomfield T, Farrar JF: Fluorescence spectra of arterial elastin. *Biochem Biophys Res Commun* 1967; 26:346–351.
8. Chang-Tung EG, Mountain CF, Chin RD, et al: Lung cancer detection using laser induced autogenous fluorescence spectroscopy. *Lasers Surg Med* 1987; 7:106.
9. Clarke RH, Isner JM, Gauthier T, et al: Spectroscopic characterization of cardiovascular tissue. *Lasers Surg Med* 1988; 8:45–59.
10. Crea F, Abela GS, Fenech A, et al: Transluminal laser irradiation of coronary arteries in live dogs: An angiographic and morphologic study of acute effects. *Am J Cardiol* 1986; 57:171–174.
11. Deckelbaum LI, Lam JK, Cabin HS, et al: Discrimination of normal and atherosclerotic aorta by laser-induced fluorescence. *Lasers Surg Med* 1987; 7:330–335.
12. Deckelbaum LI, Lam JK, Cabin HS, et al: Discrimination of normal and atherosclerotic aorta by laser induced fluorescence. *Clin Res* 1986; 34:292A.
13. Geschwind HJ, Dubis-Rande JL, Shafton EP, et al: Spectroscopic guidance of pulsed laser assisted balloon angioplasty (LABA). *Circulation* 1988; 78:II–504.
14. Gijsbers GH, Breederveld D, Vangemert MJ, et al: In vivo fluorescence excitation and emission spectra of hematoporphyrin derivative. *Lasers Life Sci* 1986; 1:29–48.
15. Grundfest WS, Litvack F, Sherman T, et al: Delineation of peripheral and coronary detail by intraoperative angioscopy. *Ann Surg* 1985; 202:394–400.
16. Hoshihara Y: Influence of tissue hemoglobin on argon laser induced fluorescence of gastrointestinal mucosa. *Jpn J Gastroenterol* 1985; 82:1853.
17. Isner JM, Donaldson RF, Funai JT, et al: Factors contributing to perforations resulting from laser coronary angioplasty: Observations in an intact human postmortem preparation of intraoperative laser coronary angioplasty. *Circulation* 1985; 72:191–199.
18. Kessel D, Sykes D: Porphyrin accumulation by atheromatous plaque of aorta. *Photochem Photobiol* 1984; 40:59–61.
19. Kittrell C, Willett RL, Santos-Pacheo C, et al: Diagnosis of fibrous arterial atherosclerosis using fluorescence. *Appl Optics* 1985; 24:2280–2281.
20. Laifer LI, O'Brien KM, Stetz ML, et al: Etiology of the fluorescence difference between normal and atherosclerotic arteries. *Circulation* 1988; 78:II–448.

21. Leon MB, Almagor Y, Bartorelli AL, et al: Fluorescence-guided laser angioplasty in patients with femoropopliteal occlusions. *Circulation* 1988; 78:II–294.

22. Leon MB, Lu DY, Prevosti LG, et al: Human arterial surface fluorescence: Atherosclerotic plaque identification and effects of laser atheroma ablation. *J Am Coll Cardiol* 1988; 12:94–102.

23. Lindgren I, Raekallio J: Accumulation of tetracyclines in atherosclerotic lesions of human aorta. *Acta Pathol Microbiol Scand* 1966; 66:323–326.

24. Lipson RI, Baldes ET: The photodynamic properties of a particular hematoporphyrin derivative. *Arch Dermatol* 1960; 82:508–516.

25. Litvack F, Grundfest WS, Forrester JS: Effects of hematoporphyrin derivative and photodynamic therapy of atherosclerotic rabbits. *Am J Cardiol* 1985; 56:667–671.

26. Lu DY, Leon MB, Smith PD, et al: Atherosclerotic plaque identification using surface fluorescence. *Clin Res* 1986; 34:630A.

27. Mackie RW, Orme E, Fox J, et al: Dihematoporphyrin ether photosensitizer enhanced laser angioplasty in yucatan miniswine: Histology and stenosis reduction or irradiated vessels. *Circulation* 1988; 78:II–505.

28. Mehta A, Richards-Kortum RR, Kittrell C, et al: Real time determination of artery wall composition and control of laser ablation using laser induced fluorescence. Conference on Lasers and Electro-optics, Baltimore, Md, April 26–May 1, 1987.

29. Murphy-Chutorian D, Kosek J, Mok W, et al: Selective absorption of ultraviolet laser energy by human atherosclerotic plaque treated with tetracycline. *Am J Cardiol* 1985; 55:1293–1297.

30. Papazoglou TG, Grundfest WS, Papaioannou T, et al: Detection of arterial wall layers during ablation by time resolved fluorescence and reflection measurements. *Circulation* 1988; 78:II–503.

31. Pettit GH, Pini R, Tittel FK, et al: Excimer laser induced autofluorescence from arteriosclerotic human arteries. *IEEE J Quan Elec,* submitted for publication.

32. Pollack ME, Hammer EJ, Wilson M, et al: Photosensitization of experimental atheroma by porphyrins. *J Am Coll Cardiol* 1987; 9:639–646.

33. Prevosti LG, Wynne JJ, Becker CG, et al: Laser-induced fluorescence detection of atherosclerotic plaque with hematoporphyrin derivative used as an exogenous probe. *J Vasc Surg* 1988; 7:500–506.

34. Prince MR, LaMuralgia GM, Teng P, et al: Preferential ablation of calcified arterial plaque with laser-induced plasmas. *IEEE J Quan Elec* 1987; 23:1783–1786.

35. Sartori M, Bossaller C, Weilbacher D, et al: Detection of atherosclerotic plaques and characterization of arterial wall structure by laser induced fluorescence. *Circulation* 1985; 74:II–7.

36. Sartori M, Henry PD, Roberts R, et al: Estimation of arterial wall thickness and detection of atherosclerosis by argon ion laser induced fluorescence. *J Am Coll Cardiol* 1986; 7:207A.

37. Sartori M, Sauerbrey R, Kubodera S, et al: Autofluorescence maps of atherosclerotic human arteries: A new technique in medical imaging. *IEEE J Quan Elec* 1987; 23:1794–1797.

38. Sartori M, Weilbaecher D, Henry P: Laser induced autofluorescence of human arteries. *Circ Res,* 1988; 63:1053–1059.

39. Sherman CT, Litvack F, Grundfest W, et al: Coronary angioscopy in patients with unstable angina pectoris. *N Engl J Med* 1986; 315:913–919.

40. Spears JR, Serur J, Shropshire D, et al: Fluorescence of experimental atheromatous plaques with hematoporphyrin derivative. *J Clin Invest* 1983; 71:395–399.

41. Vincent GM, Hammond ME, Fox JB, et al: Deposition of silver-hematoporphyrin in atherosclerotic plaque is homogeneous, intercellular, and confined to plaque. *J Am Coll Cardiol* 1987; 9:178A.

Chapter 15

Perspectives for Development of Angioplasty Guidance Systems

Rodney A. White, M.D.

George E. Kopchok, B.S.

York Hsiang, M.D.

Carol Guthrie, M.D.

Philip D. Colman, M.D.

David Rosenbaum, M.D.

Geoffrey H. White, M.D.

Precise guidance of intraluminal angioplasty devices, particularly through high-resistance, completely occlusive lesions is a limiting factor that must be addressed by future development. Recanalization of distal, small diameter vessels and coronary lesions requires control with a sensitivity of approximately 100 μm since the thickness of vessel wall that must be preserved to prevent perforation or false aneurysms is in the range of 150 to 300 μm. Thus, methods that permit reproducible concentric recanalization of the vessel yet preserve a relatively uniform thickness of the media and adventitia of the wall is the challenge.

Angioscopy and spectroscopy have been addressed as methods of guidance in the previous chapters and will be considered here only as they relate to the present topic. Improvements in fluoroscopic equipment, particularly as it relates to enhanced visualization in the operating room, and intraluminal ultrasound will be discussed in this section as part of an attempt to define the state of the art and outline the needs for future development.

FLUOROSCOPIC GUIDANCE

Fluoroscopy is readily available and is the standard method to quantitate the luminal anatomy of arterial disease. It provides a detailed outline of the location and severity of

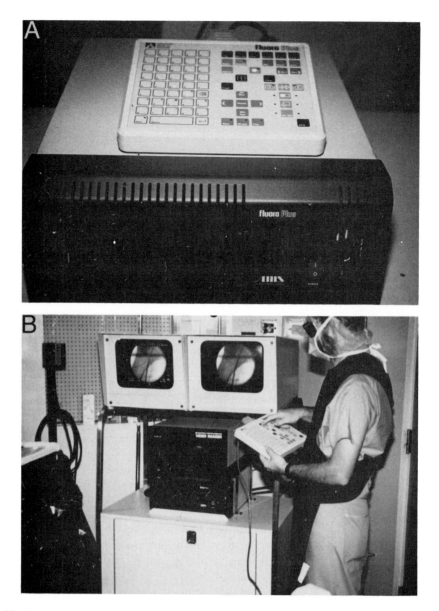

FIG 15–1.
Computerized image processing system (**A**) mounted beneath the fluoroscopy screens (**B**) enables addition of digital touch pad control to obtain contrast enhancement, image holding, and road-mapping to C-arm systems.

stenoses and occlusions and is uniformly used, as has been described in the preceding chapters, as the method to monitor the guidance of devices and determine the success of interventional procedures. There is no doubt that more elaborate systems such as those that are state of the art in new catheterization laboratories with high-resolution images, freeze-frame, and roadmapping capabilities enhance the success of transluminal interventions. Unfortunately, this equipment is extremely expensive and is not available in many facilities, particularly operating rooms. In many operating rooms, fluoroscopy is limited to C-arm images that provide less than optimal guidance for difficult angioplasty procedures. Recent advances in computerized image processing systems (Fluoro Plus, Advanced Medical Systems, Inc., Millburn, NJ) extend the advantages of digital technology by enabling modular addition of contrast enhancement, image holding, and roadmapping to C-arm fluoroscopy. The systems are relatively low-cost, easily installed, and can be mounted on a cart with the portable fluoroscopy screen display (Figs 15–1 and 15–2). Figure 15–3 displays the utility of the frozen image and roadmap capability during an angioplasty procedure.

INTRALUMINAL ULTRASOUND

A comparison of the utility of angioplasty devices including balloons, atherectomy devices, and lasers reveals that all are highly successful with partially obstructing lesions. The major advance that has been demonstrated with laser angioplasty is that lasers can recanalize a higher percentage of occluded vessels and extend the ability to disobliterating long lesions that cannot be treated by other means. Preliminary studies have indicated that lesions favorable for intraluminal therapy are concentric or have thickened or calcified arterial walls that enhance guidance of the instruments through less resistant lesions in the lumen (Table 15–1). Unfavorable lesions are those that are eccentric or have firm or calcified luminal lesions that lead to perforations or vessel dissections in a significant number of cases (Fig 15–4).

In order to enhance the guidance of devices reliably through all lesions, particularly

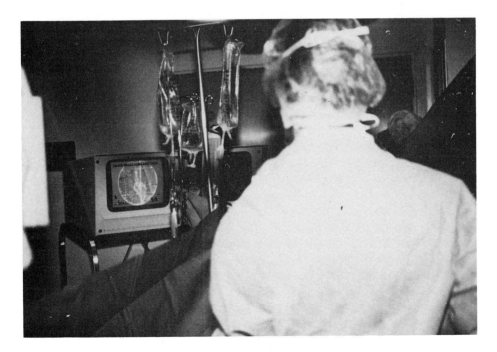

FIG 15–2.
Contrast-enhanced roadmaps are easily observed from the operating table by the surgeon performing the angioplasty.

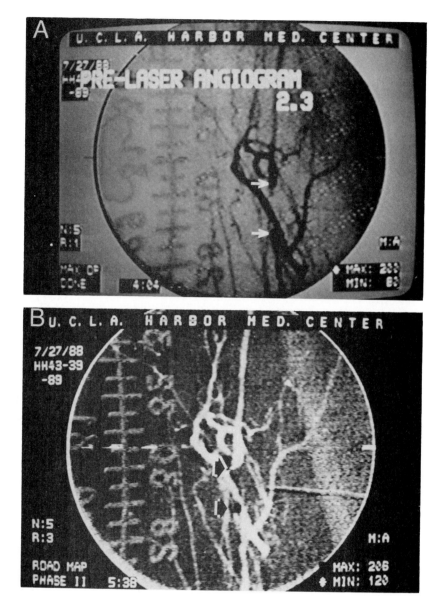

FIG 15–3.
Image enhanced roadmap of an occlusion *(arrows)* in the superficial femoral artery **(A** and **B)**.
Facing page, laser thermal probe *(arrow)* crossing the occluded lesion **(C)**. Completion angiogram
of the recanalized segment **(D)**.

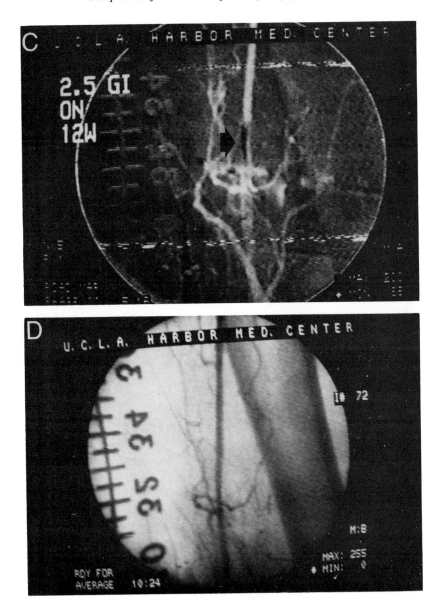

through difficult lesions that are not visualized by conventional methods, intraluminal ultrasound offers a promising way to improve recanalizations (Table 15–2). Ultrasound systems currently under development produce images by various methods. Figure 15–5 demonstrates images prepared using a phase array signal generated on the end of 3 to 8 F catheters (Endosonics, Inc., Rancho Cucamongo, Calif). Figure 15–6 displays a system that produces a high-resolution, high-frequency A-scan (Summit Technology, Watertown, Mass). The images produced by these devices outline the luminal and adventitial surfaces of normal arterial segments and show the potential to discriminate between normal and diseased vessel walls. We have observed that the ultrasound determines the dimensions of the luminal diameters of normal or minimally diseased arteries accurately within 0.05

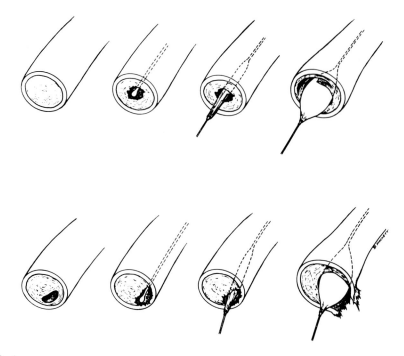

FIG 15—4.
Favorable location of concentric lesions *(top)*; enhanced potential for perforation or dissections of eccentric lesions *(bottom)*. (From White RA, et al: Laser thermal probe recanalization of occluded arteries. *J Vasc Surg*, in press. Used by permission.)

mm.[1] Outside diameter of the vessels is less accurate, with a margin of error up to 0.5 mm. Pandian et al.[2] and others[3, 4] have reported similar findings. The systems have also been used to identify intimal flaps and dissections[4, 5] and as a diagnostic tool to differentiate normal artery from plaque.[1, 6] With further development, intraluminal ultrasound may provide the enhanced guidance required to precisely steer endovascular surgical instruments concentrically through the lumen of occluded vessels. The ultimate intraluminal system may be a combination of angioscopy, spectroscopy, and intraluminal ultrasound to provide accurate three-dimensional guidance through lesions.

TABLE 15—1.
Predictive Factors for Laser Recanalization

Favorable	Unfavorable
Concentric lesions	Eccentric lesions
Thickened or calcified arterial wall	Heavily calcified areas within the lumen

TABLE 15–2.
Comparison of Intraluminal Guidance Methods for Identifying, Characterizing, and Quantitating Disease

	Localization of Disease	Assessment of Luminal Dimensions and Morphology	Characterization of Components of the Plaque	Measurement of Vessel Wall Dimensions*	Inspection of Distal Vessel "Runoff"
Fluoroscopy	"Gold standard" applicable to all levels and diameters	Yes	No	No	Yes
Angioscopy	Excellent identification, limited to segments with diameter larger than scope	Yes	Only as suggested by visual assessment	No	Limited to view within 3–5 cm of the scope
Spectroscopy	Localization on a microscale only	No	Yes	No	No
Ultrasound	Diagnostic ability promising; limited to segments with diameters larger than the delivery catheter	Yes	Possible diagnostic ability (normal vs. abnormal) plus precise localization of lesion	Yes	No

* Determination of both inside and outside diameters of the vessel wall.

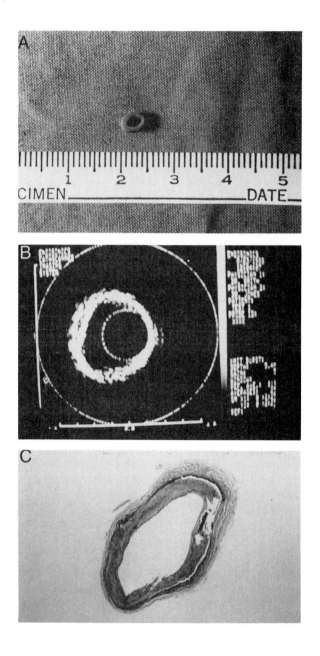

FIG 15–5.
Intraluminal ultrasound image of a human hepatic artery produced by phase array signals generated on the end of a 5.5 F catheter. **A,** gross appearance of the vessel. **B,** intraluminal ultrasound image of the artery. **C,** histologic section of the artery (Verhoeff–van Gieson's stain, × 4).

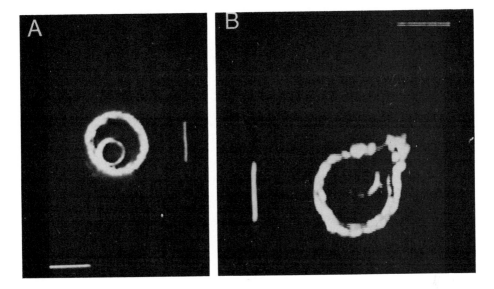

FIG 15–6.
Intraluminal ultrasound image of the same vessel as Figure 15–5 produced by a high-resolution, high-frequency A scan. Ultrasound image at a location comparable to that shown in Figure 15–5 (**A**) and at the origin of a branch artery (**B**).

REFERENCES

1. Kopchok GE, White R, Guthrie C, et al: Intraluminal vascular ultrasound: Dimensional and morphologic accuracy. *Circulation* submitted for publication.
2. Pandian NG, Kreis A, Brockway B, et al: Ultrasound angioscopy: Real-time, two dimensional, intraluminal ultrasound imaging. *Am J Cardiol* 1988; 62:493–494.
3. Hodgson J, Eberle MJ, Savakus AD: Validation of a new real time percutaneous intravascular ultrasound imaging catheter. *Circulation* 1988; 78(suppl 2):21.
4. Uchida Y, Kawamura K, Shibuya I, et al: Percutaneous angioscopy of the coronary luminal changes induced by PTCA. *Circulation* 1988; 78(suppl 2):84.
5. Pandian N, Kreis A, Brockway B, et al: Intraluminal ultrasound angioscopic detection of arterial dissection and intimal flaps: In vitro and in vivo studies. *Circulation* 1988; 78(suppl 2):21.
6. Yock P, Linker D, Seather O, et al: Intravascular two-dimensional catheter ultrasound: Initial clinical studies. *Circulation* 1988; 78(suppl 2):21.

Balloons and Mechanical Devices

Albert K. Chin, M.D.

Thomas J. Fogarty, M.D.

HISTORY OF TRANSLUMINAL ANGIOPLASTY

It was no accident that the earliest attempts at intravascular treatment of atherosclerotic disease employed mechanical devices and balloons. Mechanical displacement of stenotic material, although conceptually primitive, proved simple and effective. Dotter and Judkins introduced the concept of transluminal dilatation in 1964, using coaxial passage of tapered catheters.[1] The following year, they pioneered the procedure of balloon angioplasty by successfully dilating an iliac lesion with a Fogarty embolectomy balloon.[2] Although these early cases served as an introduction to a new era in cardiovascular therapy, much improvement was required in the instrumentation applied by Dotter. Coaxial tapered catheters generally proved too traumatic, resulting in an unacceptably high incidence of vessel injury and distal embolization. A long tapered coaxial catheter system developed by Van Andel[3] still finds application in transluminal angioplasty when placement of a balloon angioplasty catheter is difficult due to the severity of the disease. The elastomeric balloon employed by the Fogarty catheter functions well for arterial embolectomy, but the pliability of the balloon hindered the application of force to the plaque while increasing the chance for overdistention of adjacent normal artery.

Gruntzig's development of a constant volume balloon catheter provided the breakthrough needed for successful transluminal angioplasty (Fig 16–1). With a correctly sized balloon, controlled radial displacement of the diseased artery may be achieved, resulting in a safe increase in lumen size. The Gruntzig balloon succeeded in balloon angioplasty where other balloon dilatation concepts failed. Porstmann attempted to surround a latex balloon catheter with a Teflon cage to increase its strength and prevent overdistention.[4] The uneven surface characteristics of this balloon traumatized the arterial wall during catheter passage and balloon inflation. The smooth polyvinyl chloride Gruntzig balloon permitted placement of the dilating medium with limited morbidity. The original polyvinyl chloride balloons were later replaced with polyethylene balloons. Polyethylene is less elastomeric than polyvinyl chloride, allowing higher inflation pressures with minimal

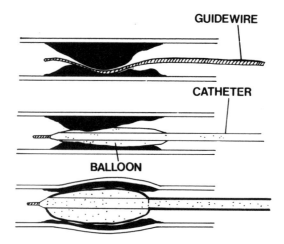

FIG 16–1.
The Gruntzig catheter. A polyethylene balloon is placed in a coaxial configuration about the catheter body.

increase in balloon diameter. When overinflated, balloons made with either of these two materials tear rather than shatter, as may be the case with latex balloons. There is decreased chance of balloon material embolism with the plastic angioplasty balloons.

The Gruntzig balloon catheter found use in both the peripheral vascular and the coronary systems. The initial efforts were directed at occlusive disease in the peripheral vasculature. Application of this new technology was aided by the simplicity of the iliofemoral system. The small size and tortuosity of coronary vessels demanded further refinements in angioplasty instrumentation. Simpson et al. contributed to this endeavor with their introduction of a percutaneous coronary angioplasty catheter with an independently movable guidewire.[5] This concept imparted maneuverability to the coronary balloon dilatation system, simplifying selective cannulation of coronary vessels.

The above described systems employ a coaxial arrangement of the angioplasty balloon around the shaft of the dilatation catheter. An alternate system introduced by Fogarty and Chin in 1981 uses an angioplasty balloon that is initially inverted within the lumen of the catheter (Fig 16–2).[6] The catheter is advanced 1 cm short of the stenosis and pressurized to extrude the balloon through the occluded segment, achieving dilatation. The linear extrusion catheter was originally introduced for intraoperative use, as prior guidewire passage is not required, and placement of the dilating element within the stenosis does not depend on fluoroscopic guidance. The unrolling balloon front decreases the propensity for catheter dissection to occur during dilatation of tight lesions. Tortuous segments are traversed in a simplified manner, as the extrusion balloon follows the contours of the artery. Shear forces exerted by the catheter on the arterial wall are also decreased. In tight stenoses, the difference in shear force between placement of a coaxial balloon catheter and placement of the linear extrusion balloon may approach a factor of 40 times.[7] In a recent study involving electron microscopic examination of rabbit arterial lesions following balloon angioplasty with the linear extrusion catheter, a flattened layer of endothelial cells was demonstrated in eight of ten cases.[8] This was in contrast to endothelial strippage seen in all cases during passage of a coaxial balloon catheter. For guidewire applications, an everting through lumen catheter is used (Fig 16–3). This catheter contains an inner tube that runs the length of the catheter and connects to the everting balloon, allowing passage of a guidewire or injection of contrast material.

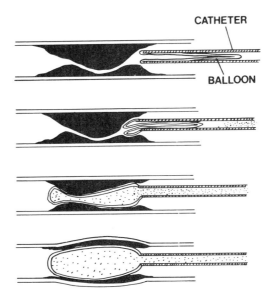

FIG 16–2.
The Fogarty-Chin catheter. A polyethylene balloon initially inverted within the lumen of the catheter is unrolled through the stenosis upon inflation.

Further advancements in balloon angioplasty catheters include decreased catheter profiles to allow placement in tight lesions. Dilatation balloons placed on guidewire bodies are available for initial enlargement of the arterial lumen, followed by coaxial introduction of a full-sized angioplasty catheter. Other areas of advancement include hydrophilic coatings for the dilatation balloon, catheter body, and guidewires. Such coatings absorb water during intravascular use, resulting in a slippery surface for improved passage. The reduced shear forces from hydrophilic-coated catheters and guidewires should decrease the incidence of endothelial trauma during arterial instrumentation.

Another area of transluminal angioplasty research involves the application of heat to the arterial surface during balloon inflation. Surface heating during dilatation is an attempt to remodel the plaque and tack down flaps formed by the angioplasty procedure. Laser

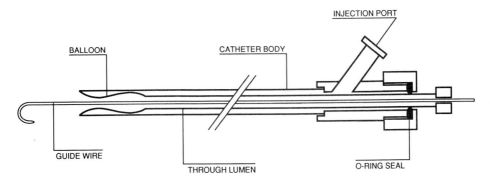

FIG 16–3.
The through-lumen everting catheter. An inner lumen runs the length of the catheter, allowing introduction of a guidewire.

energy applied through the transparent balloon of a coaxial dilatation catheter is one method of generating heat for surface treatment.[9] The short-term and long-term effects of this therapy are not established at present.

MECHANISM OF TRANSLUMINAL ANGIOPLASTY

Transluminal angioplasty involves radial displacement of the plaque material during balloon inflation. Previous studies show that very little remodeling or compaction of the plaque occurs during dilatation.[10, 11] Rather, the force exerted by the balloon causes the formation of cracks and tears in the plaque material and arterial wall. The plaque is separated from the underlying arterial wall, allowing a fusiform distention of the artery with a resultant increase in lumen size. The majority of cracks and tears occur in a longitudinal direction. Tears in this orientation are less apt to be lifted by the restored blood flow, accounting for the relative scarcity of intimal flap formation and early occlusion following balloon angioplasty. These observations are in contrast to the earlier notion of plaque as a compressible material that may be permanently deformed by the application of force.

The linear extrusion balloon achieves dilatation using the same mechanism employed by coaxial balloon angioplasty catheters, resulting in similar plaque separation and arterial cracking. However, with the linear extrusion catheter, the forces exerted on the plaque and artery remain radial to the contours of the lumen, even during placement of the dilating element within the lesion. The advancing front of the balloon dilates the artery sufficiently to allow the remainder of the balloon to pass forward. There are minimal shear forces tending to dislodge the plaque from the arterial wall during catheter use.

LIMITATIONS OF BALLOON ANGIOPLASTY

With the advent of low profile coaxial balloon catheters and the linear extrusion balloon catheter, access into tight stenoses or total occlusions has been facilitated. Although not every lesion may be crossed with a balloon catheter, most stenoses of medium and short length may be treated with transluminal angioplasty. The present limitations of balloon angioplasty are related more to the mechanism of transluminal dilatation and the occurrence of restenosis. The rough surface that remains following transluminal angioplasty alters the flow characteristics through the dilated segment, perhaps contributing to the 30% to 50% incidence of coronary restenosis cited.[12–14] The displacement mechanism of balloon angioplasty does nothing to remove the offending plaque, and in certain lesions this characteristic results in treatment failure. If the lesion is fibroelastic, the angioplasty balloon may not achieve permanent dilatation. Instead, the rubbery plaque returns to its original conformation once the balloon is deflated. Restenosis following an initially successful dilatation is determined by the healing response to the dissection caused by the angioplasty balloon. Aggressive formation of myointimal hyperplasia has been identified as the cause of restenosis upon biopsy examination of these lesions.[16]

In order to address the problem of restenosis, two additional mechanical devices are being studied. These two devices include atherectomy catheters and arterial stents. Atherectomy devices also attempt to improve the ability of catheters to gain access through tight lesions or total occlusions. Arterial stents are implantable devices that serve as structural support for the artery following dilatation. These two classes of mechanical therapy will be discussed in turn.

ATHERECTOMY DEVICES

Simpson Atherectomy Catheter.—The Simpson atherectomy catheter, developed in 1987, involves cutting and removal of atheromatous plaque.[15] The system consists of a cylinder with a cutout along one side (Fig 16–4). The cylinder houses a cutting element that rotates at 2,000 rpm. A nonelastomeric balloon situated opposite the opening in the cylinder is inflated to push the cylinder against the plaque. The rotating cutter is advanced forward within the cylinder to slice a section of plaque and to impact the section in the distal portion of the cylinder. Torque is applied to the catheter to rotate the cylinder and to center the opening over the desired area of removal. Repeated passes are performed with the cutter until the storage chamber is filled. The catheter is then removed to empty the biopsied shavings prior to continued atherectomy.

The Simpson atherectomy device leaves a smooth surface following plaque removal. Its use in peripheral arteries has been relatively safe, with a low incidence of distal embolization and angiographically detected arterial dissection. A high restenosis rate (52% at 6 months for all sites) occurs if residual stenoses greater than 30% are allowed to remain. This restenosis rate drops to 18% if aggressive atherectomy is performed, with all stenoses reduced below 30%.[16] This device is being applied to coronary artery lesions, and follow-up studies from these cases will be forthcoming. The Simpson atherectomy catheter is currently the most widely applied atherectomy device.

The advantages of the cylindrical atherectomy device include a high degree of safety and the ability of the device to remove sectioned plaque. The eccentrically placed balloon inflates to force the cylinder against the artery, straightening the artery in the process. The cutter removes only the material protruding into the cylinder. This design minimizes the possibility of cutter perforation. Sectioned plaque is trapped within the storage section of the cylinder, decreasing the likelihood of distal embolization. The retrieved biopsy specimen may be studied to yield information regarding plaque composition and restenosis morphology following previous balloon or mechanical intervention.

The limitations of this device include its inability to gain access through tight lesions and the need for multiple catheter withdrawals to remove collected plaque. The side-biting configuration of the Simpson atherectomy catheter requires positioning of the cylinder within the lesion for successful plaque removal. In tight lesions, a front-acting atherectomy device may be preferable. Alternatively, a linear extrusion balloon may be used to gain access and enlarge the lumen sufficiently to allow atherectomy catheter placement.

Auth Atherectomy Device.—This instrument consists of an oval diamond studded burr that spins at high speed, grinding away plaque (Fig 16–5).[17] The burr rotates at speeds of 100,000 to 120,000 rpm, driven by a compressed air turbine via a flexible saline-cooled shaft. The burr may be advanced coaxially over a previously placed guide-wire, imparting directionality to its passage.

At the high rate of rotation achieved by the atherectomy burr, preferential removal of hard calcified plaque occurs. Elastic tissue tends to be deflected by the burr during its passage through the vessel. Histologic examination of atherosclerotic human cadaver and animal arteries following atherectomy with the Auth device reveals a smooth polished intraluminal surface, without the intimal flaps demonstrated on balloon angioplasty.

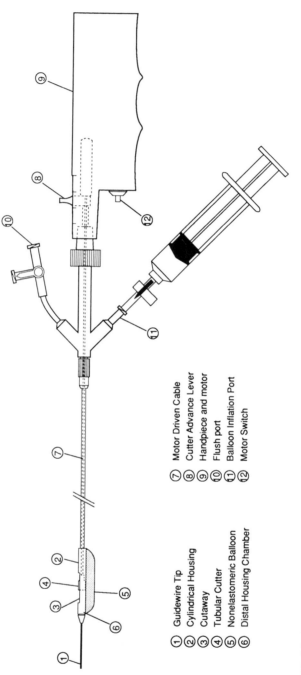

1. Guidewire Tip
2. Cylindrical Housing
3. Cutaway
4. Tubular Cutter
5. Nonelastomeric Balloon
6. Distal Housing Chamber
7. Motor Driven Cable
8. Cutter Advance Lever
9. Handpiece and motor
10. Flush port
11. Balloon Inflation Port
12. Motor Switch

FIG 16–4.

Simpson atherectomy catheter. The nonelastomeric balloon (5) pushes the cutaway (3) against the plaque. The tubular cutter (4) shaves a section of plaque and impacts it in the distal chamber (6).

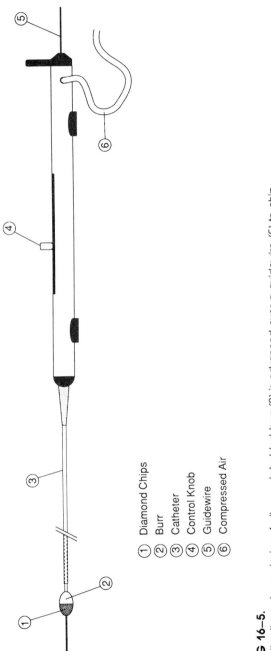

1. Diamond Chips
2. Burr
3. Catheter
4. Control Knob
5. Guidewire
6. Compressed Air

FIG 16–5.
Auth atherectomy device. A diamond-studded burr (2) is advanced over a guidewire (5) to chip away small particles of plaque.

Atherectomy particles collected during the procedure have been analyzed by a Coulter counter, and particles vary in size from 1 to 35 μm with the majority of particles in the 5- to 10-μm range. Radionuclide scans of technetium-labeled atherectomy particles in the canine model show that most particles accumulate in the lung, with lesser amounts in the liver, spleen, and extremities.

Advantages of this system include safety and maneuverability due to tracking of the device over an independent guidewire, the ability of the instrument to remove plaque in a forward direction, and the speed of plaque removal during the treatment of long-segment stenoses. Disadvantages of this design include difficulty with guidewire passage through total occlusions and difficulty with recanalization through elastic chronic thrombotic occlusions.

The Auth device is currently undergoing clinical trials and early results should be available soon.

Kensey Catheter.—The Kensey catheter is also a front-acting, high-speed, rotational plaque removal device.[18] An electric motor and step-up transmission drive a torsion cable at speeds approaching 100,000 rpm. The cable rotates a cam at the distal end of the polyurethane catheter, resulting in disruption of plaque on contact (Fig 16–6). Fluid is pumped through the catheter, cooling the torsion cable and exiting in a fine jet at the base of the cam. This system does not track over a guidewire.

Advantages of this system include the forward plaque-removing action of the cam and the possibility of recanalizing total occlusions. Elimination of guidewire use may be an advantage during attempted passage through total occlusions. However, this feature may increase the possibility of arterial perforation during catheter use. Another limitation of this device is the release of emboli. Studies employing diseased cadaver superficial femoral arteries interposed as xenografts in canine carotid and aortorenal positions revealed the presence of emboli in the brain and kidney. The significance of emboli and microemboli produced by the Kensey catheter is being evaluated through clinical trials.

STENTS

Mechanical devices that support the arterial lumen following balloon angioplasty are being analyzed (Fig 16–7). Some of these stents are expandable stainless steel coils or fenestrated tubes placed over the dilatation balloon and fixed in the vessel upon balloon inflation.[19] An alternate design uses a self-expanding stainless steel meshwork, initially elongated over a delivery catheter and held in its compressed state by an overlying sheath.[20] Withdrawal of the sheath delivers the stent in an expanded configuration. Special wire titanium-nickel alloy stents with a temperature dependent memory are also under investigation.[21] These alloy wires start out in a long thin configuration prior to release in the vascular system. At body temperature, the wire proceeds through its transition state to change its shape, forming an expanded stent.

Relevant questions regarding stents include those concerning the long-term safety and efficacy of these devices. Possible complications include early migration of the stents or erosion of the stents through the vessel wall following a period of implantation. Restenosis tends to occur at the interface of the stent and the adjacent unstented artery, sometimes requiring serial lengthwise stent placement.

In a 1-year follow-up of 37 patients who had 44 coronary stents placed during 40 interventions, examination at a mean interval of 16 weeks showed no significant stenoses

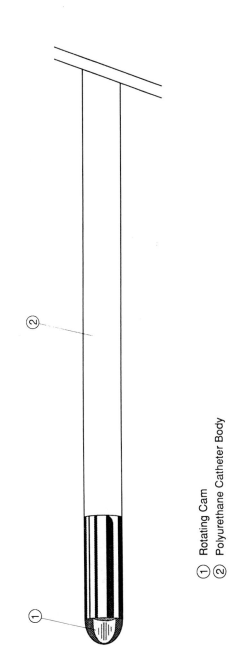

① Rotating Cam
② Polyurethane Catheter Body

FIG 16–6.
Kensey catheter. A rotating cam placed at the end of a catheter body spins at high speed to remove plaque.

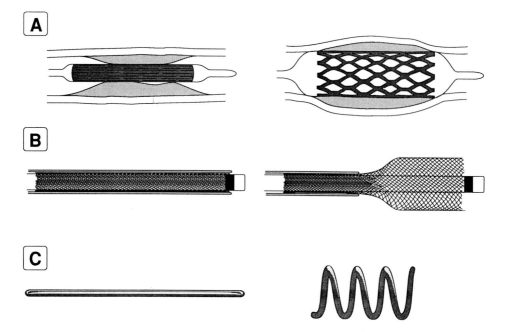

FIG 16–7.
Mechanical stent designs. **A,** an expandable framework of stainless steel is placed over an angioplasty balloon and opened to support the dilated arterial segment. **B,** a self-expanding stainless steel meshwork is constrained over a delivery catheter and released to stent the vessel. **C,** a straight segment of Nitinol wire initially cooled in ice water is introduced into the artery and transformed into a coil stent upon warming to body temperature.

within the stented segments.[22] Complications occurred in 17 cases (17 of 40 = 42.5%), and 2 deaths occurred (5.4%). The complications included local hematoma, false aneurysm of the puncture site, temporary occlusion, permanent thrombosis, coronary spasm, and myocardial infarction. With continued advancements in stent instrumentation, the future data will hopefully reflect a sustained increase in the patency rates and an improvement in the complication rates.

CONCLUSION

The varied pathology in arterial occlusive disease demand a spectrum of therapeutic modalities. Mechanical displacement, plaque removal, and stenting are three techniques used in addressing the problem of atherosclerotic narrowing. A combination of these approaches will be required to treat the range of patients with coronary and peripheral artery disease adequately. Continued research will be required to determine the optimal therapy for this important disease entity.

REFERENCES

1. Dotter CT, Judkins MP: Transluminal treatment of arteriosclerotic obstruction: Description of a new technic and a preliminary report of its application. *Circulation* 1964; 30:654–670.
2. Dotter CT: Transluminal angioplasty: A long view. *Radiology* 1980; 135:561–564.